The Complete Guide to Whole Foods and Health

Nourish and Energize Your Body and Mind

Manfred Urs Koch

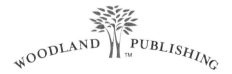

WOODLAND PUBLISHING

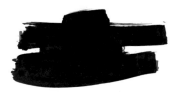

2007 U.S. Edition Published by Woodland Publishing

Published by special arrangement with Manfred Urs Koch, Renaissance World Publishing, Ulmarra, Australia.
renaissanceworld@hotkey.net.au

For permissions, ordering information, or bulk quantity discounts, contact:
Woodland Publishing, 448 East 800 North, Orem, Utah 84097

Visit our Web site:
www.woodlandpublishing.com
Toll-free number: (800) 777-BOOK

The information in this book is for educational purposes only and is not recommended as a means of diagnosing or treating an illness.
All matters concerning physical and mental health should be supervised by a health practitioner knowledgeable in treating that particular condition.
Neither the publisher nor the author directly or indirectly dispenses medical advice, nor do they prescribe any remedies or assume any responsibility for those who choose to treat themselves.

Cataloging-in-Publication data is available from the Library of Congress.
ISBN: 978-1-58054-487-0
Printed by Everbest Printing Co., China
www.everbest.com

PREFACE

Mr. Manfred Urs Koch first published this book titled Laugh with Health in Australia in 1981.

Initally, four years of intense research into nutrition was required to understand the subject and to develop the basic outline of the book.

During the winter months, Manfred travelled north to warmer parts of Australia and spent many days at a time in recluse areas, with his fully restored Holden car as a mobile office.

The first edition was hand-folded by volunteers from a yachting village in Victoria, named Metung. Local people came to the 'wood cottage' for 2 weeks and finally the 234,000 folded sheets were taken to Melbourne for binding and cover placement. From the first edition of 1,000 books, 500 were given away to friends, shops and the numerous helpers. One year later, book shops asked for more copies and the 2nd. printing took place.

In 1983 the book was published in the U.S.A. & also in the U.K. In 1993 the book format changed and was totally revised. The book has been self published for 14 printings by the author and 6 printings by other publishers in Australia.

Manfred has also self published two other books one titled the Health Index, in 1983 and the other book titled Natural to Juice, in 2000.
The total revision of this book commenced in 2000 and included the color photos and new charts, plus a complete rewrite of the entire contents. The color edition was released in 2002 and sales have been increasing on a monthly basis.

This book is a best seller throughout health shops in Australia and it is used as a reference book for school students and also for naturopaths. It is also endorsed by the medical profession and naturopaths.

In Australia, 73,000 copies have been sold with no promotion. A total of 140,000 copies of this book have been sold worldwide. The book has progressed from the original idea of a small handbook into the complete guide to health, diet, nutrition and natural foods.

T A B L E O F C O N T E N T S

QUESTION 1

What is Nutrition?

Nutrition is the supply of the essential nutrients from foods.

QUESTION 2

What foods supply the essential nutrients?

A variety of the 13 main food groups will supply all the essential nutrients.

QUESTION 3

What are the 13 main food groups?

1 - Grains
2 - Legumes
3 - Fruits
4 - Vegetables
5 - Nuts
6 - Seeds
7 - Sprouts
8 - Fish
9 - Seafood
10 - Meat
11 - Poultry
12 - Eggs
13 - Dairy

QUESTION 4

Are all the 13 groups natural foods?

Yes

QUESTION 5

What are the essential nutrients?

1 - Carbohydrates
2 - Proteins
3 - Fats & Oils
4 - Minerals
5 - Vitamins
6 - Water

NOTE: All amounts in this book are measured in milligrams (mg) per 100 grams, unless stated otherwise.

What food groups supply the essential nutrients?

The chart below shows the 13 main food groups and their *average* supply of the five essential nutrient groups. It is clear from this chart that a variety of food groups are required in order to obtain a complete supply of nutrients. This chart is only a general guide, as within each food group there are variations with the supply of essential nutrients. Throughout this book, over 100 individual natural foods are described and evaluated for their unique nutritional benefits. Natural foods provide all the essential nutrients.

NATURAL FOODS & ESSENTIAL NUTRIENTS CHART

FOOD GROUPS	CARBOHYDRATES	PROTEIN	LIPIDS	MINERALS	VITAMINS
GRAINS	excellent	fair	fair	fair	fair
LEGUMES	excellent	good	poor	good	fair
FRUITS	excellent	poor	poor	good	excellent
VEGETABLES	excellent	poor	poor	excellent	excellent
NUTS	fair	excellent	excellent	excellent	good
SEEDS	fair	excellent	excellent	excellent	good
SPROUTS	good	fair	poor	good	good
FISH	poor	excellent	excellent	fair	fair
SEAFOOD	poor	good	good	fair	fair
MEAT	poor	good	fair	fair	poor
POULTRY	poor	excellent	poor	fair	poor
EGGS	fair	excellent	fair	fair	fair
DAIRY	fair	good	good	good	fair

What foods do not provide the essential nutrients?

As can be seen from the chart above, numerous food groups are a poor source of some essential nutrient groups. Also, many processed and refined foods that line supermarket shelves, even though some contain 'added nutrients', most are often *deficient in many of the essential nutrients.* A prolonged deficiency of individual nutrients can lead to various types of illness, as detailed in the mineral and vitamin chapters. Refer to chart 17, page 15 for information regarding the various types of food processing. For a 'balanced diet', refer to charts: 7, 8 & 9 on pages 9 and 10 and pages 30, 42, 60, 77, 211- 213. Humans need 48 individual essential nutrients as shown on page 6. A varied diet including all natural food groups is the best way to ensure the supply of every nutrient. Cooking also depletes the heat sensitive nutrients: refer to the vitamin and mineral food charts. Various trace minerals and many vitamins are not available from processed and cooked foods.

How many essential nutrients do we need?

The human body needs a total of 48 individual essential nutrients.
Each of the essential nutrients perform specific functions as detailed throughout this book. In addition, the 4 elements are required as part of water (hydrogen & oxygen) and as components of the 3 main food groups: carbohydrates, proteins and lipids and also as part of minerals and vitamins. Physical exercise is also required to keep the body active and strong. Balance your life with natural foods and regular daily exercise. A regular intake of water is also essential, refer to page 8 for details.

The chart below provides a complete list of the essential human nutrients, however, within individual natural foods there are numerous other elements, substances, antioxidants, fibre and enzymes that may not be termed essential, but, they add great benefit to the diet for health and healing. Only natural foods can provide the correct balance for complete human nutrition. Everyday the body needs nutrients and over a period of a week, all nutrients are required for optimum health.

2	INDIVIDUAL ESSENTIAL HUMAN NUTRIENTS	
CARBOHYDRATES	**Glucose** Glucose is composed of; Carbon, Hydrogen & Oxygen.	1
PROTEIN (amino acids)	**Arginine -** (essential for children). **Phenylalanine, Isoleucine, Leucine, Lysine, Valine, Tryptophan, Threonine, Methionine.** Protein is composed of; Carbon, Hydrogen, Nitrogen &Oxygen.	9
LIPIDS (fats & oils)	**Linolenic acid - Omega 3 Linoleic acid - Omega 6** Lipids are composed of; Carbon, Hydrogen, Oxygen.	2
MINERALS	**Calcium, Chlorine, Copper, Fluoride, Iodine, Iron, Manganese, Magnesium, Phosphorus, Potassium, Silicon, Sodium, Sulphur, Zinc.**	14
TRACE MINERALS	**Cobalt, Chromium, Molybdenum, Selenium, Vanadium.**	5
VITAMINS	**A, C, D, E, F, K, P, B1, B2, B3, B5, B6, B12, Biotin, Choline, Folate, Inositol.**	17
TOTAL ESSENTIAL NUTRIENTS		48
ESSENTIAL ELEMENTS	**Carbon, Hydrogen, Nitrogen & Oxygen.** As in water H_2O and the nutrients above.	4

What quantity of nutrients does the human body require?

In the past 50 years, statistics for human nutrient requirements have been evaluated by the US Department of Agriculture, American Academy of Sciences and these are now termed as the; (R.D.I.) Recommended Dietary Intakes, previously termed the (R.D.A.) Recommended Daily Allowances. The chart below displays the approx. R.D.I. amounts for the main food groups: carbohydrates, proteins and lipids. For the average person, these figures may seem complex at first, but hopefully this information will help to provide a guide to the main nutrients required for human health and nutrition. For details on the (R.D.I.) of minerals and vitamins, refer to chart: 13, page 96. Everyday we need nutrition and science proves we need natural foods, they are the foundation of all nutrients.

Natural foods give full value per gram and provide a balance of the essential human nutrients for daily health and prevention of illness. For details on the balanced diet, refer to page 9. All the essential nutrients can be obtained within a balanced dietary intake of carbohydrate, protein and lipid foods.

ESSENTIAL HUMAN NUTRIENT (R.D.I.) CHART

NUTRIENTS & ELEMENTS	ALL AMOUNTS DEPENDANT ON AGE, GENDER, HEALTH, PHYSICAL ACTIVITY LEVELS AND CLIMATIC CONDITIONS.	grams	calories
CARBOHYDRATES	Adult male 280 - 400 grams per day approx. Adult female 230 - 340 grams per day approx. Children 160 - 380 grams per day approx.	160- 400 per day. approx.	650 - 1600 per day. approx.
PROTEIN	Adult male 58 - 63 grams per day approx. Adult female 44 - 50 grams per day approx. Children 20 - 69 grams per day approx.	20 - 63 per day. approx.	80 - 260 per day. approx
LIPIDS (fats & oils)	Adult male 51 - 65 grams per day approx. Adult female 40 - 60 grams per day. Children 28 - 64 grams per day approx.	28 - 70 per day. approx.	252 - 630 per day. approx.
MINERALS	Calcium, Chlorine, Copper, Fluoride, Iodine, Iron, Manganese, Magnesium, Phosphorus, Potassium, Silicon, Sodium, Sulphur, Zinc.	measured in milligrams - mg and micrograms mcg per day. Refer to page 96.	
TRACE MINERALS	Cobalt, Chromium, Selenium, Molybdenum, Vanadium.		
VITAMINS	A, C, D, E, F, K, P, B1, B2, B3, B5, B6, B12 Biotin, Choline, Folate, Inositol.	measured in mg, mcg, plus I.U., TE. & R.E. units. Refer to page 96.	
WATER (H_2O)	Hydrogen & Oxygen	3 - 5 litres per day approx. refer to water chart page 8.	
OXYGEN	Approx. one fifth of air is composed of the vital element oxygen.	14,000 litres per day approx.	
CARBON	Obtained from carbohydrates, protein and lipids.	no value determined.	
HYDROGEN	Obtained from carbohydrates, protein and lipids.	no value determined.	
NITROGEN	Obtained from protein foods.	no value determined.	

QUESTION 10

How much water do I need everyday?

Water is essential for life and regular intakes of pure water, daily, is vital for good health. Chart four provides a list of the daily requirements for water plus a variable amount for different types of work plus climate variations. In a hot climate a person needs over three times the water intake compared to a person in a cold climate. You can calculate the approx. amount of water required for your lifestyle and work requirements, plus climate, to be sure your daily intake of water is adequate. Chart five shows the average amount of water intake per day for different body weights. Refer to chart: 11, page 11 for your approx. ideal body weight to height ratio, on the *body mass index* chart. Chart six provides a list of fresh fruits and vegetables with their beneficial supply of water which can also be included as part of the daily water requirement. Herbal teas and freshly extracted juices are also beneficial forms of water intake. Ideally, obtain half the daily requirement as pure water.

4

DAILY WATER USE	COLD climate	WARM climate	HOT climate
During sleep	300 ml.	500 ml.	1 litre
Evaporation	500 ml.	2 litres	4 litres
Food oxidation	300 ml.	300 ml.	300 ml.
Filter kidneys	1 litre	1 litre	1 litre
ESSENTIAL WATER	2.1 litres	3.8 litres	6.3 litres
ADD <u>ONE</u> OF THE FOLLOWING FOR TOTAL			
Sedentary work	300 ml.	500 ml.	1 litre
Moderate work	500 ml.	1 litre	2 litres
Hard physical work	1 litre	2 litres	4 litres
TOTAL DAILY WATER	2.6 litres	4.8 litres	8.3 litres

5

Kilograms	COLD climate	WARM climate	HOT climate
40 kg.	1.6 litres	2.9 litres	5.0 litres
45 kg.	1.8 litres	3.3 litres	5.7 litres
50 kg.	1.9 litres	3.6 litres	6.3 litres
55 kg.	2.1 litres	4.0 litres	6.9 litres
60 kg.	2.3 litres	4.4 litres	7.6 litres
65 kg.	2.6 litres	4.8 litres	8.3 litres
70 kg.	2.7 litres	5.0 litres	8.6 litres
75 kg.	3.0 litres	5.5 litres	9.5 litres
80 kg.	3.2 litres	5.9 litres	10.2 litres
85 kg.	3.3 litres	6.2 litres	10.7 litres
90 kg.	3.5 litres	6.6 litres	11.4 litres
95 kg.	3.7 litres	6.9 litres	11.9 litres
100 kg.	3.9 litres	7.3 litres	12.4 litres

6

WATER CONTENT OF FRESH FRUITS, VEGETABLES, LEGUMES & HERBS							
APPLES	85%	MANGO	82%	ASPARAGUS	93%	LETTUCE	95%
APRICOT	86%	NECTARINE	91%	BEANS	91%	OKRA	89%
BANANA	75%	OLIVES	70%	BROCCOLI	88%	ONIONS	88%
CANTALOUP	93%	ORANGES	86%	BRUSSEL SPROUTS	85%	PARSLEY	81%
CHERRIES	82%	PAPAYA	88%	CABBAGE	95%	PEAS	78%
CURRANTS	80%	PEACHES	87%	CARROTS	89%	POTATO	80%
DATES	23%	PEARS	84%	CAULIFLOWER	91%	PUMPKIN	92%
FIGS	79%	PINEAPPLE	85%	CELERY	94%	RADISH	95%
GRAPEFRUIT	89%	PLUMS	83%	CUCUMBER	96%	SPINACH	92%
GRAPES	81%	STRAWBERRY	89%	EGGPLANT	92%	SQUASH	95%
LEMON	90%	TOMATO	94%	GARLIC	61%	SWEET POTATO	71%
LYCHEE	82%	WATERMELON	93%	LEEKS	87%	ZUCCHINI	95%

QUESTION 11	*What is the Balanced Diet?*

The Laugh with Health diet balanced diet suggests approx. 50 % Carbohydrate foods, 30 - 40 % Protein foods and 15 - 20 % Lipids. A variety from each main food group is required in order to obtain a complete supply of the essential minerals and vitamins. The chart below shows the main types of food within each of the three main food groups and the proportion of foods recommended for a balanced diet. It is best to consider the balanced diet over a period of one week in order to obtain a full variety of natural foods.

CARBOHYDRATES

GRAINS
LEGUMES
FRUITS
VEGETABLES

LIPIDS

VEGETABLE OILS
OLIVE OIL
BUTTER,
CHEESE,
AVOCADO,
NUTS, SEEDS,
DAIRY FOODS
BACON, MEAT,
MARGARINE

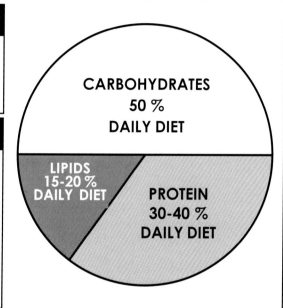

CARBOHYDRATES
50 %
DAILY DIET

LIPIDS
15-20 %
DAILY DIET

PROTEIN
30-40 %
DAILY DIET

PROTEIN

WHOLE GRAINS
LEGUMES
NUTS
SEEDS
SPROUTS
EGGS
FISH
SEAFOOD
POULTRY
MEAT
CHEESE
MILK
YOGHURT

QUESTION 12	*What is the Food Pyramid?*

The Food Pyramid was designed by the (USDA), US Department of Agriculture to provide a simple guide to the requirements for a balanced diet. The Australian Healthy Eating Guide is also a simple way to show the proportions of the main food groups required for a well balanced diet. On pages 30, 42, 60, 77 & 104, a more detailed guide to the balanced diet and the intake of food groups is provided. The Laugh with Health diet is also compared on the pages mentioned, plus on pages 211 - 220 in the summary section.

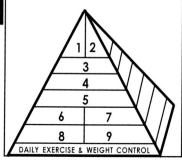

DAILY EXERCISE & WEIGHT CONTROL

1 - Red meat, butter.	SPARINGLY
2 - White rice, White bread, Potatoes, Pasta & Sweets.	SPARINGLY
3 - Dairy or calcium supplement.	1 - 2 serves
4 - Fish, Poultry or Eggs.	0 - 2 serves
5 - Nuts, Legumes.	1 - 3 serves
6 - Vegetables	ABUNDANCE
7 - Fruits	2 - 3 serves
8 - Whole grain foods	MOST MEALS
9 - Plant oils: olive, canola, soy, sunflower, peanut.	MODERATE
10. Daily Exercise & Weight Control.	REGULAR

QUESTION 13

How do I obtain a balanced daily calorie or kilojoule intake?

The balanced daily calorie / kilojoule intake is based on the ratio of 50% carbohydrate, 30-40% protein and 15-20% lipids. The charts below are designed to show (1) the proportion of calories per day from each main food group, (2) the variety of foods within each group, (3) the proportion of individual food groups in daily percentages, (4) the amount of calories per individual food group, plus, (5) the serves per day from each food group. See chart: 10 below for details on serve sizes. In basic terms, use the chart below to balance your daily intake of calories with natural foods. Refer to the Food Combination Chart on pages 208 -210 for details on the best way to combine foods and to the Diet Ideas Guide on pages 214 -219 for numerous simple, balanced recipes based on a variety of natural foods. A proper calorie balance will promote weight control and an abundance of energy and health. Also refer to pages 30, 42, 60, 77, 211 & 212 for more details on the balanced diet.

9

SERVES PER DAY US. FOOD PYRAMID	50% DAILY DIET CARBOHYDRATES MALE 18-50 years (1,450 k.calories daily) 6,069 k.joules daily			SERVES PER DAY US. FOOD PYRAMID	30-40% DAILY DIET PROTEIN Male 18-50 years (870 k.calories daily) 3,641 k. joules daily			SERVES PER DAY US. FOOD PYRAMID	15-20% DAILY DIET LIPIDS (fats & oils) Male 18-50 years (580 k.calories daily) 2,428 k.joules daily		
2 - 4	Fruits	15%	290 c. 1,214 k.j.	2 - 3	Grains	5%	44 c.	SPARINGLY	Dairy foods	20%	116 c.
	Fruit Juice	5%			Legumes	15%	130 c.	1 - 2	Nuts	30%	174 c
3 - 5	Vegetables	15%	290 c. 1,214 k.j.	1 - 2	Nuts	15%	130 c.	1 - 2	Seeds	10%	58 c.
1	Veg. Juice	5%			Seeds / Sprouts	12%	105 c.	1 - 2	Avocado	10%	58 c.
4 - 8	Grains	15%	507 c. 2,122 k.j	1 serve per DAY	Fish / Seafood	25%	217 c.	1	Olive oil	10%	58 c.
	Bread / Pasta	20%			Meat	5%	44 c.	USE SPARINGLY	Margarine	5%	29 c.
1 - 2	Legumes	20%	363 c. 1519 k.j.		Poultry / Eggs	15%	130 c.		Cooking oil	5%	29 c.
	Sprouts	5%		1	Dairy	8%	70 c.		Other foods	10%	58 c.
	TOTAL	100%	1450 K.c. 6,069 k.j.		TOTAL	100%	870 K.c. 3,641 k.j.		TOTAL	100%	580 K.c. 2,428 k.j

SERVES PER DAY US. FOOD PYRAMID	50% DAILY DIET CARBOHYDRATES Female 11-50 years (1100 K.calories daily) 4,605 k. joules daily			SERVES PER DAY US. FOOD PYRAMID	30-40% DAILY DIET PROTEINS Female 11-50 years (660 K.calories daily) 2, 763 k.joules daily			SERVES PER DAY US. FOOD PYRAMID	15-20% DAILY DIET LIPIDS (fats & oils) Female 11-50 years (440 K.calories daily) 1,841 k. joules daily		
2 - 4	Fruits	15%	220 c. 921 k.j.	2 - 3	Grains	5%	33 c.	SPARINGLY	Dairy foods	20%	88 c.
	Fruit Juice	5%			Legumes	15%	99 c.	1 - 2	Nuts	30%	132 c.
3 - 5	Vegetables	15%	220c. 921 k.j.	1 - 2	Nuts	15%	99 c.	1 - 2	Seeds	10%	44 c.
1	Veg. Juice	5%			Seeds / Sprouts	12%	80 c.	1 - 2	Avocado	10%	44 c.
4 - 8	Grains	15%	385c. 1,612 k.j.	1 serve per DAY	Fish / Seafood	25%	165 c.	1	Olive oil	10%	44 c.
	Bread / Pasta	20%			Meat	5%	33 c.	USE SPARINGLY	Margarine	5%	22 c.
1 - 2	Legumes	20%	275 c. 1,151 k.j.		Poultry / Eggs	15%	99 c.		Cooking oil	5%	22 c.
	Sprouts	5%		1	Dairy	8%	52 c.		Other foods	10%	44 c.
	TOTAL	100%	1100 K.c. 4,605 k.j.		TOTAL	100%	660 K.c. 2,763 k.j.		TOTAL	100%	440 K.c. 1,841 k.j.

10

ONE CARBOHYDRATE SERVE SIZE	1 slice of bread	half cup cooked rice	half cup cooked pasta	1 ounce cereal
	half cup cooked beans	1 piece of fruit	3/4 cup fruit juice	half cup of vegetables
ONE PROTEIN SERVE SIZE	2 - 3 ozs fish	2 - 3 ozs. lean meat	2 - 3 ozs. poultry or1 egg	1. 5 cups cooked legumes
ONE DAIRY SERVE SIZE	1 cup milk	1. 5 ozs. cheese	1 cup yoghurt	1 cup ice cream

How many calories / kilojoules do I need everyday?

11

(RDA) KILO CALORIES PER DAY CHART / ACTIVITY EXERCISE CHART (k.calories per day approx.) * / BODY MASS INDEX CHART measured in pounds (lbs.)

(RDA) KILO CALORIES PER DAY CHART		less than 30 min.	30 -60 minutes	1 - 2 hours	2 - 4 hours	4 - 6 hours	feet & inches	normal	overweight	obese
0 - 5months	650						4'10"	118	119 - 142	143 +
5m. - 1year	850	n/a	n/a	n/a	n/a	n/a	4'11"	123	124 - 147	148 +
1 - 3 years	1300	1200	1300			1500	5' 0"	127	128 - 152	153 +
4 - 6 years	1800	1700	1800			1900	5" 1"	131	132 - 157	158 +
7 - 10 years	2000	1800	2000		2200	2300	5' 2"	135	136 - 163	164 +
MALE							5' 3"	140	141 - 168	169 +
11 - 14 years	2500	2400	2500		2700	2800	5" 4"	144	145 - 173	174 +
15 - 18 years	3000	2600	3000	3100	3200	3400	5' 5"	149	150 - 179	180 +
19 - 24 years	2900	2700	2900	3000	3200	3300	5' 6"	154	155 - 185	186 +
25 - 50 years	2900	2500	2900	3000	3200	3300	5' 7"	158	159 - 190	191 +
51 + years	2300	2200	2300	2400	2500	2700	5' 8"	163	164 - 196	197 +
FEMALE							5' 9"	168	169 - 202	203 +
11 - 14 years	2200	2100	2200		2400	2600	5' 10"	173	174 - 208	209 +
15 - 18 years	2200	2100	2200		2400	2600	5' 11"	178	179 - 214	215 +
19 - 24 years	2200	2000	2200	2400	2500	2600	6' 0"	183	184 - 220	221 +
25 - 50 years	2200	2000	2200	2400	2500	2600	6' 1"	188	189 - 226	227 +
51 + years	1900	1800	1900	2100	2200	2500	6' 2"	193	194 - 232	233 +
Pregnancy	2500	2500	2500	2600	2700	2900	6' 3"	199	200 - 239	240 +
Lactation	2700	2600	2700	2900	3000	3200				

12

CALORIES / KILOJOULES PER MINUTE / HOUR ACTIVITY CHART

ACTIVITY	CALORIES MIN.	HOUR	KILOJOULES MIN.	HOUR	ACTIVITY	CALORIES MIN.	HOUR	KILOJOULES MIN.	HOUR
SLEEPING	.9	54	3.7	222	SLOW SKIPPING	5.5	330	23	1380
LYING DOWN	1	60	4.1	246	MODERATE TENNIS	5.8	348	24.2	1452
SITTING DOWN	1.4	84	5.8	348	SURFING	5.9	354	24.6	1476
COMPUTER WORK	1.5	90	6.2	372	MODERATE SWIMMING	6.0	360	25.1	1506
IRONING	2	120	8.3	498	HORSE RIDING ACTIVE	6.1	366	25.5	1530
DRIVING	2.3	138	9.6	576	ACTIVE DANCING	6.2	372	25.9	1554
SLOW WALKING	2.9	174	12.1	726	COMPETATIVE CRICKET	6.3	378	26.3	1578
SWEEPING	3	180	12.5	750	WALKING UPSTAIRS	6.4	384	26.7	1602
LAWN BOWLS	3.5	210	14.6	876	BASKETBALL / RUNNING	6.6	396	27.6	1656
EASY GARDENING	4	240	16.7	1002	HEAVY GARDENING	7.0	420	29.3	1756
RELAXED GOLF	4.5	270	18.8	1128	FOOTBALL / RUGBY	7.5	450	31.3	1878
WASHING FLOORS	4.6	276	19.2	1152	FAST RUNNING	7.8	468	32.6	1956
MODERATE WALKING	4.8	288	20	1200	COMPETATIVE TENNIS	8	480	33.4	2004
ACTIVE GARDENING	5	300	20.9	1254	RUNNING UPSTAIRS	10	600	41.8	2508
BRISK WALKING	5.2	312	21.7	1302	COMPETATIVE SKIING	14	840	58.6	3516
SLOW BIKE RIDING	5.4	324	22.6	1356	SPRINTING	15	900	62.7	3762

How many Calories / kilojoules are in foods?

Chart 13 provides a variety of foods with their calorie/kilojoule value. The foods with the highest lipid content usually have the highest calorie value, as lipids supply 9 calories per gram, or 38 kilojoules per gram. Carbohydrates and proteins supply 4 calories per gram. Foods with a high water content usually have less calories per gram. The average person burns about 250 calories per hour. 1 Kilo calorie equals 4.186 Kilojoules (Kj.) A calorie is defined as the quantity of heat required to raise the temperature of one gram of water by one degree, specifically from 14.5 C. to 15.5 C. Natural foods provide a balance of calories plus a variety of the essential nutrients. Processed and refined foods are deficient in nutrients and fibre, they are termed 'empty calorie foods'. Chart 14 provides an average summary of the fibre and carbohydrate content of 10 main food groups. A prolonged deficiency of fibre foods can lead to various problems with the digestive and elimination system. Protect your body with fibre rich foods as part of a complete balanced daily diet.

13

FOOD CALORIES & KILOJOULES VALUE CHART

HIGH CALORIE / KILOJOULE FOODS	k.calories 100 g	k.joules 100 g	MEDIUM CALORIE / KILOJOULE FOODS	calories 100 g	k.joules 100 g	LOW CALORIE / KILOJOULE FOODS	calories 100 g	k.joules 100 g
Hamburger	856	3,583	Beef steak	437	1,829	Wheat	329	1,377
Vegetable oils	884	3,700	Pork chops	436	1,825	Rye flour	327	1,368
Potato chips	727	3,043	Soy flour	419	1,753	Honey	322	1,347
Butter/Margarine	727	3,043	Soy beans	416	1,741	Tuna	288	1,205
Macadamia nuts	718	3.005	Rolled oats	389	1,666	Sausages raw	275	1,151
Pine nuts	700	2,930	Ham	389	1,666	T. bone rare	258	1,079
Pecan nuts	691	2,892	Sugar	385	1,611	Chicken fried	243	1,017
Pine nuts	673	2,817	Swiss cheese	378	1,582	Rye bread	237	992
Bacon grilled	661	2,766	Pasta	371	1,553	Wheat bran	225	941
Brazil nuts	656	2,746	Rice brown	370	1,548	Chestnuts	224	937
Walnuts	654	2,737	Corn flakes	370	1,548	Carob flour	222	929
Hazel nuts	628	2,628	Sweet corn	365	1,527	Wheat bran	216	904
Almonds	578	2,419	Lamb chops	355	1,486	Fish baked	202	845
Sesame seeds	573	2,398	Chick peas	364	1,523	Roast chicken	199	833
Tahini	570	2,386	Cream	364	1,523	Salmon	182	762
Peanuts	567	2,373	White bread	361	1,511	Avocado	171	716
Cashews	566	2,369	Wheat germ	360	1,506	Tuna in water	167	699
Sunflower seeds	560	2,344	Lamb chops	355	1,486	Boiled egg	120	502
Pistachio nuts	557	2,331	Coconut meat	354	1,481	Rice boiled	120	502
Pepitas	554	2,277	Barley	354	1,481	Cottage cheese	106	443
Chocolate milk	538	2,252	Maple syrup	348	1,456	Ice cream low fat	104	435
Chocolate dark	534	2,235	Mung beans	347	1,452	Ricotta cheese	100	419
Cashew nuts	566	2,369	Cream cheese	345	1,444	Prawns	85	355
Linseed	498	2,072	Buckwheat	343	1,435	Oysters raw	68	284
Bacon raw	458	1,917	Green beans	343	1,435	Cows milk	67	280
Cheddar cheese	450	1,883	Muesli	340	1,423	Fresh fruits average	50	209
Cheddar cheese	450	1,883	Lima beans/ lentils	340	1,423	Vegetables average	45	188

14

FIBRE & CARBOHYDRATE NATURAL FOODS COMPARISON CHART

100 g.	FRUITS	VEG.	GRAINS	LEGUMES	NUTS	SEEDS	MEAT	POULTRY	FISH	MILK
FIBRE	5	5	15	12	15	12	0	0	0	0
CARB.	10	10	75	65	25	25	0	0	0	4

CARBOHYDRATE INTRODUCTION

QUESTION 16	What is a Carbohydrate?	An energy producing organic compound of carbon oxygen and hydrogen.
QUESTION 17	How are Carbohydrates made?	Carbohydrates are mainly produced by plants.
QUESTION 18	What are the main types of carbohydrates?	Sugars & Starches
QUESTION 19	How does the body use carbohydrates?	Carbohydrates are converted into glucose which is used by the brain and muscles for energy.

POLYSACCHARIDES   **DISACCHARIDES**   **MONOSACCHARIDES**

1 CELLULOSE & LIGNINS

2 uncooked STARCH cooked

3 GLYCOGEN

4 PECTIN & GUMS

5 SUCROSE CANE SUGAR — invertase →

6 MALTOSE MALT SUGAR

6 LACTOSE MILK SUGAR

amylase →

ptyalin →

converted by the liver →

invertase →

maltase →

lactase →

lactase →

8 FRUCTOSE FRUIT SUGAR

GLUCOSE

9 GALACTOSE SIMPLE SUGAR

1. Cellulose and lignins are both termed insoluble fibres. They protect against digestive problems.

2. There are two types of starch;

Amylose: takes longer to convert to glucose, it has a lower G.I.

Amylopectin: converts quickly into glucose, has a high G.I.

refer to page 16 for G.I. values.

3. Glycogen is stored in the liver and muscles and converted into glucose when the body requires extra energy.

4. Pectin and gums are water soluble fibres. They bind cholesterol and prevent it's absorption.

5. Sucrose, the common sugar.

6. Maltose, malt from grains.

7. Lactose is hard to convert for many people, due to a lack of the enzyme lactase.

8. Fructose, a simple sugar from fruits, it is easy to convert.

9. Galactose, part of milk sugar.

10. Glucose, the primary energy

NOTE: All amounts in this book are measured in milligrams (mg) per 100 grams, unless stated otherwise.

13

QUESTION 20	*What are the Carbohydrate food groups?*	**F R U I T S V E G E T A B L E S G R A I N S L E G U M E S**

QUESTION 21	*What do carbohydrate foods provide?*	**CARBOHYDRATES PROTEIN, LIPIDS, WATER, MINERALS, VITAMINS, FIBRE, ENZYMES & ANTIOXIDANTS.**

Carbohydrate foods provide the greatest supply and variety of nutrients. Throughout the following chapter, a detailed summary of the main nutrients with individual carbohydrate foods is provided. As can be seen from chart 15, fruits and vegetables have a low protein content and calorie content with a high water content. Grains and legumes supply protein and a generous calorie content compared to the fruits and vegetables.

The amounts on the charts are based on the average food group values and for more details on the exact value of individual carbohydrate foods, plus their mineral and vitamin content, refer to the individual foods throughout the following carbohydrate chapter. Carbohydrate foods can provide nearly all the essential nutrients, however, for a well balanced diet, the other nine natural food groups, refer to page 4, are required. The amounts below are all based on 100 grams. Chart 16 provides a list of the individual foods within each main carbohydrate food group.

15 CARBOHYDRATE FOOD GROUPS	CARB. %	PROTEIN %	LIPIDS %	WATER %	CALORIES	KILOJOULES
Whole grains	75 grams.	12 grams.	2 grams.	11 grams.	330	1,381
Legumes (beans & peas)	65 grams.	21 grams.	2 grams.	12 grams.	340	1,423
Fruits	10 grams.	0.5 grams.	0.2 grams.	90 grams.	40	167
Vegetables	10 grams.	6 grams.	0.2 grams.	83 grams.	45	188

QUESTION 22	*What are the individual Carbohydrate foods?*

16	NATURAL FOODS & INDIVIDUAL FOOD GROUPS	
	WHOLE GRAINS	Barley, Bulgur, Corn, Millet, Oats, Rice, Rye, Sorghum, Triticale, Wheat.
	LEGUMES (beans / peas)	Carob, Green, Kidney, Lima, Mung, Soy, Chick pea, Lentils, Peas, Peanut.
F R U I T S	**SUB ACID FRUITS**	Apples, Apricot, Cherries, Grapes, Papaya, Peaches, Pears, Mango.
	SWEET FRUITS	Banana, Date, Fig, Prunes, Raisins, Sultanas, Dried Fruits.
	ACID FRUITS	Grapefruit, Kiwi fruit, Lemons, Limes, Mandarin, Oranges, Passionfruit, Tomato.
	MELONS	Cantaloup, Casaba, Honeydew, Watermelon.
VEG.	**STARCH VEGETABLES**	Artichoke, Beetroot, Carrot, Parsnip, Potato, Pumpkin, Radish, Turnip.
	LEAFY VEGETABLES	Lettuce, Cabbage, Celery, Silverbeet, Spinach, Watercress.
	FLOWER VEGETABLES	Asparagus, Broccoli, Cauliflower, Brussel sprouts.
	OTHER VEGETABLES	Capsicum, Cucumber, Egg plant, Mushrooms, Okra, Onions, Zucchini.

7

QUESTION 23

Are all carbohydrate foods natural?

Carbohydrate foods all originate as natural foods, from plants, trees and grasses. The chart below provides a *basic visual guide* to the common types of processing that occurs to some natural carbohydrate foods and it is clear that the grains incur the most processing. Generally speaking, each processing stage reduces the nutritional quality of the natural food. Processing was originally designed to promote the 'shelf life' of a food. Today, additives are often used to promote the appetite and some foods are 'so tasty', they easily take first place, on the plate, compared to the unique flavours of natural foods. The black squares indicate the food has obtained 'processing', as mentioned on top of the chart.

CARBOHYDRATE FOODS		ADDED SALT	ADDED SUGAR	ADDITIVES	CANNING	REFINED FLOUR	FREEZING	BAKING	COOKING OR HEAT
GRAINS NATURAL	WHOLE GRAINS								
	ROLLED OATS								
	BROWN RICE								
	SWEET CORN								
GRAINS PROCESSED	WHOLEGRAIN BREAD	■	■	■				■	
	WHOLEMEAL BREAD	■	■	■		■		■	
	WHITE / BROWN BREAD	■	■	■		■		■	
	BREAKFAST CEREALS	■	■	■		■		■	
	PASTRY & CAKES	■	■	■		■		■	
	BISCUITS	■	■	■		■		■	
	CORN CHIPS	■		■		■		■	
	RICE CRACKERS	■		■		■		■	
	CANNED CORN	■	■	■	■				■
	PASTA	■		■		■			■
LEGUMES NATURAL	ALL WHOLE: BEANS: CAROB, GREEN, KIDNEY, LIMA, MUNG, SOY. PEAS: CHICK, LENTILS, PEAS. PEANUT, FRESH PEANUT BUTTER.								
LEGUMES PROCESSED	PEANUT BUTTER.	■	■	■					■
	CANNED BEANS / PEAS.	■		■	■				
	FROZEN BEANS / PEAS.						■		
FRUITS & VEGETABLES NATURAL	ALL FRESH FRUITS & VEGETABLES FRESHLY EXTRACTED JUICES. NATURALLY DRIED FRUITS & VEGETABLES.								
FRUITS & VEGETABLES PROCESSED	CANNED FRUITS		■		■				■
	CANNED VEGETABLES	■			■				■
	FRUIT CORDIALS		■	■					■
	FRUIT & VEG. JUICES	■	■	■					
	JAMS & SPREADS	■	■	■					■
	FROZEN FRUITS & VEG.						■		■

15

What is the Glycemic Index?

The Glycemic Index is a measure used for carbohydrate foods to assess the supply of glucose and the subsequent rise in blood glucose levels. The glycemic index was originally designed for diabetics. Foods with a high or very high glycemic index cause a rapid rise in blood sugar levels. Factors such as refinement and the dominant type of starch structure of foods determines the glycemic index value. Sugar, lollies and soft drinks, plus the cup of tea or coffee with sugar routine and alcohol drinks all provide a high glycemic index. Use the chart below to balance meals and your daily carbohydrate intake. Fats, protein and fibre lower the glycemic value of a meal. Protect your body from sudden sugar hits.
This chart is based on the reference measure of glucose at 100 glycemic index points.

18

VERY LOW GYCEMIC INDEX (below 11)	MAIN GROUPS	G.I. HINTS
broccoli, cabbage, lettuce, mushrooms, onions, capsicum, almonds, brazil, cashews, pecan, macadamia, walnut, pepitas, sunflower seeds.	**VEGETABLES** **NUTS & SEEDS**	Add plenty of these foods to your meals.
LOW GLYCEMIC INDEX FOODS (12 - 40)	MAIN GROUPS	G. I. HINTS
barley, fettucine, wholegrain spaghetti, vermicelli, red lentils, soy beans, kidney beans, lima beans, navy beans, peanuts, mung beans, tomato, apples, cherries, grapefruit, plums, peaches, tomato soup, apple juice, prunes, rice bran, milk, soy milk, flavoured milk, yoghurt.	**LEGUMES** **PASTA** **CITRUS FRUITS** **MILK & DAIRY** **APPLES** **SOUP**	Ideal for most diabetics and for regular use. Combine these foods with moderate or high G.I. foods.
MODERATE GLYCEMIC INDEX FOODS (40 - 60)	MAIN GROUPS	G. I. HINTS
baked beans, oatmeal, muesli, white spaghetti, apricots, banana, grapes, kiwifruit, brown rice, mango, papaya, pear, carrots, sweet corn, oats, orange juice, pineapple juice, custard, dried apricots, potato chips, strawberry jam, honey, basmati rice, macaroni, oat bread, yam, pita bread, sourdough bread, pumpernickel, bran, carrots boiled, peas, chocolate bar.	**BROWN RICE** **WHOLE GRAINS** **SOUR DOUGH &** **FIBRE BREADS** **OATS** **FRUITS** **FRUIT JUICES**	Add any of these foods to your diet in place of moderate or high G.I. foods. Add vegetables, nuts or seeds to these foods if compatable.
MODERATELY HIGH G.I. FOODS (60 - 80)	MAIN GROUPS	G. I. HINTS
whole grain cereals, puffed wheat, shredded wheat, croissants, rye bread, beetroot canned, corn chips, pea soup, bagels, hamburger bun, muffins, pizza base, white bread (70), raisins, wheat (68), pineapple, millet, table sugar, white rice, cola drinks, ice cream vanilla, melon, mashed potatoes, most breakfast cereals, most bakery products.	**WHITE RICE** **CEREALS** **WHITE BREAD** **BAKERY** **PRODUCTS** **ICE CREAM** **SOFT DRINKS** **SUGAR**	Add milk, cream, nuts, seeds or bran to the breakfast cereal to reduce the G.I. Add lots of salad and tahini to the bread. Avoid soft drinks and added sugar.
HIGH GLYCEMIC INDEX (80 - 100)	MAIN GROUPS	G . I. HINTS
corn flakes, jelly beans, pretzels, rice cakes, parsnips, french baquette, baked potatoes, maltose, *(glucose (100) * reference measure).*	**SWEETS** **REFINED CORN** **BAKED POTATOES**	Combine with cream, butter or milk, or add tahini or very low G. I. foods or avoid these foods.
VERY HIGH GLYCEMIC INDEX (100-110)	MAIN GROUPS	
dates, tofu	DATES, TOFU	

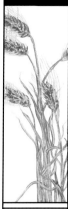

Grains have been used for thousands of years as a main provider of food, energy and nourishment.

The discovery of grains as a source of food, by primitive people, enabled them to settle in one place and rely on a food supply from the 'crop that did not wander'. People shared the task of crop cultivation until such time when machinery took over.

Nowadays, some people rarely eat whole grains. Processed and refined foods have flooded the food aisles and as they are great profit making foods, advertising becomes very competitive and compelling. Breakfast cereals are promoted to make giants out of dwarfs, biscuits can become the mother's best helper and white bread can be so spongy that the more you eat, the more flexible and active you become, well, that's advertising!

Grains are a compact carbohydrate food, an energy source.

For many people the regular diet will include only one main grain, usually wheat as in sandwiches. Rice is also a common addition to the diet, however the other grains rarely get a chance to contribute their nutritional benefits, unique taste and range of recipes.

Your health is based on the food you eat. Your diet is based on the recipes you know. Health is often poor due to the lack of knowledge on natural whole grain recipes.

The routine of modern day living can have a detrimental effect on health. Time goes so quickly in the morning before work or school that some people compensate by relying on the quickest and most convenient packaged breakfast foods.

Be prepared for breakfast and give the whole grains a chance to make your day complete.

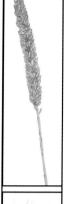

You need energy to get through a busy day and breakfast is the ideal time to obtain the stamina of whole grains. Grains supply long lasting energy. Apart from being an excellent source of carbohydrates, grains also supply a fair percentage of primary protein.

At least two meals a day should be based around whole grains. There are many forms of the whole grain, some of which are seldom included or even thought of as an excellent substitute for the commercially prepared and refined breakfast cereals. A rolled grain is a whole grain, with all the essential nutrients in proper balance.

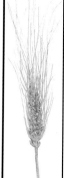

The following pages provide a detailed nutritional survey of the main whole grains: barley, corn, millet, rice, rye and wheat, providing the best attributes of each whole grain and their products, with negative factors also mentioned.

The balanced diet requires approx. 50% carbohydrates. Whole grains provide approx. 70 - 80% carbohydrate content, 10 % protein and a low fat content 5%, therefore, such foods as milk, cheese, butter, cream and oil can be added to grains, moderately, without problems.

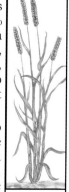

Most grains need added fats to make them appetising, such as the basic bread and cheese, in addition fats lower the glycemic index, providing a slower release of the starch content into glucose.

Refined grains lack valuable fibre and nutrients plus they increase blood sugar levels quickly, as they are mainly starch. Refer to chart page 16.

Whole grains are the ideal energy food with stamina power and a great supply of life supporting nutrients. Page 30 provides a guide to the daily intake of grains as part of a balanced diet.

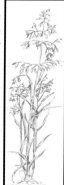

NOTE: All amounts in this book are measured in milligrams (mg) per 100 grams, unless stated otherwise.

17

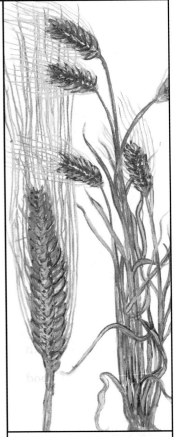

Barley has already made it's name in history, long before wheat and rye, as it was used by the Egyptians over 8,000 years ago. Barley grain was also used for the daily bread of Greek, Roman, Chinese and Hebrew civilizations from 4,000 B.C. onwards and it was also traded as payment for a day's work.

Today, barley is mainly used for the brewing of beer, vinegar and whisky. The true value of barley's unique nutritional qualities and flavour is untapped.

The best way to obtain barley in the diet is from 'barley grass juice'. It is very similar to wheat grass juice in healing power, refer to page 112.

Barley 'sprouts' have helped in the discovery of nations, as Captain Cook recognized that sprouted grains protected his hard-working men from illness, especially scurvy. Barley sprouts make an excellent addition to bread, casseroles and soups such as the classic 'Scotch broth'.

Barley flakes or rolled barley are ideal for winter porridge and when blended, for vegetarian pate . Barley provides a unique body warming effect and it was 'the fast food' for athletes and the gladiators during the Roman empire.

Barley has the ability to decrease the risk of colon cancer, as the barley fibre promotes the growth of 'friendly' bacteria in the colon. Beneficial fatty acids termed butyric acids are formed which promote colon health by stimulating cells. These beneficial bacteria also retard the action of harmful bacteria. In addition, the good supply of the mineral selenium is known to protect against colon cancer.

Barley fibre is also a good source of beta glucan which helps eliminate bile acids, produced by the liver and stored in the gall bladder to process fats. The removal of bile actually lowers blood cholesterol, as the liver will utilize stored cholesterol in the manufacture of more bile acids. Barley will provide approx. 60% of the daily dietary fibre from one cup of cooked rolled barley and nearly 20% of daily protein when combined with milk. Rolled barley is best presoaked in water overnight and cooked for breakfast with milk added. If you have to add a dash of sugar, don't worry, as the barley fibre slows blood sugar levels. However, barley is rich in maltose, or malt sugar, providing good natural sweetness.

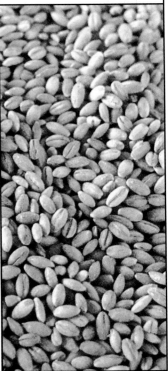

The supply of organic copper from barley is ideal for the health of the joint system, the blood vessels and the skeletal system. A one cup serve of barley provides over 25% daily copper requirements.

Compared to white bread toast for breakfast, the rolled barley breakfast will protect against rheumatoid arthritis due to a good supply of copper. The phosphorus content 296 mg is abundant and beneficial for the brain and nervous system in addition to magnesium 37 mg.

Barley water, made by boiling barley grains for 1 hour, allow to cool and drinking the water, has proved beneficial for asthmatics as it contains the substance hordenine, an antispasmodic.

Be brave, try barley for breakfast and in winter, place a pot of barley grains on the potbelly stove and get the true old fashioned slow-cooking flavour, 2 hours for soups, just add your vegies, spices and herbs in the last 20 minutes.

Barley brings a bounty of beautiful body benefits.

CORN-MAIZE *Zea mays*	GLYCEMIC INDEX: 56	C. 82	P. 7	L. 11	CALORIES - total: **365 kcal. per 100 gram** Calories from: Carb:300 Protein:26 Fat:39

Corn is the 'daughter of life' according to the American Indians and for 10,000 years it was their staple grain and also in Mexico, the daily bread 'tortilla' and in North America 'hominy'. Corn was exported to China, Africa, Japan and India during the 16th. century, but, it was 'scorned' when compared to wheat and rye for breadmaking.

Corn flour contains no gluten and it is low in 2 essential amino acids: tryptophan and lysine. In addition to this, niacin in corn flour is poorly absorbed.

There are 5 main types of corn: dent corn is used for bread making, flint corn for animal fodder, flour corn is the best quality for breadmaking, pop corn is the most popular and least nutritious, the wonderful sweet corn is by far the most nutritious and delicious. Sweet corn, also known as 'corn on the cob' is full of benefits; the folate content 19 mcg is a great bonus for children or people who don't like to eat their 'greens'. Folate is vital for growth of children, essential during pregnancy and also for the brain and nervous system.

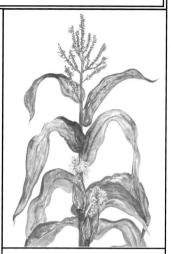

Sweet corn is the best grain source of vitamin A 400 I.U. combined with the top sulphur content of 368 mg it will protect the body against infections, especially when eaten raw or with light steaming.

The vitamin A is mainly in the form of beta-cryptoxanthin, a carotenoid. One report showed a 37% reduction in the risk of lung cancer in smokers, for those who regularly consumed beta-cryptoxanthin rich foods.

Sweet corn is a good source of potassium 280 mg and for those irritable children with a 'sweet tooth', a cob of corn for an after school snack may just 'hit the spot' and the magnesium 48 mg may be just enough to help them concentrate and be creative with homework. Sweet corn is a natural treat with a very low calorie (96) and fat content 1 g, so add a dab of butter and don't wait till summer, it is available nearly all year round, but, it's best and sweetest in summer.

The vitamin C 12 mg plus the good supply of fibre 0.07 g both add to the benefits of sweet corn. Unlike flour corn, it contains a good supply of vitamin B3 1.7 mg and combined with the phosphorus and magnesium content, sweet corn is food for the brain. Vitamin B3 is required for the synthesis of a nerve transmitter: *acetylcholine*, required for memory and protection from Alzheimer's disease, senility and age related mental function.

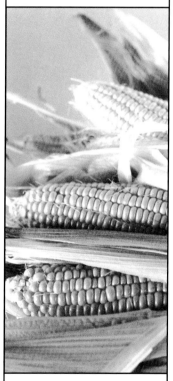

Make a corn soup for the elderly before you forget the benefits. Fortunately, vitamin B3 is stable to heat, so you can 'cook up' the benefits. Even canned corn provides a portion of the benefits.

Corn chips and tacos have become a popular snack or meal maker and even though they only provide a crunch nutritionally, on their own, it is the added ingredients that can make them a complete health meal.

I have noticed children eating lettuce, grated carrot, capsicum, kidney beans and cheese when tacos are prepared, it's a great way to help children obtain proper nutrition. The fast and simple nachos is also a delight and the crispy tortillas can be full of flavour and natural ingredients. Corn bread is now available at supermarkets. Try corn pancakes combined with steamed apples, a sprinkle of cracked almonds and a spoon of cream. 'Corn-on'!

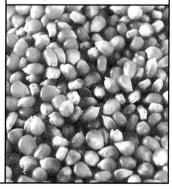

MILLET	*Eleusine coracana*	GLYCEMIC INDEX: 103	C. P. L. 80 11 9	CALORIES - total: **378 kcal. per 100 gram** Calories from: Carb:300 Protein:43 Fat:35

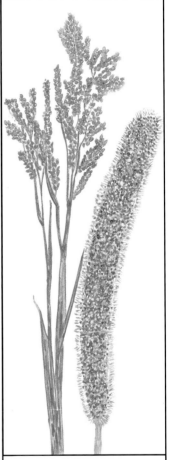

Millet is botanically speaking a mixed bag of grains: finger millet, bullrush millet, common millet and foxtail millet. The main similar characteristics are the very small grains on a drought resistant plant that can be grown in poor soils.

As half the world's soils are depleted, millet may become more a necessity in the future than it's current status in the developed world as 'bird food' or cattle feed.

Millet is cultivated on a large scale in the arid areas of India, Ceylon, Africa and Rhodesia. The finger millet in particular can be stored for up to 5 years, a great famine reserve food in the dry tropics.

Millet has four times the amount of the essential mineral silicon 160 mg compared to wheat. Silicon is required for hair growth, blood circulation, protection from mental fatigue, arthritis and infection. Millet provides over twice the iron content 3 mg. - 6.8 mg of whole wheat and four times that of rice. Millet contains the same magnesium content 162 mg as whole wheat, twice that of rice and seven times that of white bread. Magnesium is known to reduce migraine attacks and the severity of asthma plus it reduces high blood pressure and is vital for the nervous system, memory and strong bone development.

Millet will continue to have an expanding role in the future diet due to it's gluten free benefit. For people with wheat allergies, coeliac disease and other yeast intolerances, the millet grain can provide a breakfast meal that is low in fat 4.2 g, high in fibre 8.5 g or 34% d.v. and provides complete protein 11 g, a well balanced food with a great carbohydrate supply of 72 g.

The question is, how does it taste? Like any food, if it's prepared properly and you're hungry, it tastes magnificent. Rinse half a cup of millet in a sieve, place half a cup of millet, one cup of water and one cup of milk in a saucepan, simmer for 10 -15 minutes whilst stirring, add extra milk or water when required, as millet requires nearly 5 cups liquid per cup serve. Add a dash of cinnamon and nutmeg, serve in a bowl with stewed apples, slivered almonds and a dribble of sweetened cream, a breakfast that will beat any processed cereal nutritionally. Millet can take the place of rice with vegetable dishes, add it to muffins and don't forget the famous Metung millet cookies, in the previous editions. Refer to page 216 for a few simple millet recipes. In India, millet is made into bread called *roti* and in Africa the daily bread *injera*. For a French style recipe try Normandy millet or grind millet and add it to a bread mixture.

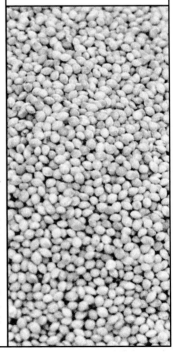

Millet is also a good source of folate 85 mcg more than cooked broccoli. During pregnancy, the combination of the great iron and folate content makes millet a sensible food to use regularly, instead of toast. Millet also provides the mineral zinc 1.7 mg required for improved immune system function, reproductive system, good skin condition and general body healing. Millet provides copper 0.7 mg or 37% d.v. More than meat, oysters or bread.

Millet provides an abundance of phosphorus 285 mg or 47% d.v. essential for the nervous system, memory and energy distribution. Millet is the ideal gluten free grain and substitute for wheat and bran. It is a non allergenic food, so don't get 'stuck in a rut' with wheat for breakfast, lunch, or the evening meal, the minute millet grain is ready any minute!

OATS *Avena sativa*	GLYCEMIC INDEX: 49	C. P. L. 70 15 15	CALORIES - total: **389 kcal. per 100 gram** Calories from: Carb:273 Protein:58 Fat:58

Oats have a short history compared to other grains, they were first cultivated about 3,000 years ago in Europe. Oats must be prepared quickly after harvesting due to a fat dissolving enzyme within the grain that causes spoilage. Only 5% of the oats produced are used for human consumption. The thoroughbreds get the balance and no wonder they are winners.

Oats are now recognized as a great nutritional food. Scottish people have kept fit and strong for centuries with oats as a staple food. They even beat the Romans in battle. Oats are prepared into various forms such as oat groats which provide the whole grain benefit. Quick cooking oats are pre-cooked and finely cut. Oat bran provides numerous health benefits. The 'old fashioned' rolled oats are basically the whole grain that is steamed and flattened by rolling. Ideally, obtain the best quality rolled oats.

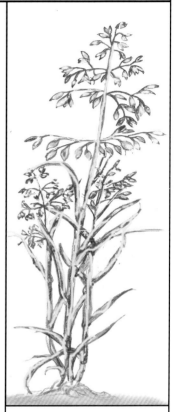

Oats for breakfast is the meal that can balance your daily energy levels. Oats contain a special ingredient in the fibre, known as beta glucan. It helps to slow the rise in blood sugar levels, ideal for diabetics. Oats are an asset for life. These days with so many foods loaded with sugar, the use of oats is more a necessity than a choice. For children, the sugar cravings and lolly eating, plus soft drink consumption can eventually trigger the onset of diabetic symptoms: hyperactivity, inability to concentrate and miserable attitudes to mention a few.

A bowl of well prepared porridge for breakfast can really balance the body for an active day. Place one cup of quality whole rolled oats in a saucepan with one cup of water and one cup of milk, slowly bring to a low simmer, whilst stirring regularly, add extra milk to ensure a s*mooth consistency*. Add a splash of cinnamon, dash of salt and serve with stewed apples and sweet cream. For adults, try raw rolled oats, soaked overnight or for at least 10 minutes in goats milk or 'pure milk', where do you get it?, well you make it.

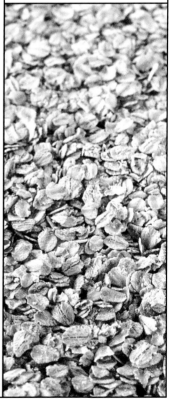

Find a top quality plain acidophillus yoghurt made from raw milk, check the labels, as only a few are made from raw milk. Mix 3 tablespoons of the yoghurt in a jar with 1 cup of pure water, stir very well, shake and pour over the raw rolled oats. Add sliced peaches, or canned apricots on top and serve with a dribble of sweetened cream, now that's the best balanced breakfast.

Apart from the stabilized blood sugar levels, the fibre, in rolled oats containing beta-glucan can reduce blood cholesterol by 8% - 23% according to one study. Oats are the best grain source of complete protein 17 g or 34% d.v. and that's from a small 100 gram serve, without the extra protein value when the milk is added, just imagine if you added a few ground almonds or sunflower seeds, obtaining over half your daily protein requirements at breakfast.

Oats are also an excellent source of fibre 10.5 g or 42% d.v. For those concerned about colon cancer, fibre is vital. The rich supply of selenium from oats 35% d.v. and oat bran 45 mcg or 55% d.v. provides an important role with *glutathione peroxidase, promoting* antioxidant power and a decreased risk of bowel cancer. White bread, meat and chicken are all common foods with one common negative factor, they provide no fibre.

An old Scottish proverb: "The whiter the bread, the sooner you're dead". Don't delay, get ya oats today!

Oats are the main ingredient in *muesli,* a recipe invented by Dr. Bircher-Benner of Switzerland in the late 1900's, the name muesli translates to mean mixture. Dr. Bircher-Benner developed a sanatorium, for healing and the muesli recipe was designed specifically as a complete health restoring meal.

The original recipe was prepared on a daily basis and it was given to the patients throughout the day or night. Initially, the method included; rolled oats soaked in pure milk overnight. Later on the recipe changed and freshly extracted fruit juice replaced the milk. In the morning, raw hazelnut or almond pieces plus an abundance of grated apple, a few grapes and berries were added.

The original muesli recipe can be refrigerated for up to 2 days. The original muesli recipe had no sugar and was ready to serve anytime, to the patients. Processed muesli formulas are often toasted and they have too many ingredients and poor combinations, causing poor digestion.

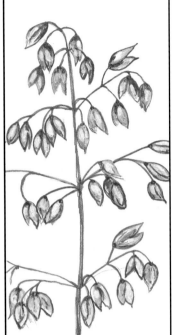

Oats are the greatest 'brain grain', the abundance of inositol 12 mg, a B complex vitamin is vital for nourishment of brain cells as it assists in the transfer of neurotransmitters between brain cells. Inositol can be manufactured by the body from glucose and with oats, the great supply of carbohydrates 66 g or 22% d.v. are converted into glucose. This provides a stable supply of brain energy, in fact the brain utilizes up to 90% of all glucose, the remainder is used by muscles during activity. The excellent supply of magnesium 177 mg or 44% d.v. adds weight to the 'brain grain' title of oats. This vital mineral is not only required for conversion of carbohydrates into glucose but it is vital for a good memory as it activates brain activity and nourishes the white nerve fibres of the brain.

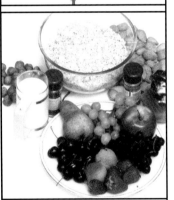

Oats are also an excellent source of phosphorus 523 mg or 52% d.v. A lack of phosphorus can lead to poor memory and poor concentration. Processed breakfast cereals are low in phosphorus plus sugar causes a depletion of this vital mineral.

Oats are an excellent source of manganese 4.9 mg or 100% d.v. 'the memory mineral'. Manganese also helps stabilize glucose levels, it is very important for people with diabetes. Manganese is essential for brain function as it coordinates nerve impulses plus it is a natural antioxidant and essential for the reproductive system.

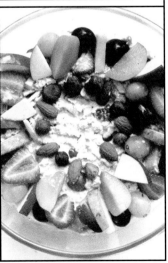

The ample supply of copper 0.6 mg or 31% d.v., assists the nervous system and it is likely to be the missing mineral causing post natal depression. Serum copper levels rise considerably during pregnancy due to elevated oestrogen levels which can take months to stabilize. The bonus with oats is the balance with the mineral zinc 4 mg or 26% d.v., as they both compete for absorption within the digestive tract.

The good iron content 4.7 mg or 26% d.v. is vital especially during menstruation, pregnancy and after childbirth. For maximum benefits, add strawberries on top of the muesli breakfast, as the added vitamin C, plus good protein from oats 17 g will greatly assist absorption of the mineral iron. The vitamin B1 0.8 mg or 51% d.v. supply is very good and it promotes mental efficiency and nerve cell function. Oats provide B5 1.3 mg, folate 56 mcg and B6 0.1 mg. The potassium content 429 mg assists muscle and nerve function. The fat content of oats is 7 g, it provides the wonderful creamy texture. Muesli is ready to make your day original!

RICE - white	*Oryza sativa*	GLYCEMIC INDEX: 72	C. 91	P. 7	L. 2	CALORIES - total: **365 kcal. per 100 gram** Calories from: Carb:332 Protein:27 Fat:6

Rice feeds half the world's population. Rice was first cultivated in China over 6,000 years ago. Rice is the only underwater grain and the old fashioned planting and harvesting were by hand and with water buffalo.

Whole rice can be stored for up to 6 months, unless it is processed into white rice. The outer layers of whole rice contain the rice bran and oil rich germ layer which are susceptible to oxidation and rancidity. There are three main types of rice: long grain, medium and short grain. They can all be eaten as either whole brown rice, or refined into white rice.

Nutritionally speaking, there is a vast difference between brown and white rice with approx. 60% loss of nearly all nutrients. White rice needs added vitamins to be approved for sale. Enriched rice has added B vitamins and iron, however over 10 other nutrients that are 'milled-out' are not replaced.

White, polished rice is basically pure granules of starch. During the Spanish colonial war, the British soldiers were fed white rice, whilst their servants lived off the rice water from cooking, the soldiers developed beriberi, a vitamin B1 deficiency. The servants worked harder and did not develop beriberi.

White rice is usually served as a base ingredient for numerous dishes that can provide a valuable variety of foods and supply of nutrients, thereby the risk of problems is reduced.

However, in some places, rice makes nearly 90% of the daily diet. Unfortunately it barely maintains life and the bonus of the whole grain brown rice can really be a deciding factor for health.

Rice was the reason behind the initial discovery of B vitamins. Dr Eijkman, in 1897 proved that men who ate whole grain rice did not contract beriberi. The Japanese navy lost thousands of sailors following the regular daily use of polished or white rice. Dr. R.R.Williams, first extracted vitamin B1 from the rice bran. His comment after receiving an award, "Man commits a crime against nature when he eats the starch and throws away the mechanism necessary for the metabolism of that starch".

Apart from the b1 deficiency in white rice, the loss of major minerals and other vitamins is obvious (refer chart) and white rice cannot be considered a nutritious food, but, if that's the only way the *children* will eat rice, be sure to use enriched rice, pile on the carrots, peas, corn, beans or cheese and make a peanut sauce. Or add a dash of vegemite, or rice bran, because b1 is vital for the children's growth, memory, concentration and appetite. A prolonged deficiency of b1 can also lead to irritability and depression.

Basically, white rice and white bread are the classic 'empty calorie' foods. They do not provide the essential nutrients to support the proper digestion and absorption of their own starch content in particular. For example, b1 is essential for proper digestion/absorption of starch, b2 essential for secretion of gastric juices and absorption of carbohydrates, b3 assists the functions of many digestive enzymes, b5 is required for enzyme development for carbohydrate utilisation. Manganese for digestive and enzyme reactions, phosphorus for energy distribution and iron for protein metabolism. All the essential fatty acids or vitamin F plus fibre are lacking from white rice. White rice is nice and filling but nasty in it's ability to give back nutrition.

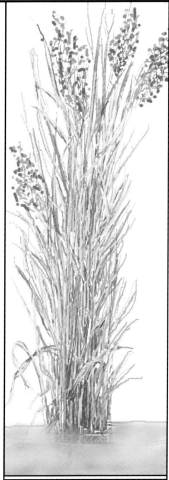

Except for calories and protein (g); all amounts are measured in mg per 100 grams, dry weight approx. * added nutrients	BROWN RICE	WHITE RICE	WHITE ENRICHED RICE	RICE BRAN	FLOUR BROWN	WILD RICE
CALORIES	359	357	363	276	292	353
PROTEIN	7.5	6.5	6.7	13	5.6	14
CALCIUM	32	17	8.7	76	8.6	19
PHOSPHORUS	256	111	108	1,386	271	432
POTASSIUM	259	110	86	1,495	233	426
IRON	1.6	0.7	* 4.3	19	1.5	1,9
VITAMIN B1	0.34	0.08	* 0.5	2.3	0.35	0.11
VITAMIN B2	0.05	0.03	* 0.04	0.25	0.06	0.02
VITAMIN B3	4.6	1.6	* 5	30	5.1	6.1

Rice as the whole grain such as brown rice is full of remarkable benefits and the alkaline balance it provides after digestion is a real bonus for health. Nearly all foods except almonds, fruits, vegetables, soy and millet are classed as acid forming foods. The ideal diet needs 75% alkaline forming foods. Brown rice is a genius in alkaline benefits and health restoring benefits due to this one factor alone. Use a rice cooker or steamer to gain a soft texture and it only takes 15 minutes longer than most white rice.

Brown rice provides complete protein 8 g and compared to all grains, it has the best percentage of available protein (70% n.p.u.). When such foods as cheese or milk are added, the protein value increases another 30% and with legumes the increase is 40%. One bowl with 200 grams of cooked brown rice with a serve of kidney beans topped with cheese will provide over half the adult daily protein requirements, plus, at one quarter the price of beef. Brown rice provides 140 % more fibre than white rice and nearly 3 times the iron 1.5 mg content. The manganese 3.7 mg content of brown rice will provide over 50% of the daily requirement 2 - 5 mg. It is essential for the nerves, hormone production and as a component of an antioxidant enzyme termed *superoxide dismutase;* required to protect against free radicals that are produced during the production of energy from cells. Brown rice is a good source of selenium 23 mcg with the R.D.I. of 70 - 85 mcg, required for protection from heart disease and free radicals.

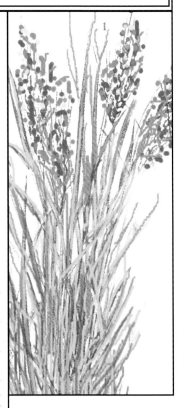

The phosphorus content 333 mg or 33% d.v. is beneficial for blood circulation, the nervous system, brain and skin system and processing destroys over half the value of this vital mineral. The magnesium content 143 mg or 36% d.v. is over 4 times that of white rice, no wonder the city stress is booming, as magnesium is essential for relaxed nerves, plus, alcohol depletes magnesium.

Brown rice is one of the easiest foods to digest (2 hrs.), it actually takes less time to digest than white rice (2 hrs. 30 m.). If you are looking for a power packed powder, try a sprinkle of rice bran on your white rice dish, or in the sauce or gravy and retrieve the abundance of missing nutrients. Rice bran provides nearly 8 times the B vitamin content of brown rice and 40 times that of white rice. Rice bran is potent in phosphorus 1,386 mg, iron 19 mg, silicon 885 mg and potassium 1495 mg, now that's nutrition. Rice bran needs to be kept in the fridge to maintain it's benefits. Try a sprinkle in sauces, breads, cookies, pancakes or on the basic breakfast cereal and whenever you have the 'nice white rice', a dash of rice bran can provide a great balance to a lot of soft white starch.

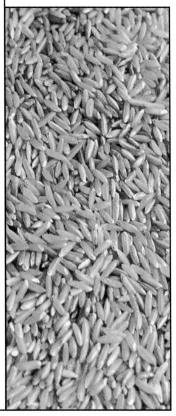

Another rice called wild rice (*Zizania aquatica)* is more expensive but prized in the best restaurants and home kitchen. The protein 14 g is double that of brown rice with a similar carbohydrate value 75 g and most nutrients approx. 20% greater value except for calcium 19 mg and a good source of iron 4.2 mg with a similar calorie value (353). Another great advantage of rice is the gluten free value especially for those with coeliac disease, yeast infections and wheat intolerances. Ideally, let brown rice replace numerous other wheat or meat meals to gain alkaline body and blood balance. If you have to take away, it's better to have rice than a hamburger. The price of brown rice is another major benefit. Yes dear, brown rice is alright tonight!

Rye is the grain that can withstand the cold, acid soil and low rainfall. Rye has been a staple grain in Europe, Scandinavia and Russia for centuries and it was first cultivated by the Romans during 400 B.C. Rye also had a dark history due to a fungus: *ergot* that attacked the grains producing a virus in humans and animals. During the Middle Ages and even up until 1953, in France, the virus caused severe conditions with the central nervous system. Modern science has eliminated this disease in the rye plant. Remember, the potato also caused problems back in the 'hay days', so don't be put off this natural whole grain.

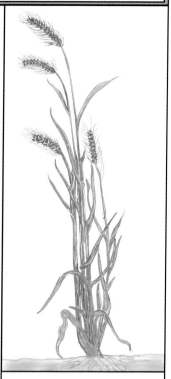

Today, rye is gaining popularity as a replacement for wheat bread and it is also used to make whisky. Whole grain rye is referred to as rye groats and they are best pre-soaked, prior to cooking, or steaming like rice and added to soups, bread or stews. The protein content 14.8 g or 30% d.v. of whole rye is a great benefit, it provides complete protein with a low fat content 2.5 g or 4% d.v. A delicious vegetable soup with rye groats, sounds unappetising, but, once soaked overnight and simmered in vegetable stock for 1 hour and cooked with winter vegetables and spices for 30 minutes; then add a splash of cream before serving, the 'rye soup' is on the way to be a great provider of flavour and nourishment.

Rye bread is available in numerous varieties and the common factor is the low gluten content, compared to wheat, however some rye breads also include either wheat flour or added gluten, to give the bread a soft and lighter texture. The ultimate rye bread is made with organic rye flour, sour rye dough, water and no yeast. Another benefit of rye bread is the excellent fibre content 14 g or 55% d.v., as the bran and germ content are difficult to separate from the grain, during milling, compared to wheat. The fibre content will help protect against colon cancer, as fibre binds with toxins in the colon to regularly eliminate possible cancer causing substances. Rye is the second best grain source of the mineral phosphorus 374 mg or 37% d.v. and when you add a slice of cheese on the rye bread, the benefits for the bones, skeletal system and nervous system are excellent.

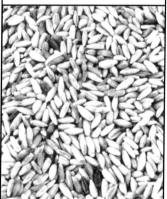

Rye also provides a source of a substance: lingan, a natural oestrogen that can be very beneficial during menopause, to stabilize the natural oestrogen levels. During menopause, normal oestrogen levels can diminish causing discomfort and hot flushes. Lignan, a natural oestrogen can also inhibit excess oestrogen production, a possible cause of breast cancer, as it blocks the oestrogen receptors. In addition the supply of manganese 2.7 mg or approx. 50% d.v. is vital for regulation of menstrual cycles and normal blood sugar levels. The good supply of magnesium 121 mg or 30% d.v. plus the valuable supply of zinc 3.7 mg or 25% d.v. and phosphorus all add up to make the rye grain ideal for strong bone development. Rye bread is full of selenium 35 mcg or 30% d.v. and that promotes the functions of the thyroid gland to regulate metabolism. White bread contains non of the above benefits or the vitamin E 1.3 mg, folate 60 mcg, potassium 264 mg or the wonderful rich flavour of freshly baked rye bread. Shop around for the best rye bread and catch the rye benefits on a shelf in your local store. Look for the worldwide variety of rye bread regularly: Rye, Rye for now!

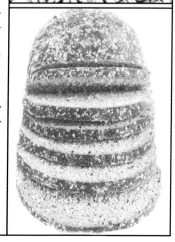

WHEAT *Triticum*	GLYCEMIC INDEX: 67	C. 78	P. 17	L. 5	CALORIES - total: **329 kcal. per 100 gram** Calories from: Carb:258 Protein:55 Fat:16

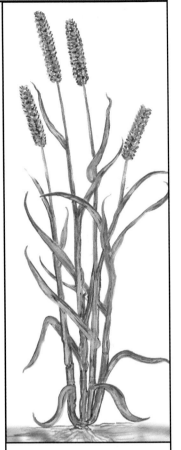

Wheat cultivation has spread the world with varieties than are grown in nearly all climates from Artic to sub tropical. The two main types of whole wheat are grouped into hard wheat and soft wheat. There are thousands of varieties of wheat from which about 300 are used commercially. Among the most common varieties are the *hard red winter wheat,* which originated in Canada and is now used worldwide. It is ideal for bread making and grows quickly and may be harvested three months after sowing. The next common variety is *white wheat.* It is ideal for pastry making and for breakfast cereals, as it is starchy and contains less gluten-protein. *Durum wheat* produces the world's best pasta, it is a very hard grain with an amber colour, it mainly grows in warm-dry climates. In England, the *Mavis Dove wheat* variety is most popular, it is a soft wheat, high in protein and classed as a winter wheat.

The whole wheat grain can be prepared into an incredible variety of recipes, products and forms. To gain the ultimate benefit from the wheat grain, there is no better than *wheat grass juice,* refer to page 112. The second best form of the wheat grain is the *sprouted wheat,* used fresh on salads, mix them in a marvellous mayonnaise and they are delightful and highly nutritious. They can also be added to breads and soups, but fresh is best.

Apart from those top value ways, wheat is also prepared into various forms such as *cracked wheat,* used in the famous and healthful *tabouli* recipe and numerous soups. It is made from whole wheat grain, cracked under pressure and it provides the full grain benefits. *Kibbled wheat* is similar, it is produced from the whole wheat grain, placed through a 'kibbler' machine that cracks the grain into tiny pieces, they are used in bread making and some breakfast cereals. The most common use of wheat is with *flour.*

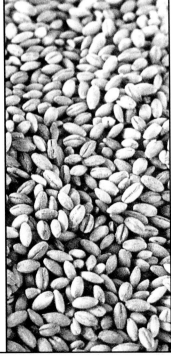

The best quality flour is made from organic whole grain wheat that is *stoneground* into a flour containing the full value of the wheat grain, including the germ and bran content. Stoneground mills do not produce excess heat and therefore the flour is of better quality. Common milling uses steel rollers that move quickly, causing the whole grain flour to heat and the wheat germ content may turn rancid, if not used promptly. *Wholegrain flour* does retain the entire wheat germ and bran layer, plus the starchy endosperm: inner portion of the wheat grain. It needs to be used soon after milling. *Wholemeal bread and wholewheat bread* varieties can vary considerably in their content, plus, they may contain all the additives that are used in the production of white bread, check the labels carefully until you find a loaf with life.

Commercial bread, even the top quality stoneground, whole wheat bread may contain a few additives, to improve shelf life, but, the less added, the better.

Due to the fact that the oil content in the wheat germ clogs-up the steel mills, it is removed for better productivity. Wheat germ is then sold separately. It is the most nutritious part of the wheat grain, but, must be kept fresh in a cool and airtight container and used within a few weeks. The *wheat bran* is also removed from the whole wheat grain, in the production of *white flour,* as it makes bread bulky. White flour is the biggest business, for bread with hundreds of different shapes, sizes and other recipes.

The whole wheat grain is ready to provide the maximum benefits.

WHEAT - BREAD	GLYCEMIC INDEX: 70	C. 80	P. 15	L. 5	CALORIES - total: **339kcal. per 100 gram** Calories from: Carb:274 Protein:49 Fat:16

For 10,000 years the wheat grain has provided the 'staff of life', the 'daily bread' and it was usually obtained in the whole grain form. The current milling of wheat produces incredibly fine white flour and wheat products. The common milling process removes all the wheat germ and bran content plus at least 40% and up to 60% of all nutrients, depending on the refinement grade of the wheat flour. Government health authorities now require '*enrichment*' of flour for mass produced bread, however, that returns only a small portion of a few B vitamins. When comparing the nutritional value of the whole wheat grain to refined flour and white bread, it is obvious, refer to the chart on page 29, that 'humans cannot live by bread alone'.

The nutritional value of whole grain wheat flour may be lowered by the presence of *phytic acid* in the bran. An excess intake of bran or whole grain products may cause problems, as phytic acid combines with minerals, especially calcium, iron and zinc forming insoluble mineral compounds that are not easily absorbed, thereby the supply of calcium 32 -100 mg in whole wheat may be of no value, but, the body can adapt to the phytic acid.

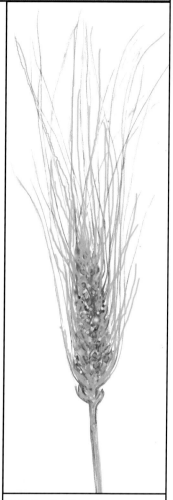

For people who eat whole grain breads as a staple food, it is more than likely their digestive system has overcome this problem. For people who are used to eating white bread, it may take a few weeks to adjust to whole grain bread and the proper absorption of calcium, iron and zinc. However, whole wheat and especially white bread are a poor source of calcium 3 - 8 % d.v., and it is best not to 'live on bread alone'. A cheddar cheese sandwich will be full of calcium 728 mg, or pasta with cheese, or tahini 420 mg on bread will all provide great portions of the daily calcium requirements 500 -1,300 mg per day.

In regards to the fair iron content 2.5 mg in both white and wholemeal bread and whole grain wheat 3 - 4.6 mg or 10 - 25% d.v., iron may bind with phytic acid in wholegrain bread which can reduce iron absorption, if your digestive system is not used to wholegrain bread. Such foods as parsley 6 mg, pepitas 11 mg, tahini 9 mg, almonds 4.7 mg, cashews 3.7 mg, sunflower seeds 7 mg and dried apricots 4.4 mg when obtained regularly, will help provide this mineral, as the daily iron requirement is 10 - 15 mg, and during pregnancy 30 mg. Such foods as beef 1.7 mg and eggs 2 mg, only add a little to the daily iron requirement. Five slices of white bread will provide approx. 3 mg of iron. With 5 slices of wholemeal bread approx. 4.5 mg of iron is provided, but, it may not be absorbed, unless it is regularly part of the diet. In regards to zinc, white bread provides 0.68 mg, wholegrain bread 1.8 mg and the daily adult zinc requirement is 10-15 mg.

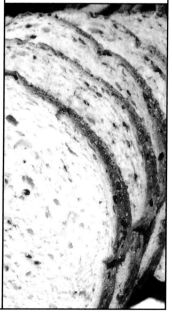

The carbohydrate content of white 72.5 g and wholegrain 72.6 g are nearly identical, same with the protein, white 12 g wholegrain 13.7 g. The main difference between the white bread 2.4 g and wholegrain 12.2 g or 50% d.v., is the fibre content, nearly 5 times the fibre content in whole grain bread.A white bread diet in combination with a regular meat diet, meat having no fibre, is a risky long term diet, especially with colon health. One study showed that the 'protective quantity' of fibre, for adults, needs to be more than 28 grams a day. That's 48 slices of white bread. Don't loaf around with no fibre.

Wheat is the main ingredient in pasta and a special type of wheat: durum wheat is used exclusively, the name implies a 'paste' with water and flour.

The main styles of pasta are: canneloni, lasagne, macaroni, rigatoni, spaghetti, tagliatelle and vermicelli. Within these styles are numerous variations in size, shape, thickness, added ingredients, plus, the plain and wholemeal versions. Some pasta has egg added to the mix 'al uovo', but generally it is made from plain durum wheat. Pasta and pizza are one of the most common meals in the family home, not just in Rome but throughout the world. It is easy to make and numerous different ingredients can be added to make each 'pasta / pizza night' different. Pasta / pizza, on it's own, has about the same protein 12.8 g or 26% d.v. as bread, same carbohydrate content 74 g and the same fibre 'problem' as white bread 2.4 g. As they have a very low fat content 1.6 g or 2% d.v., a serve of grated cheese will balance the meal plus add stacks of calcium, especially if it's parmesan 1,380 mg, but, cheese supplies no fibre, so once again, the addition of fibre foods is really beneficial. One serve of cheddar cheese 28 g or (1oz.) will add 9.4 g fat, mainly saturated 6 g, mono 2. 6 g and as the approx. daily requirement is 60 - 80 g, the cheese on top is good value for the active person.

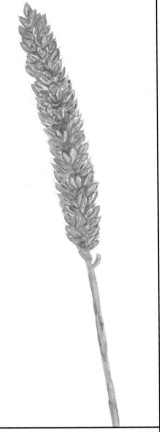

For children, pasta and cheese is great, but somehow, throughout the day, provide them with fruit, or oats or whole grain cereals, or, add some 'baby' spinach, or a dash of bran into the tomato paste mixture, or serve with 'yummy' whole grain bread and butter. The protein content of pasta 12. 8 g or 26% d.v. is good and with the added protein content of cheese 25 g the protein increases to 38 g to nearly 60% d.v. adults, children approx. 80% d.v., now that's big value for a growing family.

The main factor from pasta and pizza is the excellent carbohydrate content approx. 72 g or 25% daily value. Both pasta and bread are energy packed foods, however, as the body requires numerous nutrients, to help utilize and produce the energy, the plain white pasta, pizza or bread, on their own are fairly inadequate, due to a poor supply of essential nutrients. To overcome this problem add ingredients that are full of nutrients. The pasta with mixed vegetables, parmesan and a rich tomato sauce is basic but good nutrition.

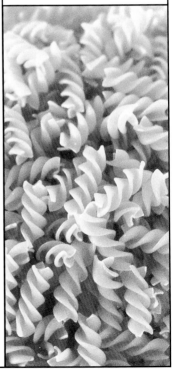

For a top quality pasta meal, add some ground pepitas on top of the cheese, now, " I'll have what she's having "! Same with the noodles, add some stir fry vegetables, blanched almonds or cracked or finely ground pepitas and you can be sure of gaining great nutrition and additional flavour.

Foods such as pasta, pizza, noodles and bread can comfortably provide one third daily energy values, another third from fruits and vegetables and the balance from the fats, oils and proteins. Pasta, bread and noodles provide approx. 72 grams of carbohydrates, per 100 gram, and, the daily average requirement for children and teenagers is approx. 300 - 350 grams, adults 300 grams. In calories per day, children (2,000), women (2,200) teenagers and men (3,000), average person (2,400 calories). Pasta or bread provide approx. 340 calories, per 100 gram serve. It's the topping that makes the bread, pasta, pizza or noodles meal healthful.

Wheat in the whole grain and as whole grain flour are a power packed food, the protein and carbohydrate value are well balanced and the supply of minerals, (except calcium), and fibre are beneficial. The main problems with the white: flour, bread, pastries, pizza and pasta products are the *low fibre content*, as mentioned, the *low calcium* and phosphorus content, essential for the nerves, brain, bones and digestion. The *low magnesium content*, as magnesium is vital for the nerves, digestion, bones and brain. The *low potassium supply*, as potassium is essential for the heart muscles, circulation and nerves. The iron content is fair, but the *manganese content*, vital for blood development, memory, glands and nerves is deficient. The *zinc content is low*, it is vital for bone strength and growth, digestion, glands and hormones. The B vitamins are 'added' to enrich the white starch-flour, but the *vitamin E content is very low*, it is vital for the heart, healing, long life, anti oxidation and fertility. The number of common ailments associated with the above nutrient deficiencies is enormous and white flour products can be a major contributor if they are the staple food in the diet. In addition, refined white bread includes additives.

Refined white flour and products cannot stand alone nutritionally, they need added ingredients to ensure proper health. In addition, the high glycemic index of especially pretzels (80), white bread and muffins (70) further adds weight to the suggestion to include beneficial foods to the white flour products. Ideally, whole grains such as oats can take the place of the breakfast toast, or add yeast extract to the bread or toast, to give it a small boost, for your nerves. The toast with tahini is great as the supply of vitamin E and minerals, plus protein is excellent.

Let your bread be delightful, but healthful, add natural ingredients to make the soft, spongy, white bread beneficial. As they say, 'child, woman or man cannot live by bread alone'. May your daily bread be loaded with benefits and flavour.

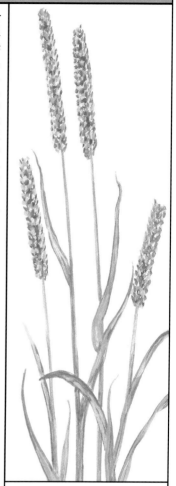

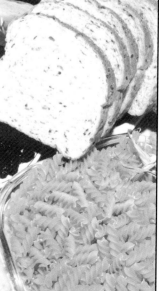

NUTRIENTS per 100 grams dry weight.	w/wheat white	w/wheat red	w/grain w/flour	white w/flour	wheat bran	wheat germ	wheat gluten	pasta	w/grain rye
Carbohydrate	75.9	68	72.6	72.5	64.5	51.8	13.8	74.7	69.8
Protein	11.3	15.4	13.7	12	15.5	23.1	75.2	12.8	14.8
Lipids	1.7	1.9	1.9	1.7	4.3	9.7	1.9	1.6	2.5
Calories	342	329	339	361	216	360	370	371	335
Fibre	12.2	12.2	12.2	2.4	42.8	13.2	.6	2.4	14.6
Calcium	32	25	34	15	73	39	142	18	33
Phosphorus	355	332	346	97	1013	842	260	150	374
Magnesium	93	124	138	25	611	239	25	48	121
Potassium	432	340	405	100	1182	892	100	162	264
Sodium	2	2	5	2	2	12	29	7	6
Manganese	3.8	4.1	3.8	.8	11.5	13.3	-	.7	2.7
Iron	4.6	3.6	3.9	4.4*	10.6	6.3	5.2	1.3	2.7
Selenium	-	-	70	39	77	79	39	62	35
Zinc	3.3	2.8	2.9	.9	7.3	12.3	.9	1.2	3.7
Vitamin b1	.4	.5	.4	.8*	.5	1.9	0	.1	.3
vitamin b2	.1	.1	.2	.5*	.6	.5	0	.1	.3
vitamin b3	4.4	5.7	6.4	7.6*	13.6	6.8	0	1.7	4.3
vitamin e	1	1	.8	.4	1.5	15.8	0	0	1.3

GRAINS SUMMARY CHARTS

WHOLE GRAINS	MAIN NUTRIENTS, ANTIOXIDANTS & PHYTONUTRIENTS	BODY SYSTEM BENEFITS
BARLEY	protects against colon cancer, arthritis, asthma, diabetes, high cholesterol	digestive, elimination
CORN - sweet	protects against infections, lung cancer, brain disorders, irritability.	respiratory, brain
MILLET	silicon, iron, gluten free, yeast free, alkaline, folate, phosphorus, zinc, copper.	digestive, repair
OATS	fibre, lowers blood sugar levels and cholesterol, ideal for diabetics, magnesium, antioxidants, protein,	digestive, blood, brain, nervous
RICE - brown	alkaline, manganese, selenium, phosphorus, gluten free, yeast free.	digestive, blood
RYE	fibre, low gluten, natural oestrogens, manganese, selenium, zinc.	digestive, glandular
WHEAT	carbohydrates, fibre, potassium, manganese, selenium, vitamin e.	muscular

GRAINS - BALANCED DIET - DAILY CARBOHYDRATE INTAKE

		ADULT MALE	ADULT FEMALE	TEENAGER	CHILDREN
TOTAL DAILY INTAKE (AVERAGE) (R.D.I) CARBOHYDRATE INTAKE		340 grams	280 grams	400 grams	270 grams
GRAINS 20 % CARBOHYDRATE INTAKE LAUGH WITH HEALTH DIET		68 grams	56 grams	80 grams	54 grams
CHOOSE ANY TWO OF THESE DAILY	100 g WHOLE WHEAT BREAD = 39 grams of carbohydrate approx.	174 grams 3 slices	143 grams 2 slices	205 grams 3 - 4 slices	138 grams 2 slices
	100 g WHITE BREAD = 51 grams of carbohydrate approx.	133 grams 2 - 3 slices	109 grams 1 - 2 slices	156 grams 3 slices	105 grams 1 - 2 slices
	100 g PASTA = 75 grams of carb. approx.	90 grams	74 grams	106 grams	72 grams
	100 g RICE = 80 grams of carb. approx.	85 grams	70 grams	100 grams	67 grams
	100 g OATS = 66 grams of carb. approx.	103 grams	84 grams	121 grams	81 grams
FOOD PYRAMID DAILY DIET		Whole grains at most meals White rice, White bread, Potatoes, Pasta: Sparingly.			
AUSTRALIAN HEALTHY EATING PLATE		6 - 12 serves	4 - 9 serves	5 - 11 serves	5 - 9 serves

1 SERVE is equivalent to: 2 slices bread (60 g), 1 cup of rice, pasta, noodles (180 g), one third of a cup of cereal (40 g), half cup untoasted muesli, quarter cup flour (40 g) 1 cup porridge (230 g).

GRAINS - BALANCED DIET - DAILY PROTEIN INTAKE

		ADULT MALE	ADULT FEMALE	TEENAGER	CHILDREN
TOTAL DAILY R.D.I. PROTEIN INTAKE APPROX.		60 grams	47 grams	65 grams	45 grams
GRAINS 5% PROTEIN INTAKE LAUGH WITH HEALTH DIET		3 grams	2 grams	3 grams	2 grams
CHOOSE ANY TWO OF THESE DAILY	100 grams of WHOLE GRAIN BREAD or 100 grams of WHITE BREAD	9 grams protein			
	100 grams PASTA	12 grams protein			
	100 grams RICE	7 grams protein			
	100 grams OATS	16 grams protein			

The above charts (and the charts on pages 42, 60, 77 & 104) are provided as a guide to the daily amount of the individual food groups that are suggested by three different dietary guidelines: 1. Laugh with Health Diet, 2. US. Food Pyramid Guide, 3. Australian Guide to Healthy Eating. These charts are provided as a guide only and are not to be considered for an exact daily intake. The main aim of these charts is to show that all the main food groups are required for a balanced diet. By referring to page 213, a summary chart with all the 13 food groups is provided. All three dietary guidelines suggest that a variety of foods be obtained on a daily basis and over a period of one week, a complete range of natural food groups can be obtained. Balance your life naturally!

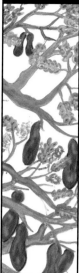

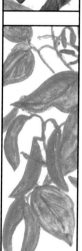

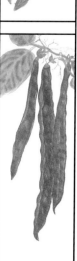

Legumes is the nutritional name used to describe the group of beans and peas, also referred to as pulses.

The following pages will provide you with information about the various types of legumes, their nutritional value, unique recipes, historical information and their various methods of preparation.

The main legumes discussed are: carob bean, chick pea, green bean, kidney bean, lentils, lima bean, mung bean, peanut, pea and soy bean. Dried legumes are one of nature's best store of nutrition. They are basically a seed and when water is added, new life will develop with every day of growth.

Pre-soaking of legumes has many advantages. For some legumes it is essential in order to convert the concentrated starches, especially stachyose and raffinose to promote better digestion, otherwise these undigested starches get attacked by intestinal bacteria, forming into carbon dioxide and hydrogen gas, causing flatulence and a great loss of nutritional benefits.

Raw-dried legumes also contain such substances as: alkaloids, glycosides and saponin and these are detrimental to digestion and are eliminated with long soaking and proper cooking. Pre-soaking for a few days will greatly enhance the digestion and nutrient quality of the associated legume. If you are short on time to prepare legumes, choose fresh beans, peas or try from a large variety of canned beans. They are very economical and can be stored in the pantry for those times when the stocks are low or you need a big boost of energy and fibre.

Legumes are waiting to be unleashed from their sleep.

Make sure that your kitchen is always well stocked with at least the essential basic legumes: chick peas, kidney beans, lentils, lima beans, mung beans and soy beans. The variety of legume produce is abundant and their popularity is increasing due to the recognition of many traditional recipes.

Legumes supply all the essential daily protein requirements and their ability to reduce blood cholesterol is a major benefit and worth hoeing in to on a regular basis.

Generally speaking, legumes are classed as a carbohydrate food. Millions of people throughout the world rely on legume produce for their daily protein requirements.

A combination of an excess intake of animal proteins and insufficient legume produce are possibly the main contributing factors towards the multitude of heart and arterial diseases that are prevalent today.

This chapter on legumes will assist you with valuable ideas on the numerous legume benefits and their method of preparation. Once you have tried a few simple recipes, you will then realise how so many people throughout the world live to enjoy their legume meals.

Legume meals could easily replace at least two animal protein meals per week. Ideally, the balanced diet requires 20% of carbohydrates to be obtained from legumes. The legume kingdom is ready now with complete protein, numerous minerals, vitamins, abundant fibre and a beneficial slow releasing energy. If you have the chance to order a legume meal at an authentic restaurant, treat yourself to the traditional and legendary legume flavours, textures and benefits.

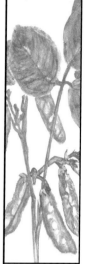

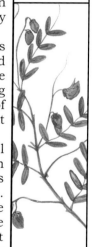

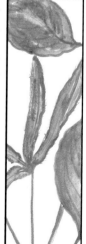

NOTE: All amounts in this book are measured in milligrams (mg) per 100 grams, unless stated otherwise.

CAROB BEANS	*Ceratonia siliqua*	C. 89	P. 8	L. 3	CALORIES - total: **222 kcal. per 100 gram**
					Calories from: Carb:198 Protein:18 Fat:6

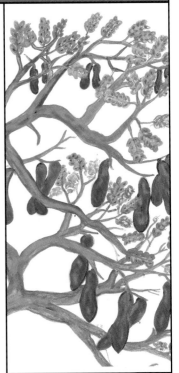

Carob beans have a remarkable history, the carob tree is said to be the oldest known fruit bearing tree in the areas of Syria, Palestine, Spain, Egypt and Sicily. Carob has provided generations with food and it has been given the title of 'bread that grows on trees', 'staff of life' and 'St John's bread', it is mentioned in the Bible as providing energy, nourishment and food for thought during times in the wilderness.

Carob is a hardy food source, it can be stored for long periods and the large 'carob pods' can be eaten as a sweet food, directly from the tree, when ripened to a very dark brown colour. One of the greatest benefits of carob is the alkaline balance it provides to the digestive system, no need for antacids, carob actually reduces stomach acidity. Carob is also an excellent source of natural pectin, vital for treatment of stomach upsets, diarrhoea and reduction of cholesterol. Pectin removes toxins from the digestive system and also promotes protein digestion as it prevents digested protein from spoiling in the lower digestive system.

Carob is a compact carbohydrate food 89% or 30% d.v. and it is full of fibre 40 g or 159% d.v., that's bulky and noticeable when making carob drinks. Ideally, for a smooth drink, allow the carob sediment to settle and then pour the liquid content into another cup. In contrast to chocolate, carob contains no caffeine, no oxalic acid and these two factors alone give carob the power to be an excellent replacement for chocolate or caffeine. For growing children especially, oxalic acid in chocolate binds with calcium and retards the absorption of this mighty mineral.

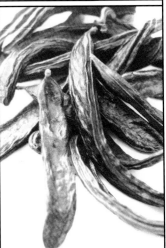

Carob is a very good source of calcium 348 mg or 35% d.v. or nearly three times that of cows milk and when combined with a milk shake, it provides a sweet flavour and does not require the loads of sugar associated with chocolate drinks. Carob provides excellent natural sweetness 49 g with the safety of B vitamins: B1, B2, B3, B5 and folate 30 mcg and a very good supply of the alkaline mineral potassium 827 mg or 24% d.v., ideal for active muscles, improved blood circulation and as potassium is heat sensitive, a carob drink will provide potent potassium, over twice that of bananas. The supply of the mineral copper 0.6 - 1 mg is only a quarter that of chocolate 3.8 g, but the recommended daily for adults is 1.5 - 3 mg, so don't overdose on copper.

Carob and chocolate both provide approx. 1 g of zinc. The fat content of carob 1 g is mainly polyunsaturated and low compared to chocolate 8.4 g which is 60% saturated animal fat. When baking cookies, carob powder with complete protein 5 g adds a sweet flavour and dark colour to cookies, make some carob crackles and be sure you're giving the children a great party food. Add a small amount of honey and ice cream to any carob milk shake or drink or recipe as it promotes a smooth consistency.

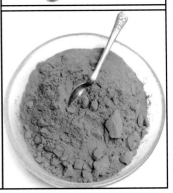

Carob also provides magnesium 54 mg, chocolate 13 mg, phosphorus 79 mg chocolate 100 mg and twelve times the iron content 3 mg of milk chocolate 0.24 mg. For adults, try carob with goats milk, soy milk or acidophillus milk. Carob snack bars are the ideal replacement for chocolate bars as they are a great calcium food plus they will promote digestion. Carob was once used to measure precious stones and gold, 'carat', it is now an easy to obtain and inexpensive, sweet and a pure snack and condiment.

NOTE: d.v. refers to daily value for woman 25 - 50 years, refer to RDI chart page 69 for adult male and children values.

Chick Peas are famous for their inclusion as the main ingredient in hummous, a common dip or spread these days and one that has supported people from the Middle East region for thousands of years. Another common name for chick peas is garbanzos, they are available in various colours such as the common light yellow, red, brown and black, all have a distinct pointed pod in which two or three peas, also with a pointed tip are located.

Another traditional product from chick peas is cous cous, used in many recipes and as a side dish. The most famous recipe is the falafel, based on chick peas, sesame seeds, potato, onions, parsley, garlic and various spices such as cayenne pepper and paprika. Next time you see falafel for sale, invest in a truly amazing meal with a tahini sauce, it is full of health benefits. If you are making hummous at home, pre soak the beans for 2-4 days, rinsing 2 times a day and you will gain an increase in the protein value and a huge decrease in flatulence, due to the starch conversion.

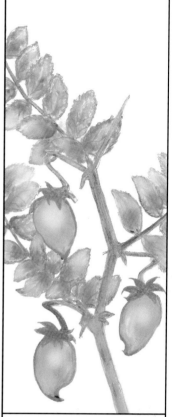

Chick peas provide complete protein 19 g or 40% d.v. and with a dab of tahini on the falafel, the protein increases greatly, due to the balance of the amino acid methionine. For a complete fibre rich food 17 g or 70% d.v., chick peas are ideal and if you need to be on a cholesterol free diet, you can gain extra benefits from chick pea fibre, as it contacts with bile to eliminate cholesterol from the body. If you need a low fat diet, chick peas supply (6 g mainly unsaturated 5 g and only 51 calories from the fat content.

Chick peas combine well with winter vegetables and for a tasty simple way to serve, after they have been cooked in water for 1 hour, place them into the oven or frypan and slightly dry roast them. Sprinkle with pure olive oil and enjoy with a fresh salad or broccoli and cheese. The calcium content 105 mg is fair and the phosphorus content 366 mg or 37% d.v. is ample to assist proper digestion of the compact nutrients. The iron content 6 mg or 35% d.v. is of great benefit during pregnancy, lactation and any time you feel weary.

Chick peas supply over three times the iron content of beef 1.9 mg. In addition, the manganese content 2 mg plus the very good copper content 1 mg or 42% d.v. are both vital for the production of new blood. Try some hummous as a dip during the week and offset those weary feelings. As with all legumes, the potassium content 875 mg is very good and once again it is a heat sensitive nutrient, so sprout them first to reduce cooking time and increase nutrient values. The magnesium content 115 mg or 29% d.v. is another activating nutrient for the nervous system and brain, plus it is required to assist enzymes for digestion and hormone production.

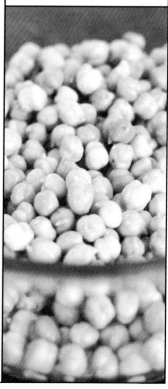

Chick peas supply five times the magnesium content of beef and milk. The supply of folate 557 mcg or 139% d.v. is excellent and vital for protection from heart attacks and for the proper functioning of the brain and nervous system. Folic acid is water soluble and required daily from the diet, for adults 200 mcg and during pregnancy 400 mcg and lactation 350 mcg. Spinach supplies only 95 mcg of folate, chick peas are the folate king. The supply of the trace mineral molybdenum is excellent, over 75% daily value from a one cup serving. Very few foods supply molybdenum, required for the nerves and brain and fat metabolism.

Chick peas are ready to please your 'nutritional appetite'.

GREEN BEANS	*Phaseolus vulgaris*	C.	P.	L.	CALORIES - total: **343 kcal. per 100 gram**
		76	19	5	Calories from: Carb:261 Protein:65 Fat:17

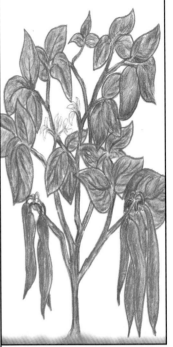

Green beans, commonly termed the French bean or string bean belong to the same botanical species as the kidney bean. During the 16th. century, the green bean was considered a luxury food for royalty and it is reported as one of the oldest known foods, dating back 7,000 years in Mexico and by the American Indians. The green bean supported the survival of early settlers in America prior to the cultivation of corn and other crops.

Green beans are a good carbohydrate food 8 g, plus a fair source of dietary fibre 3.5 g, important for elimination of waste as it binds with cancer causing toxins, usually as a by-product of meat digestion and cleanses the colon. As meat, chicken and fish provide no fibre, the addition of green beans to the menu is really a life saver, in the long term.

The good supply of folate 40 mcg is worth snapping into especially for the expectant mother, as folate is vital for infant development and the reproduction of body cells. Folate also promotes brain function and it is essential for the nervous system and prevention from nervous exhaustion. Folate is water soluble and required regularly from the diet. The supply of iron 1.1 mg plus vitamin K from the green bean 22 mcg is also important for an expectant mother, plus it is vital for the circulatory system. If you freeze your beans, the vitamin K may disappear, plus, antibiotics, aspirin, mineral oils and x rays can all deplete the body's store of this fat soluble vitamin. Green beans provide complete protein 2 g with a very low fat content 0.013 g, so you can add the butter or oil to the slightly steamed green beans and still have a well balanced food.

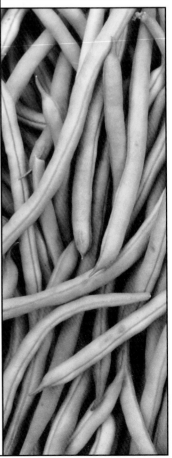

The supply of potassium 230 mg is worth picking fresh from the vine, as potassium is heat sensitive and in combination with the phosphorus content 42 mg the benefits of increased oxygen into the brain for efficient mental function are obtained. The magnesium content of 25 mg promotes nourishment to the white nerve fibres of the brain. The vitamin A content 700 I.U. is fair and with the supply of vitamin C 16 mg, the fresh French bean is an antioxidant food, able to retard the oxidation of cholesterol and subsequent arterial plaque.

The green bean is a safe food for diabetics 50 G.I., plus it is said to promote the production of natural insulin due to supply of plant hormones, in combination with the small amount of the mineral zinc 0.26 mg.

The green bean is very low in calories 34 and with the supply of fibre, you can easily eat them all day and feel satisfied that the waistline is on the decline. Slight cooking of the green bean, immersed in near boiling water for 2 minutes is ample to soften the texture, add your favourite cream sauce and serve with grilled ocean fish and roast pumpkin for a colourful healthful meal. Green beans supply a small amount of calcium 41 mg so add a sprinkle of cheese for a satisfying and bone building entree. When in season, the green bean is a very economical food and children seem to like the taste, so that's a bonus for their health as green beans are the best legume source of vitamin A, K and folate.

Whenever you see the green bean, if it snaps when you bend it, try it raw or if it's a few days old, slightly steam the green bean for an excellent addition to any protein meal such as with rice, chicken, meat or fish. The green French bean will help you stay lean.

KIDNEY BEAN	*Phaseolus vulgaris*	C.	P.	L.	CALORIES - total: 333 kcal. per 100 gram
		73	25	2	Calories from: Carb:244 Protein:82 Fat:7

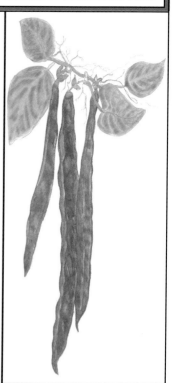

Kidney beans have numerous cousins, the navy bean, pinto bean, snap bean, Mexican black bean, cannellini bean, flageolet bean and haricot bean, plus the fresh green bean and snap bean. Originating in Peru, the Phaseolus vulgaris species spread the world.

The red kidney bean is the most famous 'canned bean' or 'baked bean' and today it lines the supermarket shelves from Ulmarra to Uganda, providing one of the cheapest and easiest to prepare meals, baked beans on toast. The kidney bean is the main ingredient in numerous Mexican dishes, the bean taco with salad and cheese is a great meal that children like and gain great benefits from the excellent protein value. On their own, kidney beans supply complete protein 24 g or 47% d.v. and with added cheese, two tacos will provide children 8 - 14 years with all their daily protein requirements. In addition, kidney beans provide calcium 143 mg and with a good sprinkle of cheese, the taco can provide all the daily calcium for growing children. The corn part of the taco shell is fairly low in nutrients but it provides the 'crunch factor' that promotes the appetite.

The carbohydrate content 60 g of kidney beans is as 'good as it gets' due to the excellent supply of fibre 25 g or 100% d.v. which helps stabilize the supply of 'blood sugar energy' gradually, in contrast to the very common 'high glycemic index' of white bread 70 and common processed potato chips 52. Kidney beans boiled have a low glycemic index of 29, canned beans 52 and corn taco shells have a high glycemic index of 72. The added cheese to the taco will greatly reduce the g.i. of the corn shell and make it a safe food for children. For a very low g.i. kidney bean meal, ideal for diabetics, use boiled kidney beans 29 with added cheese 0, onion 9, lettuce 5, tomato 35 and capsicum 8. Kidney beans are very low in fat content 1 g or with only 7 calories per 100 gram serve, so you can add the cheese and still be confident of a very lean meal, plus an excellent supply of nutrients such as the potassium content 1,406 mg or 40% d.v., a heat sensitive nutrients, so sprout your legumes first to reduce cooking time by 70% and increase their nutrient balance and promote their digestion. If kidney beans are not sprouted and or cooked properly, till soft, a toxic factor termed *haemagglutinin* will not be removed from the bean and it may lead to gastroenteritis. Sprouting alone reduces the haemagglutinin in kidney beans to a level equal to that of other legumes.

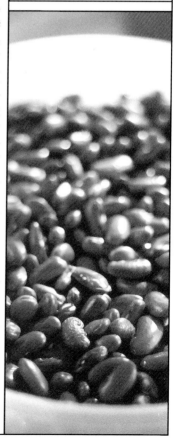

For those people too busy to sprout and cook kidney beans, or other legumes, a wide range of 'well cooked canned' legumes are available at a very low price and they should be a regular part of the shopping list, as they are quick to prepare into nourishing meals, a bean salad in summer will provide excellent folate 394 mcg or 98% d.v., lettuce only supplies 41 mcg of folate. Keep a few cans of kidney beans in your pantry, ready in minutes!

For an excellent supply of organic iron 8 mg or 46% d.v., kidney beans are really essential, supplying four times the iron content of beef and over ten times that of cheese 0.67 mg or chicken. The supply of molybdenum is excellent 80% d.v., plus the phosphorus 407 mg or 41% d.v., plus magnesium 140 mg or 35% d.v. and copper 48% d.v. If you miss out on kidney beans in your diet, you may never get the full benefit of true health. Kidney beans are very competent and keen to support your nutritional needs.

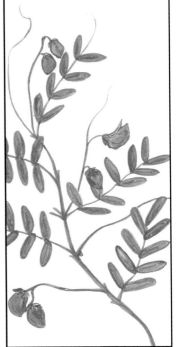

Lentils have been around for ages, they were one of the first culti-vated foods over 8,000 years ago. Lentils were also used by the Egyptians as a main food that helped build the mighty pyramids. Further proof of the power of lentils is from the Russian soldiers during both world wars, as lentils provided the major part of their battle-field diet. Two main types of lentils are available with the reddish-brown from India being common, or in China the pale green lentil. Lentils are tiny but power packed with benefits.

The protein value 28 g or 56% d.v. is complete in all the essential amino acids, however, lentils have a low net protein utilization of 30 %. From the total protein in lentils, only one third is useable, unless other foods are combined to assist in the balance of the 'limiting amino acids'. Such foods as rice or cheese, or egg are most common and can improve the lentil protein balance by 50%. The main limiting amino acids in lentils are methionine and tryptophan.

Lentils are compact and ready to provide a great supply of calories 338 or 17% d.v. with a very low fat content of 1 g. If you are a regular meat eater, the risk of cardiovascular and heart problems is likely, due to the saturated fat and cholesterol content. Lentils provide none of those nasties and in fact the excellent fibre content helps to lower cholesterol, as fibre contacts with the fat dissolving enzyme bile and helps to rid the body of the cholesterol within the bile.

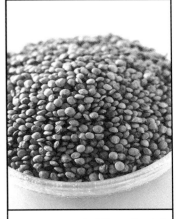

Lentils are also a good food for diabetics as the low glycemic index of 27 with red lentils and 30 with brown or green lentils is another big benefit. Lentil vegetable soup or the famous Indian dish, *dahl*, made from red lentils, onions, garlic, curry, tomatoes and a bay leaf are really low on the g.i. scale and a small dob of sour cream in the soup, or plain yoghurt makes a simple and tasty lunchtime or weekend snack or meal.

Let lentils loose in your kitchen and be amazed at their ability to make a meal, lentil burgers, are another favourite. One advantage with lentils, compared to other legumes is they require far less cooking. Ideally, place the dried lentils on a large plate and check for any cracked or damaged seeds, then rinse the good lentils and place into boiling water, allow water to reboil and then simmer the brown or green lentils for 50 minutes and red lentils for 30 minutes. Sprouting the lentils, for two days is a good idea, but not essential. Sprouting and cooking converts the starches *stachyose* and *raffinose* into a simpler starch that can be absorbed into the blood-stream. Otherwise flatulence can occur as the intestinal bacteria will convert those starches into carbon dioxide and hydrogen, a gas, especially if lentils are not part of your regular diet.

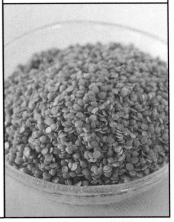

Lentils provide an excellent supply of organic iron 9 g or 50 % d.v. and that's from a small 100 gram serve, imagine if you ate a bowl of lentils, beef only supplies 2 g iron! The secret behind the power of lentils is the potent iron content, plus the supply of numerous minerals. From one cup of cooked lentils you also obtain and excellent supply of phosphorus 50 %, copper 25 %, molybdenum 90 % manganese 30 % magnesium 25 % and zinc 20 %, all based on d.v. Try getting that value from take away foods 'without gas'!

Lentils were once termed 'poor man's meat', they are now formally classified as the 'rich, red, iron food'!

LIMA BEANS *Phaseolus vulgaris*	C. 76	P. 22	L. 2	CALORIES - total: **338 kcal. per 100 gram** Calories from: Carb:258 Protein:74 Fat:6

Lima beans gain their name from the Greek word - *phases*, for aspect or appearance and 'lunatas' derived from the Latin - *luna*, meaning moon. Lima beans 'appear like the moon', does that mean they only come out at night! Try the lima bean midnight special, or invent one similar.

Considering their preparation, lima beans are best soaked overnight, to reduce the *raffinose* starch, or oligosaccharides. Buy a few cans of cooked lima beans from the local store for a quick, easy to add ingredient with many recipes. Lima beans are also termed butter beans, curry beans, pole beans and sieva beans.

Lima beans originated from Lima in Peru over 7,000 years ago and were discovered by Christopher Columbus and introduced to Europe and Asia. The protein content 21 g or 43% d.v. is complete in all essential amino acids with a very low fat content 1 g or 1% d.v. so you can add the butter to the beans, just before serving and relax about the added calories, as lima beans provide only 6 calories from unsaturated fats, butter supplies 700 calories per 100 gram or 100 calories per teaspoon. As the recommended daily adult calorie intake is 2,500 - 3,000 k.calories, the dab of butter with lima beans will easily fit into the balanced diet menu.

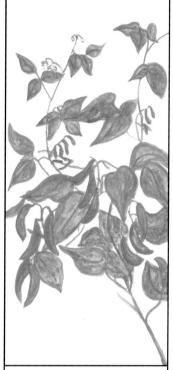

Lima beans are one of the richest potassium foods 1,700 mg equal to soy beans and more than any other legume or natural food. Potassium is heat sensitive and lima beans need to be cooked, but if pre-soaked and slow cooked, the abundance of potassium will still be supplied. The magnesium content 224 mg or 56% d.v. is not heat sensitive and same with the phosphorus content 385 mg or 38% d.v., both these major minerals are essential for the brain, nervous system and heart muscles.

The manganese content 2 mg is similar to sunflower seeds and apart from wheat germ, bran, nuts and seeds, lima beans are a very good source. Manganese works with enzymes for energy production and as an antioxidant; the enzyme *superoxide dismutase* needs manganese to destroy free radicals from within cells.

Even though they are white, lima beans are a rich source of organic iron 8 mg or 42% d.v. In addition, lima beans provide the following nutrients, from one cupful of cooked beans, molybdenum 85 % d.v., folate 40 % d.v., phosphorus 30 % and copper 20 %. Now that's a bean that's full of beans and nutrients plus *purines*, naturally occurring substances that are broken down by the digestive system into uric acid. For persons with the conditions of gout or kidney stones, it is best to avoid lima beans due to the purine content, but a healthy body can eliminate uric acid which is also a by product of meat consumption, far more than from lima beans. In addition, lima beans provide no saturated fat or cholesterol.

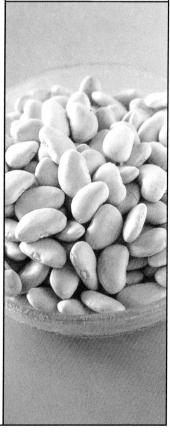

The rich fibre content in lima beans actually lowers cholesterol and also promotes a steady supply of valuable starch energy and for a price that's cheap as chips. Buy some lima beans dried, canned or frozen and gain power from the protein, strength from the iron and antioxidants from the manganese and molybdenum. Try a lima bean salad or the traditional native American dish *succotash* for a moonlight night to remember. Lima beans are available as the common white, red, brown, black and purple. Get over your weary phase, let the power of lima beans liberate your life!

MUNG BEAN	*Phaseolus mungo*	C.	P.	L.	CALORIES - total: **347 kcal. per 100 gram**
		73	24	3	Calories from: Carb:255 Protein:83 Fat:10

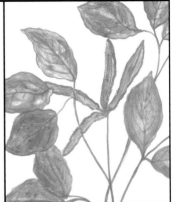

Mung beans have been around before recorded history. In India, the mung bean is made into a flour, or porridge and in China the mung bean was part of the sprouting invention, thousands of years ago. Other names for the mung bean are: golden gram, black gram and green gram, plus the Oregon pea. If you need protein, mung beans are ready to supply 24 g of complete protein, or 48 % d.v., mung bean sprouts supply 37 g protein. Mung beans are full of dietary fibre 16 g or 65 % d.v. and beneficial for elimination of toxic waste in the bowel. The iron content 7 mg or 47 % d.v. is a bonus for the blood system in addition to the manganese, 1 mg and the supply of copper 1 mg or 47% d.v.

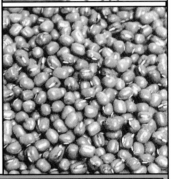

Mung beans are a very good source of magnesium 189 mg or 47 % d.v. plus phosphorus 367 mg or 37 % d.v. plus an excellent supply of folate 625 mcg or 156 % d.v. Mung beans are one of the best folate foods, essential for prevention from nervous fatigue, anaemia and blood disorders and essential for expectant mother's. Even a few cooked mung beans mixed into a soup or salad can make the world of difference to your well being. The very good supply of potassium 1246 mg or 36% d.v. plus zinc 3 mg will help protect against infections, improve blood circulation and nerve transmission. The fair amount of calcium 132 mg or 13 % d.v. will assist digestion and as mung beans provide a very lean fat content of 1%, you can easily add a cream sauce, mayonnaise or salad dressing to boost the taste of the magnificent mung bean. Refer to page 111 for mung sprouts.

PEAS	*Pisum sativum / arvense*	C.	P.	L.	CALORIES - total: **341 kcal. per 100 gram**
		82	25	3	Calories from: Carb:246 Protein:85 Fat:10

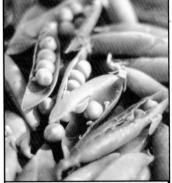

Peas are possibly the most popular legume, often considered as a vegetable but botanically they belong to the pea and pod family (Leguminosae). Peas are a great companion to numerous meals, the common steak meal, without peas is very limited in numerous nutrients and the peas actually supply more iron 4 mg than the steak 1.8 mg. Peas are an excellent source of fibre 26 g or 102 % d.v, meat supplies no fibre and very little magnesium 20 mg, peas are a good source of magnesium 115 mg or 30 % d.v. and potassium 981 mg or 28 % d.v., meat supplies 318 mg of potassium. The supply of food folate from peas is very good 274 mcg, meat supplies no folate. A deficiency of folate can reduce iron absorption and retard protein digestion as folate stimulates the production of hydrochloric acid in the stomach. Eat your peas before the meat for better

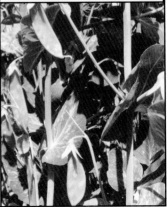

digestion. Winter is pea season so stock up on the benefits from snow peas, green peas and obtain a fair supply of vitamin K 19 mg and remember that vitamin K is destroyed by freezing, you need your greens or whites: cauliflower 150 mcg folate for blood clotting plus protection from pollution. Meat or chicken supply no vitamin K and their digestion can actually upset the intestinal bacteria that help manufacture vitamin K, plus the older we are, the more vitamin K is required. The supply of copper from peas is good 1 mg or 43% d.v., meat supplies only .007 mg of copper. Peas supply more protein 25 g or 49% d.v. than chicken 21 g or beef 24 g, so pile on the peas. Fresh peas provide a sweet flavour due to the excellent carbohydrate content 60 g and sugar content 8 g. Oh, sweet pea!

PEANUTS *arachis hypogae*	C.	P.	L.	CALORIES - total: **567 kcal. per 100 gram**
	11	**16**	**73**	Calories from: Carb:65 Protein:90 Fat:412

Peanuts are often referred to as nuts, however, they are a member of the legume family (Leguminosea). Peanuts are unique among legumes as the seed or pea grows underground.

Peanuts provide more calories than any other legume and over 70% is from the rich fat content 49 g or 76 % d.v. Peanuts provide a saturated fat content of 7 g, polyunsaturated 16 g and monunsaturated 24 g. Most of the monunsaturated oils are in the form of oleic acid 70 %, as contained in olive oil and 20 % linoleic acid or Omega 6, with only a trace of the essential and also 'hard to get' Omega 3.

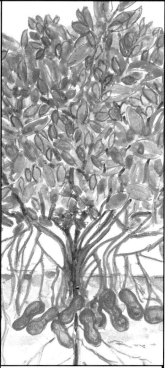

The most common use of peanuts is with the manufacture of peanut butter and the rich supply of fats makes it a tempting food. Ideally, a freshly made peanut butter: crunchy, medium or smooth can be enjoyed without any additives and obtained from the local health store. The supermarket brand does contain a lot of added salt 630 mg and sugar 8.2 g plus antioxidants 320 and only 85 % is peanuts, the balance is added oils that are hydrogenated to provide an even consistency. For the ultimate peanut butter, obtain it freshly ground and add a tbl.sp. of flax oil, mix well. When used as a spread on bread or toast, peanuts provide protein 26 g or 52 % d.v., but it is low in two essential amino acids: methionine and tryptophan. Peanuts have a net protein utilization of 43 %.

Peanuts are a very good source of B vitamins, especially biotin, a quarter cup serve supplies 26 mcg or 87 % d.v, essential for fat metabolism and sugar metabolism and it may prevent muscle cramps from excess physical exertion. For active children, the biotin in peanut butter provides power and coordination of muscles and also muscle tone. Vitamin B3 is very well supplied in peanuts 22 mg or 120 % d.v. and as it is not heat sensitive, the total value is available to assist the production of energy from carbohydrates, protein and fats. Pantothenic acid or vitamin B5 is also well supplied 2 mg or 35 % d.v., it is also required for energy production from foods but it can be depleted during processing.

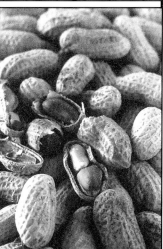

As a breakfast spread, peanut butter is great, but limit the spreading to less than 2 times per week, unless you add flax oil for the omega 3 benefits. The supply of the trace mineral copper is very good from peanuts 1.1 mcg or 57 % d.v. and peanut butter 0.5 g. Copper is essential for the metabolism of fats, isn't it remarkable how natural foods are balanced to 'self manage' their 'own' digestion! Copper is also vital for the heart muscles and the nervous system. The supply of folate 240 mcg or 60% d.v. is very good but how much peanut butter can you spread and eat, ideally for children, just enough for 2 slices of toast or approx. 20 % folate value. The folate balance required is best supplied from broccoli, legumes, vegemite or cashew nuts.

Peanuts also supply good amounts of magnesium 168 mg or 42 % d.v., phosphorus 376 mg or 38% d.v., potassium 705 mg or 20 % d.v. and zinc 3 mg or 22 % d.v. Other benefits of peanuts are from the fibre content 8 g. or 35 % d.v., vitamin E 8 mg or 28 % d.v. and manganese 2 mg or 70 % d.v. Peanuts may cause allergic reactions in some people, also the supply of oxalates may cause problems with kidney stones and gallbladder conditions. Peanuts are an acidic food and are best eaten moderately.

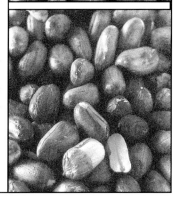

Peanuts provide protein and pure potential to promote power.

Soy beans are native to China and for 4,000 years the Chinese have produced numerous foods and products from the cultivated soy bean. Today soy beans are available worldwide and recognized as an excellent alkaline protein food 36 g or 73 % d.v. from a small 100 gram serve, now that's protein power, in fact, soy beans are the fourth best protein food after tuna, fish and eggs, refer to page 93. Soy beans require a lot of cooking time and preparation. Fortunately pre-cooked canned soy beans are very cheap. Such products as tofu - soy bean cheese are an excellent protein food, easy to add to any fried rice dish, quickly fried they acquire flavour and present well with green Oriental vegetables and a splash of soy sauce. Stock up on the soy bean benefits.

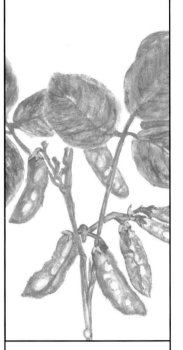

Soy beans provide the essential fatty acids linoleic acid-omega 6 and Omega 3-linolenic acid, that's a real bonus and adds to the need for more soy in the diet. The excellent supply of lecithin is vital for protection from excess cholesterol from animal product foods, soy beans supply no cholesterol and soy oil provides a fair supply of Omega 3, 7 g, but ideally add a tbl.sp of flax oil.

Lecithin is a brain food and if you are feeling fatigued, it may be a lack of iron, but add a little lecithin to your breakfast cereal, or omelette, or pancake mix and wake up your brain and nervous system. Most lecithin supplements are extracted from the mighty soy bean.

Soy beans are an excellent food for diabetics, especially non-insulin dependant, as the protein and fibre 9 g or 37 % d.v. may prevent high blood sugar levels and also keeps sugar levels stable. In some cases, regular use of soy beans has lowered the insulin medication requirements. In addition, soy beans help to lower the harmful high triglyceride levels in diabetics. For people with irritable bowel syndrome, soy bean fibre may reduce such symptoms as diarrhea and constipation. Soy beans provide a nearly unique source of genistein, an isoflavone providing protection against prostrate cancer, as genistein blocks cancer cells from reproducing.

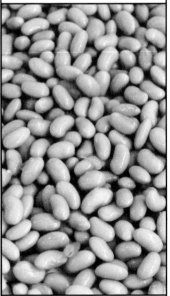

Soy milk is a common alternative to dairy milk and for those people with lactose intolerance or other dairy allergies, various varieties of soy milk are now available. Check the labels to see if the soy milk, or beans are genetically modified and if so, avoid such products as they are not time-tested to be safe.

Soy beans are an excellent source of the hard to find trace mineral molybdenum, one cup of soy beans provides nearly 80 % d.v. and it is vital for the brain and nervous system. Soy beans are a very good source of iron 8 mg plus a very good source of magnesium 280 mg or 70 % d.v. plus phosphorus 704 mg or 70% d.v. In regards to folate, soy beans 375 mg and soy flour 410 mg are a top provider.

Soy beans supply abundant vitamin K 190 mcg. It takes time to get used to soy protein power, so start off with small serves of beans or tofu and maintain a regular weekly soy meal for a protein boost that surpasses the beef that are often fed soy to promote growth. Try tofu ice cream as a dessert and make a milk shake from soy milk with a dash of ice cream for a sweet snack.

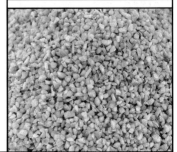

Soy is waiting to provide a range of benefits and recipes, direct from a packet, carton or can, no need to prepare.

Soy beans are small in size and superior in sustenance.

There are two types of soy beans, the edible bean and the commercial field variety. The majority of soy products are produced from the commercial field variety. Some of these products have been used for thousands of years and others have been developed only recently. Both the Chinese and Japanese have used soy products long before the western world even heard the name soy.

TOFU: Developed by the Chinese, it is prepared from ground soy beans and then powdered gypsum is added to promote a curdle effect. It can be eaten as such or fermented to produce a high protein tofu-cheese.

MISO: Used by the Japanese for over 2,000 years, it is prepared from fermented soy beans, cooked rice and sea salt. Miso preparation is a very lengthy process, the mixture is placed in large wooden vats and slowly fermented with the organism, asperigillus oryzae. Miso is available at most natural food stores. It supplies excellent amounts of protein and can be suitably combined to enhance soups, spreads, gravies or diluted and mixed with a salad dressing.

HAMANATTO: Developed in Korea, it is made from steamed soy beans, roasted wheat and then fermented. The mixture is poured into large wooden buckets and placed in the sun, salt and ginger are also added. This process takes about one year and then the mixture is placed on wooden trays and allowed to dry. Hamanatto supplies excellent amounts of protein and it combines well with most cooked meals.

NATTO: Developed by Buddhist monks over 2,000 years ago. The process includes cooked soy beans, inoculating them with 'bacillus subtilis', the mixture is then wrapped in thin sheets of pinewood and allowed to ferment for a few days.

SOY SAUCE: The most widely used soy product, it is prepared from cooked soy beans mixed with roasted wheat and then impregnated with the ferment - 'aspergillus oryzae'. The mixture is placed into wooden vats, salt is added and allowed to ferment for a minimum of six months, sometimes five years. The mixture is strained and placed in glass. Soy sauce combines very well with savoury rice dishes, salad dressings, gravies and many meals. It is full of salt, so take it easy!

TAMARI: A similar product to soy sauce, fermented for at least three years, it will enhance the taste of rice dishes, fresh garden salad or many other cooked meals. Tamari is available at most natural food stores, try the taste sometime, use as an excellent substitute for table salt. Fermented foods promote digestion and health.

SOY MILK: An excellent substitute for either powdered or pasteurised cows milk. Soy milk is prepared from pre soaked, ground soy beans. The mixture is then boiled and strained and reboiled. Commercial soy milk is available in a dry powdered form. Compared to cows milk, soy milk is not mucus forming, far richer in the mineral iron, over eight times and more compatible with human digestion. The taste is different to cows milk, try a half-half combination to start and slowly wean yourself off the cows milk and you will obtain the best of both taste and nutrients. Avoid those winter coughs and splutters, avoid cows milk.

SOY GRITS: An essential food for every kitchen, soy grits are prepared from cracked soy beans. The one advantage over the beans is that they require far less cooking time, less than half an hour moderate heat. Soy grits will enhance the protein value of all meals, small amounts could be served as a side dish mixed with steamed vegetables or combined with any soup, casserole or bean loaf or cooked mung beans.

SOY FLOUR: An excellent source of complete protein, there are three types of soy flour, full-fat, 20% fat content, medium-fat, 5% or the popular fat-free soy flour. Soy flour contains no gluten, producing a very compact home made bread. In combination with wheat, rye or triticale flour, soy flour could be used in the following proportions: 3 cups wheat (rye or triticale) with half a cup of soy flour, that will produce a light bread with an exceptional protein content. Make sure your kitchen is always stocked with some soy flour and soy oil, refer to page 143.

TEMPEH: Developed in Indonesia, it is prepared from fermented soy beans and then wrapped in banana leaves, the result is a cheese with a very distinct taste.

LEGUME SUMMARY CHARTS

LEGUMES	MAIN NUTRIENTS, ANTIOXIDANTS & PHYTONUTRIENTS	BODY SYSTEM BENEFITS
CAROB	alkaline, pectin, fibre, calcium, potassium, zinc, iron, carbohydrates.	digestive, muscular.
CHICK PEAS	protein, fibre, folate, iron, copper, manganese, potassium, molybdenum.	blood, circulatory.
GREEN BEANS	folate, potassium, fibre, vitamin a, plant hormones, vitamin k.	circulatory, digestive
KIDNEY BEANS	protein, calcium, carbohydrates, fibre, potassium, folate, iron, molybdenum, magnesium, copper,	elimination, digestive, growth, blood.
LENTILS	protein, carbohydrates, fibre, iron, phosphorus, molybdenum.	digestive, blood.
LIMA BEANS	protein, magnesium, carbohydrates, phosphorus, iron, molybdenum, fibre, folate, copper, manganese.	nervous, blood, elimination, cellular.
MUNG BEANS	protein, fibre, iron, magnesium, folate, potassium, carbohydrates.	blood, elimination.
PEAS	fibre, iron, magnesium, folate, copper, protein, vitamin k.	nervous, blood.
PEANUT	biotin, protein, vitamin b3, folate, magnesium, phosphorus, fibre, manganese, vitamin b5, copper.	nervous, muscular, growth,
SOY BEANS	protein, lecithin, fibre, genisten, molybdenum, iron, magnesium, phosphorus, folate, vitamin k, omega 6, omega 3.	growth, circulatory, blood, nervous.

LEGUMES - BALANCED DIET - CARBOHYDRATE INTAKE

	ADULT MALE	ADULT FEMALE	TEENAGER	CHILDREN
TOTAL APPROX. DAILY INTAKE (AVERAGE) (R.D.I.) CARBOHYDRATE INTAKE	340 grams	280 grams	400 grams	270 grams
LEGUMES 20 % CARBOHYDRATE INTAKE LAUGH WITH HEALTH DIET	68 grams	56 grams	80 grams	54 grams
100 g LEGUMES FRESH = 12 grams of carbohydrate approx.	425 grams	460 grams	660 grams	450 grams
100 g LEGUMES COOKED = 20 grams of carbohydrate approx.	340 grams	280 grams	400 grams	270 grams
FOOD PYRAMID DAILY DIET	3 serves	2 serves	3 serves	2 serves
AUSTRALIAN HEALTHY EATING PLATE	80 gram	80 gram	80 gram	75 gram

LEGUMES - BALANCED DIET - PROTEIN INTAKE

	ADULT MALE	ADULT FEMALE	TEENAGER	CHILDREN
TOTAL APPROX. DAILY INTAKE (AVERAGE) R.D.I. PROTEIN INTAKE	218 grams	170 grams	220 grams	160 grams
LEGUMES 15% PROTEIN INTAKE LAUGH WITH HEALTH DIET	32 grams	25 grams	33 grams	24 grams
100 grams LEGUMES FRESH = 4 grams PROTEIN approx.	800 grams	625 grams	828 grams	600 grams
100 g LEGUMES COOKED = 8 g PROTEIN	400 grams	312 grams	412 grams	300 grams
FOOD PYRAMID DIET	2 serves	1 serves	2 serves	1 serve
AUSTRALIAN HEALTHY EATING PLATE	80 gram	80 gram	80 gram	75 gram

80 -100 grams of fresh and cooked legumes is equivalent to approx. half a cup.

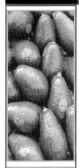
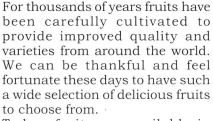
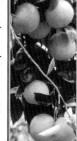

For thousands of years fruits have been carefully cultivated to provide improved quality and varieties from around the world. We can be thankful and feel fortunate these days to have such a wide selection of delicious fruits to choose from.

Today, fruits are available in shopping centres, with an incredible variety that our predecessors would have truly cherished.

To ensure maximum nutrition, the human diet needs fresh fruits. On average 20% of the daily food supply is best obtained as fresh fruits.

Fruits provide an alkaline balance to the blood which is most beneficial for healing.

Fruits assist in the proper elimination of toxins and body waste, essential for maintenance of daily health.

Fruits are the most refreshing food, especially during hot weather. Keep most fruits in the fridge for that extra crunch and freshness. Fruits are the best foods to have after a complete fast or whenever you need a 'mini-fast', to offset the effects of those complex protein meals.

The human digestive system is well suited to fruits. The digestive tract is between 12 - 14 times the height of the body, similar to most fruit eating animals. The herbivore's digestive tract is approx. 20 times the height of the body. The carnivores digestive tract is approx. five times the body height.

As our complex digestive system is best adapted to fruits, we can also expect maximum nutritional benefits from the proper combination of fruits.

There are four main fruit groups: sweet fruits, sub acid fruits, acid fruits and melons. Refer to pages 208 - 210.

Fruits provide a unique abundance of fruit sugars termed fructose, an ideal source of natural energy.

Fruits provide a variety of minerals and vitamins to assist in the utilization of their fructose content, plus, providing numerous other positive health and healing benefits.

Fresh fruits are the easiest food to digest especially when eaten either on their own, or in a fruit salad.

For information on food combining with fruits, refer to pages 208 - 210. Fruits are the best take away foods in their colourful natural packaging. Fruits are ready to go. The following pages will point out the main nutrient benefits of 32 different fruits.

All fruits have an individual set of some 'essential human nutrients'. With this information, we can reap specific health and healing benefits.

Most fruits are best when picked direct from the tree, bush, vine or plant, when ripe.

Many people live a long way from the nearest fruit tree. The shopping centre, supermarket and local fruit store do their best to supply fruits as fresh as possible.

Fruits are an excellent source of antioxidant power. We need all the anticancer and ailment prevention resources possible these days and numerous antioxidants are only available from fresh fruits. Fruits provide the greatest array of unique flavours and sweetness.

It would be a dull life without fruits.

Welcome to the fruit kingdom. Every fruit is ready to serve you with unique qualities, fit for a king or queen. Let fruits regularly provide you with their unique golden health benefits and amazing textures.

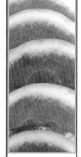
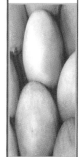
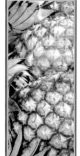
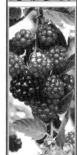

NOTE: All amounts in this book are measured in milligrams (mg) per 100 grams, unless stated otherwise.

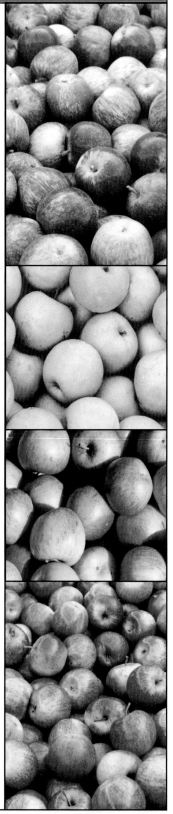

Apples are of great benefit to the digestive system. The excellent supply of pectin and malic acid both stimulate the digestive system and cleanse the digestive system by eliminating toxins from the small intestine. Whenever you have a weak digestive system, let the apple give you strength.

The green granny smith apple steamed is ideal to assist a weak digestive system, then progress to fresh ripe apples. If you can 'stomach' the apple, you're on the way to recovery and improved digestive function.

Pectin is a soluble fibre, apples contain 0.78 grams per 100 gram. Pectin slows digestion and the rise in blood sugar, plus as apples have a low glycemic index (G.I. 36), they are an ideal food for hyperactive children or diabetics. Pectin also reduces the amount of cholesterol produced by the liver and pectin may lower blood cholesterol levels and the risk of heart disease. Pectin is especially concentrated in the apple peel. Pectin removes toxins from the digestive tract by supplying a substance termed *galacturonic acid*. Pectin promotes proper protein digestion, as it prevents digested proteins in the small intestine from spoiling.

The malic acid content of apples prevents liver disorders and promotes better digestion, plus the alkaline elements increase the flow of saliva, for carbohydrate digestion.

The red apples contain anthocyanins which are powerful antioxidants and in addition, all apples contain flavonoids such as catechins and quercetin which increase the antioxidant qualities of the fruit. One study showed a decrease in mental deterioration due to the flavonoids and another study stated flavonoids protect against the effects of tobacco carcinogens in cases of bladder cancer. Apples, the richest fruit source of the flavonoid quercetin, were found to protect against lung cancer and reduce the risk of thrombiotic strokes. The bioavailability of quercetin, in apples, is amongst the best and *even a day after eating an apple*, the level of quercetin in the blood was still considered effective. A National cancer Institute stated that quercetin helps to prevent the growth of prostrate cancer cells.

Research has shown that the phytochemicals in the apple skin restricted the growth of colon cancer cells by 43 %, however, as the average consumption of apples is one apple every five days, don't expect great results, unless, you eat an apple a day, now it seems more crucial than ever. Other apple research discovered benefits such as; reduced type 2 diabetes, reduced incidence of asthma and reduction of cholesterol with apples and apple juice, due to the supply of phytonutrients.

A study at the University of California showed that having two apples a day, or apple juice, reduced the oxidation of cholesterol, the buildup of arterial plaque and the risk from pulmonary disease in smokers was reduced by half.

Apples also provide potassium 110 mg, vitamin A 90 mg and trace amounts of B1, B2 & B3, plus biotin, folate, vitamin C and vitamin E 0.71 mg.

The apple is the 'queen of hearts' and if you have an apple a day, who knows what else may stay away! Keep red and golden delicious apples in the fridge for a cool crisp crunch and try an apple and pineapple juice soon.

APRICOTS *Prunus armenica*	GLYCEMIC INDEX: 57	CALORIES - total: **74 kcal. per 100 gram** Calories from: Carb:62 Protein:7 Fat:5

Apricots provide an excellent supply of carotene 2,985 I.U. with a majority in the form of beta carotene 1,696 mcg, beta cryptoxanthin 161 mcg and lutein and zeaxanthin 138 mcg. Fresh and dried apricots are of great benefit for the respiratory system. Beta carotene protects the lungs and respiratory system from infections. Beta carotene is also vital for healing damaged skin and it promotes skin cell life by it's antioxidant effect on free radicals. The potassium content of fresh apricots is very good with 400 mg. Dried apricots supply 1,510 mg. The combination of potassium and carotene make apricots a healing food. Potassium repairs muscles, improves blood circulation and blood condition. Apricots are waiting to be appreciated.

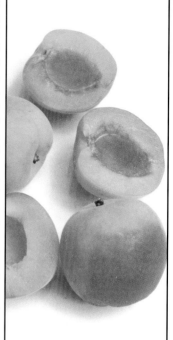

The good supply of silicon promotes skin rejuvenation plus it cleanses the blood. Apricots are ideal for the blood, skin and eyes. The supply of lutein and zeaxanthin, plus silicon protects against lens deterioration and potassium promotes nerve transmission to the brain and retards the process of ageing.

Apricots supply copper 0.4 mg and they are a good source of the trace mineral molybdenum, required for elimination of body waste. Apricots provide antioxidant power from the very good supply of flavonoids. There are two main types of dried apricots: sun dried and sulphur dried. Sulphur dried apricots are treated with sulphur dioxide and may be a problem for asthmatics. Sun dried apricots provide the maximum nutritional value and they are a safe food for children, ideal as a teething aid and energy source.

AVOCADO *Persea Armenica*	GLYCEMIC INDEX: 0	CALORIES - total: **160 kcal. per 100 gram** Calories from: Carb:31 Protein:7 Fat:123

The avocado is fruit from a tree that belongs to the Laurel family (Lauraceae), the Persea Americana. The Aztect originally cultivated the avocado. Now there are numerous varieties throughout the world. The Hass and Fuerte are common varieties, plus the Gwen, Bacon, Pinkerton, Zutano and Reed.

Avocados provide a small amount of the essential fatty acid, omega 3. The fact that avocado is eaten raw, promotes maximum benefits. About 77% of the avocado is in the form of lipids: 70% are mono unsaturated with 12 % poly unsaturated and 15% saturated. The rich oleic acid content is beneficial for reduction of blood cholesterol, plus avocados contain lecithin that further reduces blood cholesterol levels. For more information on avocado oil, refer to page 140.

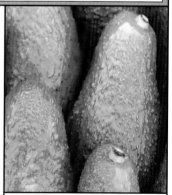

The avocado is a good source of potassium 485 - 600 mg, a heat sensitive nutrient, vital for the heart muscles. The very good supply of chlorine 645 mg and sulphur 505 mg, assists digestion of the fats plus they promote body cleansing. Avocados are a safe food for diabetics, with a zero glycemic index, plus the supply of potassium is very beneficial. The good supply of folate 58 mcg helps prevent cardiovascular disease. The avocado is nourishing to the nervous system with magnesium 29 - 45 mg plus phosphorus 52 mg. The avocado contains no cholesterol, it is not a fattening food, as the mono unsaturated fats are easily used by the body for energy. Few foods can spread so many amazing benefits as the outstanding avocado. Treat your body to an avocado dip today or on the next picnic!

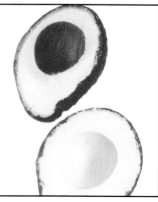

BANANA *Musaceae*	GLYCEMIC INDEX: 55	CALORIES - total: **89 kcal. per 100 gram** Calories from: Carb:83 Protein:4 Fat:3

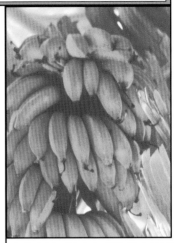

Bananas are big in carbohydrate value with a low 89 calorie value and only 0.3 grams of fat per 100 gram, thereby you can eat them all day long and never put on weight. Due to the fact that bananas are mainly eaten raw, the full value of the potassium content 370 mg, or the average banana 467 mg is available and that is of great benefit for the muscular system and the heart muscles, plus the skeletal system. Potassium rich foods counteract the problems with excess intake of common salt, such as the loss of calcium from the bones.

Bananas are rich in potassium and low in organic sodium 1 mg which promotes an alkaline condition in the blood, essential for healing and proper calcium metabolism.

Bananas contain serotonin and norepinephrine and these natural hormones can help to reduce depression.

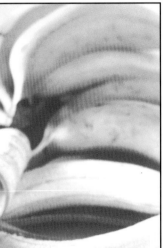

If you are an active person, the banana will easily support your energy requirements and keep your body flexible and running smoothly. For children the banana smoothie is a great supplier of nutrients with natural sweetness and protein. Get your share of the banana benefits at morning tea time before the chip cravings begin. The banana will help your body bend into shape, just like the monkeys do.

Bananas benefit the digestive system due to their pectin content, plus they supply iron 0.7 mg, chlorine 270 mg, sulphur 120 mg and bromine 0.54 mg all essential for the glandular and blood system. You have to hand it to bananas, they really give the sweetest energy. A cavendish banana with a dash of green near the stem is best for digestion. Lady finger bananas need to be fully ripe for the best taste and texture.

If you have a digestive problem or lack energy and can't put your finger on the problem, ask yourself, 'have I had a banana recently'. Bananas have a moderate glycemic index. The cavendish and lady finger bananas are ready, set, go, to supply a big bunch of benefits.

BERRIES	*Rubus ulmifolius* *Rubus loganbaccus*	GLYCEMIC INDEX: <65	CALORIES - total: **56 kcal. per 100 gram** Calories from: Carb:52 Protein:3 Fat:1

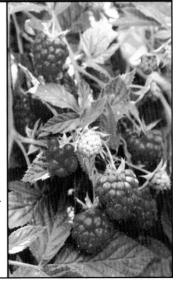

Berries of the Rubus family include: blackberry, boysenberry, dewberry, cloudberry, loganberry, raspberry and wineberry. The loganberry and raspberry are the most popular commercially grown Rubus berries. Red berries contain phytochemicals: lycopene and anthocyanins. Lycopene is a very potent antioxidant, plus it helps protect against skin damage from sunlight.

The blue, purple and blackberries contain antioxidants such as anthocyanins and phenolics. In a list of the top antioxidant foods, measured as the *oxygen radical absorbace capacity* (O.R.A.C.) as units per 100 grams, blackberries measured 2,036, raspberries: 1,220 and blueberries: 2,400, far more than any vegetable, for example, spinach is the highest common vegetable 1,260, or broccoli 890. Berries are a potent source of valuable antioxidant benefits. They reduce the risk of various types of cancer, improve the health of the circulatory system and reduce the problems of excess cholesterol. Buy or grow the beautiful big berry benefits. Refer to page 58 for the strawberry benefits. Try berries and ice cream for a cool and fabulous party dessert!

BLUEBERRIES	*Vaccinium corymbosum*	GLYCEMIC INDEX: <65	CALORIES - total: **56 kcal. per 100 gram** Calories from: Carb:52 Protein:3 Fat:1

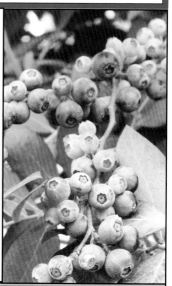

Blueberries, bilberry and cranberry belong to the family Vaccinium. These berries contain a remarkable supply of antioxidants, more specifically phytonutrients or anthocyanins. These are in the blue-red pigment of the fruit. They promote a reduction of free radicals that can damage cell structure causing conditions such as heart disease, glaucoma and cataracts.

Blueberries protect the brain from oxidative stress and may retard the onset of such conditions as dementia. Another antioxidant in blueberries is ellagic acid which has the ability to inhibit the formation of cancer and in combination with the good supply of vitamin C, blueberries really have true blue value. The bilberry is a great food for the eyes, it is usually taken as an concentrated extract and may benefit in cases of glaucoma, cataracts and diabetes. Cranberries provide antibiotic qualities against E.coli, combat urinary infections and protect against plaque and tooth decay. Try blueberry jam with pancakes and cream for a simple and nourishing breakfast or brunch. Three cheers for the beaut berry benefits!

CANTALOUP	*Cucumis melo*	GLYCEMIC INDEX: 65	CALORIES - total: **34 kcal. per 100 gram** Calories from: Carb:30 Protein:3 Fat:2

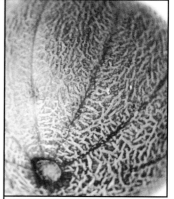

Cantaloup or rockmelon belong to the same family as pumpkin, cucumber and marrows, the 'Cucurbitaceae'. Cantaloup are a very good source of vitamin A 3,382 I.U. nearly all in the form of beta carotene, 2,020 mcg. This is a vital nutrient for the optic system and in particular for protection from cataracts. In combination with the good supply of vitamin C 37 mg the cantaloup, or Charentais, as called in France, provides antioxidant power that has the potential to activate white blood cells against infections and bad bacteria. A fully ripened cantaloup provides a very sweet meal, ideal as a breakfast entree on a hot summer's day. The potassium content of 267 mg is fully available as the fruit is eaten raw. Potassium promotes muscle power and healthy heart function. The supply of the trace mineral bromine is excellent and this is vital for the glandular system, in particular, prior to and during menopause. A decrease in bromine level occurs with age and the bromine levels in the pituitary gland needs to be replenished in order to avoid emotional disorders, depression and premenstrual tension. Also, during the 'mid-life-crisis' a regular dose of bromine may offset emotional depression in males. Bromine is present in the bloodstream and body tissues, it is vital for the coordination of numerous glands. Bromine is not considered an essential mineral, but it's benefits are so keep your emotional life 'rock- solid' with the regular supply of rockmelon, the food for a peaceful balanced life. Cantaloup also provides folate 21 mcg, ideal for those people who don't like their greens. Cantaloup are best eaten alone, before a main meal, otherwise they can ferment in the stomach. Melons require hardly any digestion so give them the 'right of way' in the busy traffic of your complex digestive system. Cantaloup are the ideal food for the elderly, as they are very easy to chew and they provide an abundance of life promoting 'happy health' benefits. Choose a fully ripened fruit for complete flavour. Roll out the rockmelon and feel on top of the world, at the start of a day.

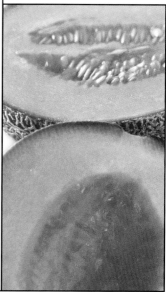

CHERRIES *p. cerasus*	GLYCEMIC INDEX: 22	CALORIES - total: **63 kcal. per 100 gram** **Calories from:** Carb:58 Protein:4 Fat:2

Cherries provide a very low glycemic index, an ideal fruit for diabetics and those hyperactive children, exceedingly better than lollies and they really are the 'lolly-look-alike' in fruits. Cherries are packed with pain killing power due to their supply of anthocyanins, in the natural pigments. A quantity of 20 cherries supplies 25 mg anthocyanins per 100 gram. Anthocyanins are as effective as aspirin or ibuprofen in cases of headaches, gout or arthritis, as they retard the enzymes that cause tissue inflammation. Cherries contain the flavonoids: isoqueritrin and queritrin plus the plant phenolic: ellagic acid, a potent anti-carcinogenic and antimutagenic compound. In addition, cherries are packed with perrillyl alcohol which stunts the growth of cancer cells and then flushes them out of the body. Cherries provide significant amounts of melatonin, also produced by the pineal gland to promote sleep. Cherries are a blood builder, plus they supply vitamin A 213 I.U. plus potassium 220 mg. If you think cherries are expensive, the trees take years to grow and the fruit is hand picked, plus they have a very short summer season. As they say 'you get what you pay for'. Have a good night's sleep, reduce pain and cherish the cheerful cherry benefits!

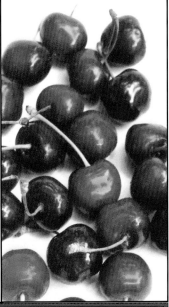

CURRANTS *Var. corinthiac*	GLYCEMIC INDEX: 50	CALORIES - total: **63 kcal. per 100 gram** **Calories from:** Carb:55 Protein:5 Fat:3

Currants are available as red, black or white. Blackcurrants are the most common and they provide the maximum vitamin C content with 155 -215 mg. White and red currants provide 41 -81 mg, dried currants provide only 3 mg per 100 grams. The recommended dietary intake of vitamin C for adults is approx. 30 -40 mg per day and during pregnancy 60 mg are required. Black currants are the third best food source of natural vitamin C and the benefits for the immune system and other body systems are numerous. Refer to page 163 for details. Vitamin C is required everyday. It is an antioxidant and it protects tissues from free radical damage. Vitamin C promotes fat metabolism and it is vital for the eyes, teeth and bones. A handful of blackcurrants will provide an incredible boost to your immune system. Blackcurrant syrup will be a good provider of the vitamin C benefits and possibly the other benefits below, but check the label for additives.

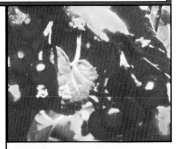

Blackcurrants provide exceptional antioxidant activity, they supply nearly double the value of blueberries in anthocyanin content and polyphenols, with the colour to match the power. The anthocyanin power of currants, especially blackcurrants will destroy free radicals and protect the immune system. Anthocyanins are very effective in locating free radicals and destroying their functions. Anthocyanins also reduces the risk of cholesterol particles attaching to arterial walls, that can eventually lead to high blood pressure and strokes. For smokers, blackcurrants or syrup is very beneficial. Blackcurrants are also an excellent source of flavonoids, they supply a fair amount of iron 2.3 mg, calcium 87 mg (dried) and vitamin A 230 I.U. carotene power and potassium 322 mg. Dried blackcurrants are a great sweet. Blackcurrants are pure antioxidant power, count on it, ready when you are, coming ready or not, to rid the body of free radicals!

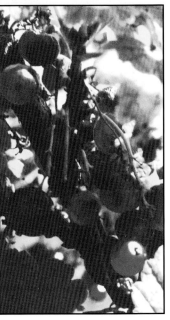

DATES	*Phoenix dactylifera*	**GLYCEMIC INDEX: 103**	CALORIES - total: **282 kcal. per 100 gram** Calories from: Carb: 270 Protein:8 Fat:3

Fresh and dried dates are a compact energy food with 75% carbohydrate content and 8 grams of fibre, that's bulky. If you lack energy and need a quick snack, dates are ready any time to boost your whole body. The muscular system will be given 650 - 730 mg of potassium, per 100 grams, to improve blood circulation, prevent hardening of the arteries, assist body healing and with the iron content 1 mg, both minerals help to utilize oxygen and normalize heart muscle action.

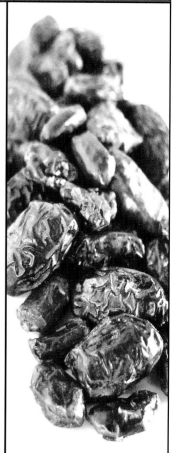

Dates are also a fair source of magnesium 43 mg, calcium 39 mg and phosphorus 62 mg, all essential for bone strength, healthy nerves and brain function. Dates provide complete protein, in small amounts, 2 grams. There is no doubt that you could survive in the wilderness with fresh dates for a long time, as they provide the energy and a wide variety of nutrients.

The very high glycemic index of dates needs to be considered. They can be beneficial in cases of low blood sugar, or, for 'instant energy' after a physical or mental work-out. Approx. 90% of all glucose or blood sugar is required for efficient brain functioning. For diabetics, dates are best avoided. Ideally, dip dates into tahini for a lower glycemic index and a magnificent snack. Dates are known to strengthen the muscles of the uterus during pregnancy and they are an ideal snack during lactation, as they alleviate depression. Dates also supply: copper 0.29 mg and manganese 0.30 mg. Dates provide 2.8 % total mineral content, nearly top of the list with all foods. Dates are usually obtained as sun dried, but fresh dates are best by a mile!

Dates are a great food for hitch hikers, bush walkers and they were given to warriors, to stimulate their muscles due to the enormous supply of potassium. Try a date slice once in a while and pick up a few fresh dates, next break. Dates are the super sweet!

FIGS	*Ficus carica*	**GLYCEMIC INDEX: 61**	CALORIES - total: **249 kcal. per 100 gram** Calories from: Carb:230 Protein:11 Fat:8

Figs provide more minerals than dates, with a far lower G.I. index. Figs are the best fruit source of calcium 162 mg, fresh figs 35 mg. For a totally huge calcium treat, dip figs into tahini. Figs also provide an abundance of potassium 680 mg and this improves calcium balance especially for people whose diet includes added salt, extra potassium is required.

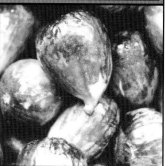

A small serve of figs supplies nearly half the essential dietary fibre. Research has shown that high fibre foods reduce the appetite and may assist weight loss. Figs can be combined in cookies and they make an ideal mid morning snack with a cup of tea, especially for the busy houseperson.

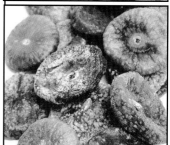

Figs supply a good amount of organic iron 2.2 mg plus manganese 0.38 mg and copper 0.30 mg, a great combination for blood building and for protection against fatigue, especially with the great supply of carbohydrates. Figs also supply magnesium 58 mg, phosphorus 67 mg plus silicon 240 mg. If you're feeling teary or weary, call figs to the rescue. Potassium provides muscle power to overcome the obstacles of a messy house and chlorine 100 mg and sulphur 270 mg will ensure that your inner house is also cleansed. Fresh figs are a most delightful fruit. Forget fatigue with figs!

| GRAPEFRUIT | *Poncirus trifoliata* | GLYCEMIC INDEX: 25 | CALORIES - total: **39 kcal. per 100 gram** |
| | | | Calories from: Carb:36 Protein:2 Fat:1 |

Grapefruit are the largest citrus fruit, with the white, pink or ruby flesh to choose from. Their bitterness is due to: liminoid a phytochemical, plus, avoid unripe grapefruit. To dull the bitter taste, add honey on top, or mix with strawberry juice. Liminoids promote the formation of a detoxifying enzyme: glutathione-S-transferase, that inhibits tumour formation especially in cases of oral, pancreatic, colon or stomach cancer. Grapefruit also contains lycopene which provides similar antitumour and antioxidant activity to fight against atherosclerosis, cataracts, arthritis and other diseases caused by oxidative stress. Lycopene provides the colour pigment to fruits. Grapefruit also contain salicylic acid, which dissolve inorganic calcium, a cause in the condition of arthritis. Grapefruit reduces body acidity and protects against kidney stone development. Grapefruit provide vitamin C 38 mg and their biotin 3 mcg content promotes fat reduction in combination with a low calorie count and their supply of vitamin B5, 0.28 mg. Get used to the grapefruit to reduce body weight, acidity and to protect against tumours. Grapefruit are a great fruit!

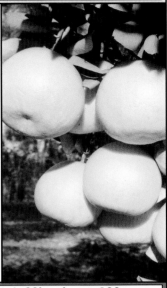

| GRAPES | *Vitis - rotundifolia - labrusca - vinifera* | GLYCEMIC INDEX: 46 | CALORIES - total: **20kcal. per 100 gram** |
| | | | Calories from: Carb:37 Protein:4 Fat:1 |

Grapes are one of the most cultivated fruits, mainly for the wine industry with numerous varieties that rarely reach the local fruit store. Keep a look out for the blue, red, green and yellow grapes and take a bunch home.

The benefits from fresh grapes are for the blood system. If you need a natural blood transfusion, eat a bunch of grapes a day, for a week, or make a fresh grape juice daily and avoid all the pips. The manganese 0.8 mg content from one cup of grapes supplies 20% of the daily requirement. Imagine if you ate a bunch of grapes! Manganese is vital for red blood cell development, a good memory and it is required allot during lactation. Grapes supply tartaric acid which stimulates the intestines. Red, blue and purple grapes contain saponin, a glucose based compound, it helps lower cholesterol by reducing oxidation and it also reduces inflammation. Plus, grapes contain the antioxidant quercetin, refer to apples.

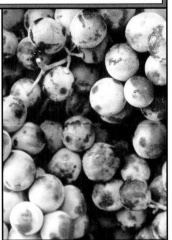

Grapes also contain a natural antibiotic, found in the skin of grapes: trans-resveratrol. It fights prostate and lung cancer. Trans-resveratrol inhibits carcinogens from binding to cell receptors and it can stop the spread of cancer. In addition, it may also promote longevity and decrease the risk of heart disease. Grape skin also contains phenolic compounds, these compounds inhibit enzymes that cause blood vessels to constrict and reduce the supply of oxygen to the heart. Grapes increase the level of nitric oxide produced by the body to protect against blood clot formation in arteries, plus it increases vitamin E levels in the blood. Nitric oxide is an antioxidant with the power to reduce oxidation of blood plasma and cholesterol. Grapes are in season for a few months, so hoe into them for great blood building and protective qualities for the immune system. Make grape juice regularly and when out of season, try good quality grape juice, it provides most of the benefits and the 'glass of red before bed' provides a good night's sleep, plus the natural antibiotic qualities. Grapes are great, mate!

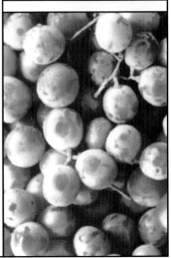

GUAVA *Psidium guajava*	GLYCEMIC INDEX: <50	CALORIES - total: **20kcal. per 100 gram**
		Calories from: Carb:37 Protein:4 Fat:1

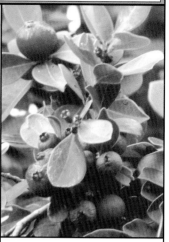

The green and strawberry guava has been named a gold medallist in one survey that included 4 nutrients: vitamin C, carotenoids, folate, potassium, plus fibre. The guava heads the list with a score of over 400, far greater than any other fruit, with watermelon second with less than half the value of guava.

There is no doubt that the vitamin C content of fresh guavas is excellent with over 200 mg. per 100 grams, approx. 4 times that of oranges. The guava is the richest natural vitamin C food apart from the very hot red peppers and how many of those can you eat in one day!

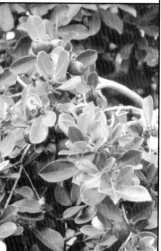

If you are a smoker, you need to replenish the vitamin C every few hours, as each cigarette takes about 30 mg. of vitamin C out from the body. A box full of guavas every week may be the best advice till you quit. The contraceptive pill and antibiotics also deplete vitamin C. If you look at the computer screen, television or video, then extra vitamin C will be required just to prevent eyestrain. The lens of the eye is dependant on a regular supply of vitamin C, that means at least twice daily and for smokers it increases with every puff.

Keep your eyes open for guava season and treat your life to the most abundant supply of vitamin C that nature can provide.

Vitamin C is the 'anti stress' vitamin, mainly because it is stored and required by the adrenal glands constantly in case of emergencies, a shock, unexpected noises or bad news. The adrenal glands produce a hormone: adrenaline for digestion, glucose production, heart rate, nervous system and conditions of stress, fear and excitement. Don't miss out on all the excitement.

Guava also provide a fair amount of vitamin A 625 I.U. nearly all in the form of lutein and zeaxanthin 5,000 mcg, vital for protection from ultraviolet radiation, especially in the eyes.

Even one guava a day can give your eyes great protection, especially for the over 50's who view the computer, play station or wide screen for hours. Guava is the tropical fruit to set your sights on!

KIWIFRUIT *Actinidia chinesis*	GLYCEMIC INDEX: 52	CALORIES - total: **61 kcal. per 100 gram**
		Calories from: Carb:54 Protein:3 Fat:4

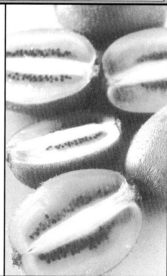

Kiwifruit are best recognized for their decorative appearance on desserts such as the pavlova. The kiwifruit is a fair source of vitamin A 175 I.U. in combination with the excellent supply of vitamin C 75 - 97 mg, which is more than oranges. The kiwifruit is a great alternative for people who dislike citrus fruits. One kiwifruit can provide twice the basic daily vitamin C requirement for adults. Let the kiwifruit balance and protect your immune system.

Kiwifruit also provides the trace mineral copper 0.16 mg. a fair iron content 0.41 mg plus a good supply of potassium 330 mg and a small supply of calcium, 26 mg. Kiwifruit contain phytonutrients that protect the development of new cells from oxidation in addition to the action of vitamin C. For children, kiwifruit has proved beneficial in cases of respiratory problems such as night-coughing and wheezing. Try kiwifruit in the next tropical fruit salad, or try an apple and kiwifruit juice combination. The gooseberry or kiwifruit when taken regularly can be an ideal natural way to help relieve the children's cough!

LEMONS Citrus limon LIMES C.aurantifolia	GLYCEMIC INDEX: <20	CALORIES - total: **29 kcal. per 100 gram** Calories from: Carb:23 Protein:4 Fat:3

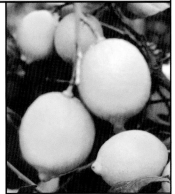

Both lemons and limes are full of citric acid, approx. 6 % and one benefit is that citric acid preserves vitamin C activity. Many people reach for a lemon or lime when they have a cold, sore throat, conjestion and many cold tablets use lemon or lime extracts, but without doubt the freshly squeezed lemon will provide the maximum benefits. Citric acid does relieve conjestion but in addition the sulphur content 125 mg makes all the difference, as it dissolves mucous in the respiratory system, cleanses the body of toxins and has an antiseptic and cleansing effect for the digestive system.

The vitamin C content 50 - 75 mg is a great bonus during times of fever, in combination with sulphur.

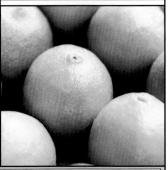

Lemons and limes provide an alkaline balance to the stomach, as potassium carbonate in the lemons and limes forms to neutralizes stomach acids, reach for a lemon or lime. In places where cholera, typhoid and diptheria are prevalent, lemons and limes, taken daily, have proved beneficial in preventing the contraction of these conditions. Lemons are also preventative to some forms of cancer, due to their powerful detoxifying and antioxidant abilities. Lemons and limes reduce uric acid in conditions such as gout, rheumatism and gall stones. Lemon or lime juice can destroy over 90% of bacteria in seafood within 15 minutes. If you need a quick, cheap detox, squeeze a lemon or lime, just add water and be on the way to recovery, a bitter price for better healing.

MANGO Mangifera indica	GLYCEMIC INDEX: 55	CALORIES - total: **65 kcal. per 100 gram** Calories from: Carb:61 Protein:2 Fat:2

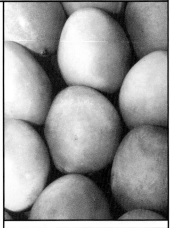

Mangoes are the golden tropical treat and most people need no convincing to eat a fresh ripe mango. The benefits are really worth discovering and the most obvious is the rich vitamin A, beta carotene content, 445 mcg.

One large mango will provide the total vitamin A required for one day per average adult. Vitamin A can be stored by the body, in the liver, however the body will utilize vitamin A, especially during times of infection, viruses, pregnancy, lactation and the 'pill' also depletes the reserves of vitamin A. Mango is a good source of the mineral chlorine, it is vital for normal blood pressure, purifying the blood, body cleansing and it assists digestion of protein foods. Slices of mango make an ideal pre dinner aperitif, or, breakfast starter, or the most delicious fresh juice combination with orange, strawberry and pineapple. The Mango provides a rich flavour for any meal or dessert, try mango sauce on baked fish, or fresh mango with ice cream, it's a dream dish.

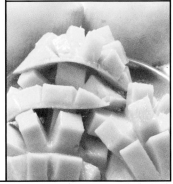

Mango also provides fair amounts of vitamin C 28 - 35 mg, potassium 156 mg, magnesium 9 - 18 mg and a very low fat content with only 0.2 grams per 100 gram and a low 65 calories. Your skin system will treasure the balance of nutrients in the mango. Keep some pocket money aside and make your next skin treatment appointment with the mango. The beta carotene content of Mango, plus the vitamin C and chlorine content will all provide a cleansing and antioxidant effect on the blood system. Beta carotene is required for growth, strong bones and teeth, healthy skin, hair and for the eyes. Mango is magnificent in flavour and it is the ideal fruit for any celebration.

MELONS *Cumus melo*	GLYCEMIC INDEX: 72	CALORIES - total: **30 kcal. per 100 gram**
		Calories from: Carb:27 Protein:2 Fat:1

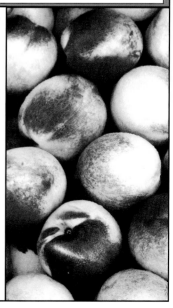

Melons are the biggest fruit and the variety is enormous, including numerous local melons with their own name, such as our local Tyndale-tiger, or the following: cassaba, canary, cranshaw, galia, honeydew, musk melon, ogen, persian, prince, santa claus and the cantaloup and watermelon. One of the main features of melons is the alkaline balance they provide to the diet. Most foods are acid forming and ideally 75% of the diet needs to be based on alkaline foods. Melons are here to rescue the body from a state of acidity, as the body cannot heal properly if the blood is always in an acid condition. Melons are approx. 90% natural mineral water. Relax with a big slice of melon and balance your body with alkaline benefits. Melons need no digestion in the stomach and if they are eaten after a meal, the problems of flatulence and intestinal aches can easily develop. There is no point in eating melon if it ferments in the digestive system and destroys the valuable supply of nutrients. Eat melons before other foods.

Melons are an excellent source of the trace mineral bromine which is most valuable for the glandular system. Bromine is one of the 'unknown' minerals, generally speaking, however it is required constantly in the bloodstream and controlled by the pituitary gland, the master gland. Bromine is vital for the health of the glandular system and for regulating emotions. It is required especially as we get older and in particular during menopause for women. Let the melon balance your emotions and also protect against those male mid life crisis situations. Melons provide a very low calorie value, ideal for anyone who likes to eat big but not put on weight. Try a melon fast once a week during summer and notice the new life that melons provide from the enzymes. Cooked foods provide no enzymes, melons are full of enzymes and a fair source of vitamin C, potassium and vitamin A.

Melons provide a mighty spark to a dull diet.

NECTARINE *Prunus persica*	GLYCEMIC INDEX: 54	CALORIES - total: **44 kcal. per 100 gram**
		Calories from: Carb:38 Protein:4 Fat:3

The nectarine is like a cousin to the peach, in fact there is only one gene difference, the gene that gives peaches their outer skin 'velvet' texture. Generally the nectarine has the same nutritional value as the peach. The potassium content of the nectarine is 200 mg, the peach supplies 190 mg. The benefits of potassium are for general body healing, movement of oxygen into the brain, regulating the body's water balance and the elimination of blood impurities via the kidneys. Potassium is an alkaline mineral and often destroyed by heat and cooking, plus excess salt depletes potassium from the body. Both alcohol and caffeine deplete potassium reserves, it is easy to see that the average diet may need more fresh potassium foods and the nectarine is a delightful choice. Nectarines are a real bonus for the respiratory system with 332 I.U. vitamin A, in the form of beta cryptoxanthin 67 mcg and beta carotene 162 mcg. The supply of lutein and zeaxanthin 130 mcg is most important for the health of the optic system, especially the retina and lens.

Slip a nectarine into your next fruit salad. Nectarines are ready to help your twin kidneys keep clean. Nectarines make a delightful snack with almonds.

OLIVES *Olea europaea*	GLYCEMIC INDEX: <5	CALORIES - total: **115 kcal. per 100 gram**
		Calories from: Carb:23 Protein:3 Fat:89

Black and green olives both supply approx. 80 % fat content with the majority of oil being mono unsaturated 9g, polyunsaturated 1g and saturated 1g. Refer to pages 131-135 for details on olive oil.

Olives straight from the tree are very bitter as they contain oleuropin, mainly contained in the olive skin. To remove this compound, olives need to be processed, otherwise they are inedible. Green olives are picked as an unripened fruit, black olives are usually fully ripened on the olive tree and then shaken off the tree, often collected on large sheets. There are four main processes for olive preparation and they all take many months of soaking plus with the *water cured* olives, numerous stages of rinsing.

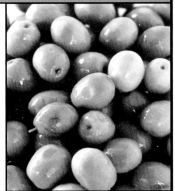

Most olives are processed in a *brine or salt solution* for one to six months, same time as with oil cured olives. Green olives are soaked in a solution of lye, thoroughly washed and then placed in salt-brine. Black olives go straight into the brine which promotes lactic acid fermentation and they are later treated with lye to remove the oleuropein.

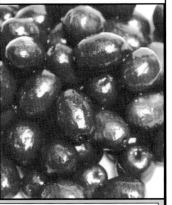

Olives are the most processed fruit and the high sodium content 800 - 2,000 mg can be a problem, especially for people with heart problems or circulatory problems. Olives supply some calcium 60 mg, potassium 55 mg, iron 1.6 mg, vitamin A 400 I.U., plus trace amounts of other minerals. Olives are an ideal addition to pizza, or anytime you need a salt flavour for a salad or meal, a few olives is all it takes, *instead of the salt shaker*. Enjoy your olives, once in a while and use olive oil regularly with salads.

PAPAYA *Carica papaya*	GLYCEMIC INDEX: 58	CALORIES - total: **39 kcal. per 100 gram**
		Calories from: Carb:36 Protein:2 Fat:1

Papaya are an incredible fruit and one of the best all round healing foods. The golden fruit contains numerous active enzymes that are most valuable for the digestive system. In particular, the enzyme papain is beneficial as a protein digestive aid and if you have a weak stomach, the ripe golden papaya will be the easiest food to digest. Papaya is an almost unique food source of two enzymes: carpain which is beneficial for the heart and also fibrin, for the process of blood clotting. Papain and the enzyme chymopapain are both of great benefit for the healing of burns and for the reduction of inflammations. Papaya also supply vitamin E 1 mg and an excellent vitamin C content of 62 mg plus a fair amount of vitamin A 1095 I.U., in the form of beta cryptoxanthin 761 mcg, beta carotene 276 mcg and lutein and zeaxanthin 75 mcg. As lutein is heat sensitive, the papaya provides the full benefit. The optic system is well rewarded with the excellent vitamin C plus lutein and zeaxanthin content. If you need to prevent eye deterioration, papaya is pleased to participate. The high beta cryptoxanthin content may help the healing of colon cancer and lung cancer. Papaya is the perfect food for the elderly and young children as it is very easy to digest, no chewing and it provides a wealth of healing and digestive benefits. Papaya and it's skin can be used directly over wounds, for healing, or, try papaya gel/ointment anytime the skin is damaged. If you need healing, don't forget papaya power. Papaya has proven healing benefits and if it's sore, ask for help from the paw paw!

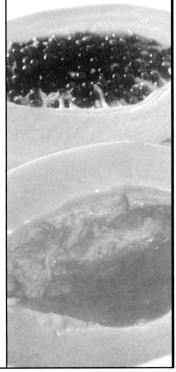

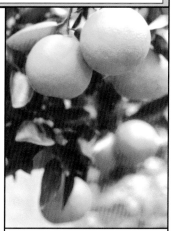

Oranges are the most convenient form of fruit drink available today. Slice an orange in half and you have an instant nature drink for two. The benefits of freshly squeezed orange juice are far above that of the commercially prepared substitutes. Most commercial orange juice is water added to orange concentrate, so why pay extra for that and all those artificial preservatives, sugar, colourings and fancy packages. Have a freshly squeezed juice and obtain all the benefits. Even the 100% juice may contain added water and 5% sugar, according to the 'production rules' without stating such on the container.

The vitamin C content 53 mg of fresh oranges is the most common understood nutritional fact for the general public, but, does it survive the processing and time lapse between drinks, not really. In addition, vitamin P is also abundant in fresh oranges, but in very limited amounts from orange juice. In fact, approx. only 10% of the vitamin P value compared to a whole orange, from *unstrained* juice. Vitamin P is located in the white pith of citrus fruits and capsicum, it is essential for strong blood capillaries, protection from varicose veins and it is 'vital' for the efficient functioning of vitamin C. Now it becomes clear, why, processed juices are not ideal to rely on for daily vitamin C. Buy 'in season' oranges next time they are available and make a freshly squeezed orange juice daily. Ideally, organic or home grown oranges are superior in flavour as they do not contain an artificial dye: citrus red number 2, that is injected into some commercial oranges, to obtain a uniform 'orange colour'. Try a natural drink. A fresh organic orange juice is full of natural life.

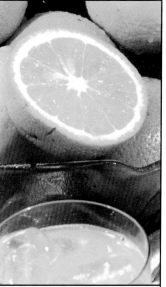

Oranges are one of the best fruit source of the main mineral calcium 40 mg, that in combination with the minerals phosphorus 20 mg is also beneficial for protection from infections and viruses. Orange juice is beneficial for maintenance of healthy skin and hair, as vitamin P and C work together to produce collagen, the substance that joins skin tissues.

Oranges supply magnesium 10 mg and this gives oranges their revitalising power, in addition to the citric acid, vitamin C and enzymes. A glass of freshly made orange juice is the quick way to start the day. If you smoke, drink alcohol and tend to be nervous, orange juice will provide good natural balance, plus, you will need extra vitamin C daily to counteract their negative effects.

Oranges provide a good source of phytonutrients and one in particular, unique to oranges is hesperidin. It has proved effective in lowering blood cholesterol and blood pressure, in animal studies, plus it provides anti-inflammatory power and once again, it is located in the white pith or pulp of the whole orange. The fibre content of one whole orange provides 10 - 15% of the daily dietary requirement and it helps reduce cholesterol and protects against colon cancer, as fibre attaches to cancer causing elements in the digestive system.

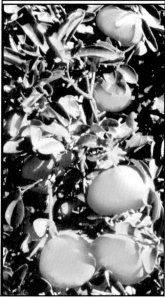

The mandarin is often the 'forgotten fruit' in most health and nutrition books but it really provides a delicious and unique flavour with a great supply of vitamin P and all the benefits of the orange. The mandarin makes a delightful juice when combined with strawberries. Give the mandarin a quick peel next time they are in season. Oranges and mandarins are handy take away treasures of precious phytonutrients and antioxidants.

PEACHES *prunus persica*	GLYCEMIC INDEX: 42	CALORIES - total: **39 kcal. per 100 gram** Calories from: Carb:34 Protein:3 Fat:2

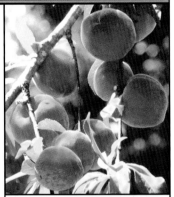

Peaches are a most delicate and delicious fruit and valuable source of vitamin A 300 - 500 I.U. with beta carotene 162 mcg, beta cryptoxanthin 67 mcg and lutein and zeaxanthin 91 mcg. Fresh peaches are an excellent food for a healthy skin condition due to the carotene content but mainly due to the good source of the mineral sulphur, one of the most important cleansing minerals. Sulphur foods prevent infection, such as acne and they improve the complexion by cleansing the body of acid poisons and by cleansing the blood.

Peaches contain antioxidants such as polyphenols, flavonols, procyanidins and hydrocinnamic acid. Peaches provide an alkaline balance to the blood and assist the cleansing of the kidneys and bladder. The triple combination of carotene, sulphur and polyphenols in peaches is ideal for prevention from infections such as bronchitis and gastritis. The potassium 190 - 210 mg is fair and it also helps remove blood impurities via the kidneys. Peaches supply hardly any vitamin C, 7 mg and a small source of vitamin E 1.2 I.U. and this gives the peach the ability to be a skin rejuvenating food, in combination with the nutrients already mentioned. Peaches supply more vitamin E than cashews, macadamia or coconut and for the maximum vitamin E snack treat, try a handful of almonds with a fresh ripe peach, it is 'out of this world in flavour', and vitamin E content, as almonds are a big 'E' food 50 I.U.

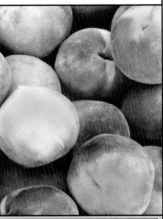

Try a fruit salad with peaches, nectarines, strawberries and mango. Fresh peaches 'in season' are worth their weight in flavour, plus, receive a bonus of a rejuvenated skin complexion. Reach for a peach as a real treat and beat the boring bicky habit!

PEARS *Pyrus communis*	GLYCEMIC INDEX: 38	CALORIES - total: **58 kcal. per 100 gram** Calories from: Carb:56 Protein:1 Fat:1

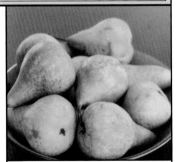

There are over 50 varieties of common pears throughout the world with the green, yellow and brown fruit as the basic difference. The Williams, Bartlett, Packam, Josephine, Thompson and Bosc pears are well known.

Raw pears in particular provide a very good fibre content, one pear supplies 20% daily fibre. This abundance of fruit fibre is delicate on the digestive system compared to the common use of wheat bran. The fibre in pears can bind with toxins in the colon and reduce their effectiveness, thereby helping to protect against colon cancer. In addition, pears supply a fair amount of the trace mineral copper 0.12 mg. Copper has proved to be deficient in people with colon cancer and the combination with the good fibre content gives pears the tag of being a top preventative food for people prone to colon cancer. A low copper intake can increase free radical production within the colon. Pears are a very simple food to digest, especially a nice ripe pear, or the steamed pears are ideal for babies, children and the elderly. Pears supply potassium 120 mg, iron 0.25 mg and a good amount of silicon, also vital for protection from cancerous tissue development and body cleansing. The folate 7.5 mg also helps, in combination with fibre, to protect from gastrointestinal disorders, constipation and diarrhoea. Once again, the 'pear get's rid of bad air'. If you have problems 'down below' reach for a pear and keep the bad bugs at bay. Pears are waiting to attack the enemy.

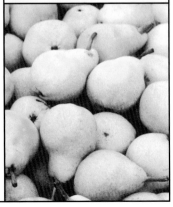

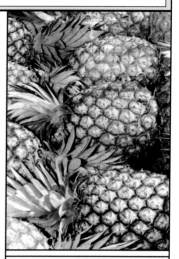

Pineapples are a versatile fruit for numerous recipes. One of the main health benefits is for the respiratory system, due to the good supply of both chlorine and sulphur, both cleansing minerals and best obtained from fresh foods, as they are both heat sensitive minerals. Sulphur protects against accumulations of mucus in the respiratory system and digestive system. Chlorine 30-46 mg reduces congestion and bronchial problems. Both these minerals are available from freshly made pineapple juice and they provide relief from bronchitis and even tuberculosis, the pineapple is tops in natural healing power. Fresh pineapple will cleanse the respiratory system when taken regularly, fresh juices are best. The fair vitamin A 56 I.U, protects against respiratory infections and the fair vitamin C 36 mg content also protects against infections. The pineapple is a great choice when the common cough is busy in the office or workplace. Pineapples are the best fruit source of the mineral manganese 1.7 mg, often termed the 'memory mineral' as it helps nourish the nervous system and brain. The manganese content is most valuable for mothers during times of lactation as it stimulates gland secretions that promote the development of mothers milk. Freshly made pineapple juice is one of the best drinks for women, especially those with menstruation problems. Manganese is destroyed by processing, however, wheat germ and bran are an excellent source.

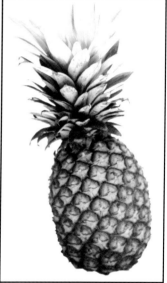

Pineapples are a natural blood thinner and that can prevent the development of blood clots but they must be restricted for people with liver or kidney disease or haemophilia. Pineapple juice is the ideal drink to have before and during a long airflight, to avoid blood clots. Pineapples are a unique provider of bromelain, an enzyme that promotes protein digestion and just as important is the natural anti- inflammatory properties of bromelain, especially for conditions such as gout and rheumatoid arthritis.

Pineapple will balance your blood acid - alkaline levels due to the great supply of bromelain and also promote hormone production particularly for the pancreas which produces amylase to process uncooked starch, lipase to convert fats and trypsin for protein conversion. To obtain the maximum bromelain value, eat fresh pineapple alone, between meals, or as a fresh breakfast juice. In addition, the supply of organic acids: citric, malic and tartaric acid also promote digestion. Malic acid stimulates production of digestive enzymes. Pineapples supply fair amounts of: iron 0.5 mg, copper 0.07 mg, selenium 0.6 mg and zinc 0.25 mg and when obtained fresh with a juice, the pineapple can be tops in reducing fever especially during those mid winter blues. Canned pineapple provides a small portion of the benefits, both sulphur and chlorine will be depleted by the canning process, plus vitamin C, and, often syrup or sugar is added. For pizza's, pineapple is a favourite and as it promotes protein, fat and carbohydrate digestion, it makes sense to put pineapple on pizzas as they are a 'busy meal' to digest. The silicon content 11 - 70 mg also assists body cleansing and blood and skin cell development.Pineapples have antioxidant power as manganese is a key ingredient in the production of enzymes that defend our cells from free radical damage.

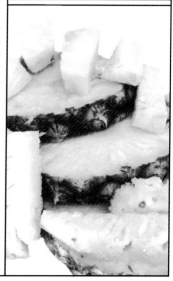

Pineapples are pleased to provide, promote, purify and protect!

PLUMS-PRUNES *Prunus domestica*

GLYCEMIC INDEX: 39

CALORIES - total: **46 kcal. per 100 gram**
Calories from: Carb:41 Protein:2 Fat:2

Plums and dried plums, or prunes are packed with phytonutrients with great antioxidant power, especially, protection from free radicals as a result of cooked fats. Prunes in particular are the greatest antioxidant food based on the ORAC comparison, the measure of total antioxidant potential of a food. Prunes were top of the list with 5,770 orac units per 100 gram, more than double of blueberries 2,400 and plums 949. Due to the dehydrated weight of prunes, they measure higher, so blueberries are top of the list.

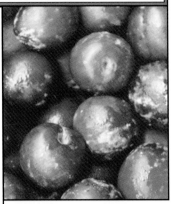

Plums contain neochlorgenic and chlorogenic acid, or phenols that can protect against the free radicals termed superoxide anion radicals. The phenols contained in plums and prunes have also shown to be effective in neutralizing the free radicals that can damage the fats within the structure of brain cells. Plum sauce is a good addition to those heavy fat based meals, as it provides antioxidant power to help protect from cholesterol and excess triglycerides. Plums provide vitamin A 345 I.U, trace amounts of iron 0.1 mg, copper 0.04, manganese 0.04 and a fair supply of potassium 157 mg. Plums supply 9mg of vitamin C and a fair supply of lutein and zeaxanthin 73mg plus beta carotene, all benefiting the optic system.

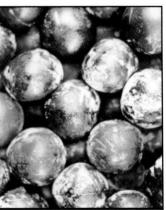

Prunes are a compact energy food with a low glycemic index (39). Prunes are well known as a natural laxative, the high level of sorbitol, a sugar alcohol, plus the high potassium 810 mg content and fibre content are the main laxative factors. Prunes and plums are packed with power to protect against fatty oxidation problems and to promote proper elimination.

STRAWBERRIES *Fragaria virginia*

GLYCEMIC INDEX: 40

CALORIES - total: **32 kcal. per 100 gram**
Calories from: Carb:27 Protein:2 Fat:3

Strawberries are a worldwide favourite, especially with cream. Strawberries contain vitamin P, also known as rutin. It is a valuable blood thinner and it increases the strength of blood vessels, plus it promotes circulation. Fresh strawberries taken regularly will promote reduced blood pressure and improved eyesight and possibly prevent the development of glaucoma.

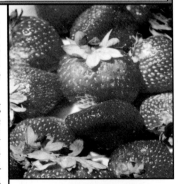

Strawberries are a good food for the blood due to the fair iron 1mg content plus the sulphur content promotes blood cleansing, the manganese content 0.28 mg plus copper 0.37 mg helps build blood cells. Strawberries with their good silicon content in combination with the sulphur content and the excellent vitamin C 57 mg, are a skin and beauty treatment and for the price of one facial, you can purchase about 20 punnets of the delightful red berries. Strawberries are full of antioxidants such as anthocyanins that give the bright red colour. They protect body cells by preventing oxygen damage. Strawberries are an anti-inflammatory due to the ability of the phenols such as anthocyanin and ellagitannins to reduce the activity of enzymes that cause inflammation.

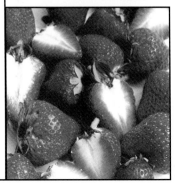

Strawberries also supply vitamin K, F, potassium 153 mg and folate 24 mcg. A regular intake of strawberries will do wonders for the skin and eyes plus strengthen and protect the immune system and help to make some of the millions of blood cells. Strawberries are ready for your next transfusion!

| TOMATO | *Lycopersicum esculentum* | GLYCEMIC INDEX: 38 | CALORIES - total: **18 kcal. per 100 gram** Calories from: Carb:14 Protein:2 Fat:2 |

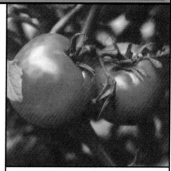

Tomatoes are an acid fruit and they provide citric acid 0.38 mg, malic acid and oxalic acid in small amounts. The tomato is the best food-source of natural chlorine 1,800 mg. Chlorine has numerous functions, it stimulates the liver to filter-out waste products, it stimulates the production of gastric juices for protein digestion and it assists weight reduction by maintaining correct fluid level retention of body cells and reduction of excess blood fat. Organic chlorine is a heat sensitive mineral and these benefits do not refer to cooked tomatoes but with a fresh tomato juice, the cleansing power is red hot.

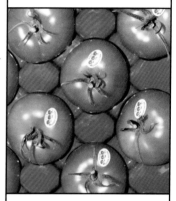

One major benefit obtained from both cooked and fresh tomatoes is the excellent supply of lycopene 2,570 mcg, a carotenoid, part of the vitamin A family. Lycopene has proven to be protective against breast cancer, prostrate and lung cancer, due to the antioxidant power and protection of white blood cells.

Tomatoes may also protect against stomach and colon cancer if taken on a regular basis. Tomatoes protect against sun damage, as lycopene is part of the skin adipose tissue protective structure. Tomatoes are a very good source of sulphur 500 mg, also an acid mineral, it assists the liver to secrete bile and has a cleansing and antiseptic effect on the digestive system, bloodstream and skin.

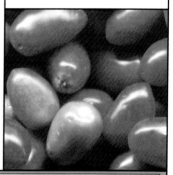

Sulphur is a heat sensitive nutrient. Other minerals also well supplied by the tomato are the heat sensitive potassium 244 mg and silicon 175 mg. The vitamin C 23 mg is fair and the very low calorie count (18) is ideal for weight watchers, plus the low glycemic index (38) makes it safe for nearly everybody. The raw tomato will provide all the benefits, the cooked tomato or sauce will provide the lycopene and that is a bonus for numerous cooked meals, pies and pasta sauces.

Tomatoes also provide a fair supply of vitamin K, 8 mcg, vitamin E, 1mg and a good supply of biotin 1.5 mcg. One tomato can supply nearly half the daily biotin requirement, vital for energy exertion and prevention from cramps in combination with the good potassium 237 mg content. A tomato a day can help you play, reduce, cleanse and protect from those nasty free radicals. The tomato is one of the easiest fruits to grow at home.

| WATERMELON | *Citrullus vulgaris* | GLYCEMIC INDEX: 72 | CALORIES - total: **30 kcal. per 100 gram** Calories from: Carb:27 Protein:2 Fat:1 |

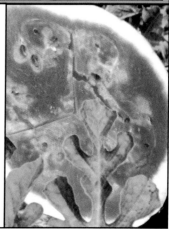

Watermelon are the greatest fruit in size and for summer satisfaction. Chill the big red melon pieces and serve just before the children ask for a fizzy drink. For women, melons are the ideal food for emotional balance due to the super supply of bromine, required by the pituitary gland to control the glandular system. In countries where melons are consumed regularly, depression and menopausal problems are uncommon. The melon can also help dad's through their mid life crisis and with the relaxing power of melons, even the children may slow down. Have a great summer holiday, but don't forget the melon. The G.I. is high but the carb. content is low. Watermelon will promote cleansing of the kidneys. It is low in most nutrients except vitamin A 590 1.U., especially lycopene 4,532 mcg nearly twice the amount of tomatoes. Melons are a great antioxidant, alkalinizer, balancer and relaxant.

FRUITS SUMMARY CHART

FRUITS	MAIN NUTRIENTS, ANTIOXIDANTS & PHYTONUTRIENTS	MAIN BODY SYSTEM
Apples	alkaline, pectin, malic acid, antioxidants, quercetin,	digestive
Apricots	beta carotene, potassium, lutein, zeaxanthin, silicon, molybdenum.	respiratory
Avocado	omega 3, lecithin, potassium, folate, phosphorus, magnesium,	circulatory
Banana	potassium, seratonin, norepinephrine, pectin, chlorine, sulphur.	muscular
Berries	lycopene, anthocyanins, phenolics, ellagic acid, vitamin c, vitamin p.	immune
Cantaloup	vitamin a, vitamin c, potassium, bromine, folate.	skin
Cherries	anthocyanins, isoqueritrin, queritrin, ellagic acid, perrillyl alcohol melatonin, vitamin a, potassium.	immune
Currants	vitamin c, anthocyanin, vitamin a, potassium,	immune
Dates	fibre, potassium, iron, magnesium, calcium, phosphorus, copper	muscular
Figs	calcium, potassium, fibre, iron, manganese, copper, magnesium phosphorus, silicon, chlorine, sulphur	blood
Grapefruit	liminoids, lycopene, salicyclic acid, vitamin c, biotin, b5,	joint
Grapes	manganese, saponin, trans-resveratrol, phenolic compounds,	blood
Guava	vitamin c, lutein, zeaxanthin,	immune
Kiwi fruit	vitamin c, vitamin a, copper, iron, potassium, phytponutrients.	respiratory
Lemon/Lime	citric acid, sulphur, vitamin c, antioxidants.	immune
Mango	beta carotene, chlorine, vitamin c, potassium.	respiratory
Melons	alkaline, bromine, vitamin c, potassium, vitamin a, enzymes.	glandular
Nectarine	potassium, beta cryptoxanthin, beta carotene, lutein, zeaxanthin.	respiratory
Olives	added sodium, calcium, potassium, iron, vitamin a, oleic acid.	nil.
Papaya	papain, carpain, chymopapain, vitamin c, beta cryptoxanthin, beta carotene, lutein, zeaxanthin,	immune repair, skin
Mandarin Oranges	vitamin p, vitamin c, citric acid, calcium, phosphorus, magnesium, phytonutrients, fibre,	immune respiratory
Peaches	beta carotene, beta cryptoxanthin, lutein, zeaxanthin, sulphur.	skin, elimination
Pears	fibre, copper, potassium, silicon, folate.	elimination
Pineapple	chlorine, sulphur, manganese, bromelain, vit. c, copper, selenium, zinc.	respiratory, blood
Plums	phytonutrients, phenols, vitamin a, copper, manganese, carotene.	immune, brain
Strawberries	vitamin p, vitamin c, iron, sulphur, copper, silicon, antioxidants, phenols, vitamin k, potassium, folate	circulatory, blood, skin, immune
Tomato	chlorine, lycopene, sulphur, potassium, silicon, vitamin c, biotin.	immune, skin
Watermelon	bromine, lycopene, vitamin c, vitamin a, alkaline.	glandular, urinary

FRUITS - BALANCED DIET - DAILY CARBOHYDRATE INTAKE

TOTAL DAILY (RDI) CARBOHYDRATE INTAKE	ADULT MALE	ADULT FEMALE	TEENAGER	CHILDREN
	340 grams	280 grams	400 grams	270 grams
FRUITS 15 % DAILY - LAUGH WITH HEALTH DIET	51 grams	42 grams	60 grams	40 grams
100 g FRESH FRUITS = 12 grams of carb.	400 grams	350 grams	330 grams	225 grams
100 g DRIED FRUITS = 65 grams of carb.	78 grams	64 grams	92 grams	61 grams
100 grams of fresh fruits is equivalent to any one of the following, approx.1 small apple, 3 apricots, 1 small banana, 1 cup of berries, or 12 dried dates, half grapefrut, 1 cup of grapes, 1 and half kiwifruit, half mango, 1 small orange, 1 peach, or 1 tomato.				
FRUIT JUICE 5% LAUGH WITH HEALTH DIET	17 grams	14 grams	20 grams	14 grams
100 g. FRUIT JUICE = 10 g. carbohydrate.	170 grams	140 grams	200 grams	140 grams
100 grams of fruit juice = half glass of fresh juice or 100 ml. approx.				
FOOD PYRAMID DAILY DIET GUIDE	3 serves	2 serves	3 serves	2 serves
AUSTRALIAN HEALTHY EATING GUIDE	2 serves	2 serves	3 serves	1 serve
1 serve is equivalent to: 1 medium piece of fruit: apple, banana, orange or pea, or 2 small pieces of fruit: apricot, kiwi fruit, plums (150 g) or 1 cup of diced canned fruit (150 g) or 4 dried apricots or half cup (125 ml.) fruit juice.				

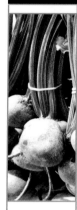

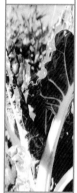

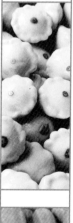

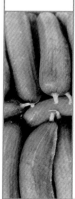

The vegetable kingdom provides incredible benefits, a full range of colours and an incredible variety of flavours, textures, shapes and sizes. Nutritionally speaking, we would be lost without vegetables, as a major portion of the essential minerals and vitamins are derived from especially fresh vegetables.

Fresh vegetables are a great provider of the heat sensitive nutrients that are required for body cleansing and numerous body system functions.

Throughout this vegetable section, the benefits of 25 vegetables are detailed and with this information you may be encouraged to reap their unique nutritional rewards.

Some vegetables need cooking, especially the starch vegetables: artichoke, parsnips, potatoes, sweet potatoes, pumpkin and turnips.

Cooking opens up the starch structure of foods and allows easier digestion of the concentrated plant starches and enables larger quantities of the food to be eaten, thereby giving longer lasting energy. Vegetables are very low in calories, compared to their almost zero fat content and on their own, they are not a fattening food. Some vegetables provide powerful protective action against free radicals and they are really essential in this era of fast fried foods, as they strengthen the immune system and counteract oxidisation.

Another nearly unique benefit from some vegetables is the supply of chlorophyll. Chlorophyll has a nearly identical structure to human blood. Chlorophyll is based on a magnesium atom, blood is based on an iron atom, apart from that, they are identical. Green leafy vegetables will help your blood system to regenerate.

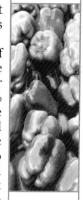

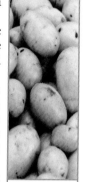

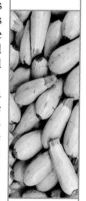

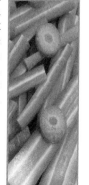

Green fresh vegetables are great blood builders, blood cleansers and body system activators.

Vegetables are a great source of organic mineral water, as the average vegetable contains over 70% water, the potato is 80% water, spinach and lettuce are 90% water. These days it is vital to obtain pure water plus organic mineral water from vegetables to supply the daily water and nutrient requirements, without the addition of *inorganic* chlorine and fluoride, as contained in some city water supplies.

Many vegetables provide organic chlorine and fluoride to provide protection against infection and tooth decay.

As the ideal daily diet requires 70% fresh foods, the garden salad is one simple way to gain the alkaline balance, plus, 75% of the daily diet needs to be from alkaline foods.

Most vegetables are alkaline but dairy, meat, fish, cheese and eggs are very acid forming. Vegetables can provide the healing balance to the diet as an alkaline blood balance promotes natural healing.

Vegetables may provide only a small amounts of complete protein but combined with grains or legumes, they help increase the protein value, plus they add a lot of flavour and colour to grain and legume meals.

Vegetables are meal-makers, even with the most basic common meals, a few vegetables are often on the plate, just to make it look nice but when eaten, they provide a valuable supply of nutrients that are lacking from the cooked animal product foods. The home vegie garden can supply an abundance of the essential basic vegetables.

Vegetables are now waiting for an invitation to your next lunch, evening meal or banquet!

NOTE: All amounts in this book are measured in milligrams (mg) per 100 grams, unless stated otherwise.

ARTICHOKE	Cynara Scolymus Helianthus Tuberosus	CALORIES - total: 20kcal. per 100 gram
		Calories from: Carb:38 Protein:8 Fat:8

There are two main types of artichoke, the Globe artichoke and the Jerusalem artichoke. They have varying nutritional values with the globe artichoke having 47 calories per 100 gram compared to 76 calories of the Jerusalem artichoke. The main common nutrient is potassium, the globe 370 mg, the Jerusalem 429 mg. The sodium content of globe artichokes is 94 mg, the Jerusalem supplies only 4 mg. They both supply approx. 77 mg of phosphorus, with the iron content of Jerusalem artichoke being very good with 3.4 mg, the globe only 1.6 mg. The vitamin A content of the globe is far better at 185 I.U. compared to 20 I.U. Artichokes have basically no protein and a very low fat content. Over 80 % of the calories are from the carbohydrate content and they are a good source of dietary fibre. One medium globe artichoke will provide over 20% daily dietary fibre, ideal for meals with chicken or meat.

Clinical trials with artichokes and their active ingredients cynaropicrin and cynarin showed patients experienced a reduction of cholesterol and low density lipids and an increase in the beneficial high density lipids. Arthichoke provide a stabilizing effect for the metabolism due to the supply of valuable oils. Artichokes are beneficial for the liver as they stimulate liver cell regeneration. They also assist reduction of water retention, oedema. The raw artichoke contains the enzyme inulase which assists conversion of the starch content. Artichoke have been used in cases of diabetes mellitus and may also benefit in cases of atherosclerosis. Artichokes are really worth the effort.

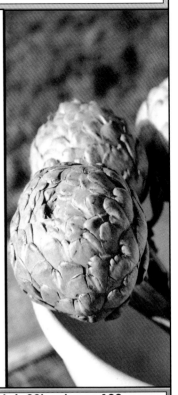

ASPARAGUS	Asparagus officinalis	CALORIES - total: 20kcal. per 100 gram
		Calories from: Carb:14 Protein:5 Fat:1

Asparagus is a member of the Lily family (Lilaceae) and has been recognized for centuries for it's distinctive flavour and therapeutic qualities. There are 3 main types: the green spears, blanched white (grown underground) and the French asparagus with a blue-violet colour and stronger flavour. The main benefit from asparagus is due to the alkaloid: *asparagine* which stimulates the cleansing of the kidneys and bladder. The strong smell once the urine passes is due to the alkaloid residue. Asparagus is a very good source of *silicon* 950 mg, healthy hair and the combination with the minerals sulphur 536 mg and chlorine 510 mg makes it ideal for skin cleansing, however, canned or overcooked asparagus may not do the trick. Blanch the stems only in boiling water for 2 minutes and 'dip the tips' in for a second, then serve for the full flavour and benefits. Both chlorine and sulphur are heat sensitive nutrients. Asparagus supply good amounts of natural fluoride for the eyesight and bromine- glandular system. Asparagus also contain glutathione, an anti-carcinogen and rutin to strengthen the blood vessels. For a 'land food' asparagus are a good source of iodine which promotes correct thyroid metabolism balance. Asparagus canned and fresh are a very good source of folate with 120 mcg, vital for the nerves and brain and during pregnancy. It also provides vitamin A, 900 I.U. plus isoleucine for the glands plus bromine for the glandular system. Asparagus may seem a luxury, but 'in season' grab a bunch and cleanse the urinary system and help balance the wonderful glandular system.

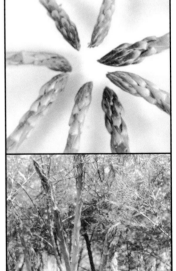

NOTE: d.v. refers to daily value for woman 25 - 50 years, refer to the RDI chart on page 69 for adult male and children RDI values.

BEETROOT *Beta vulgaris*

CALORIES - total: 42 kcal. per 100 gram
Calories from: Carb:37 **Protein:4** Fat:1

Beetroot has been considered a nutritional food since the early Roman and Greek times for reduction of fevers and for the blood. Even though the iron content is only fair at 0.91 mg, it is in a easily assimilated form due to the vitamin C plus the balance of the minerals manganese 0.34 mg and copper 0.007 mg.

The supply of organic sodium 72 mg and potassium 325 mg is one reason for the blood cleansing abilities of beetroot and in particular fresh beetroot juice.

The cleansing power of beetroot continues with the excellent supply of chlorine 295 mg, sulphur 50 mg, both are 'heat sensitive' so the canned beetroot may not be the way to go for body cleansing. Sulphur *cleanses the digestive system* and protects against infections. Chlorine purifies the blood, *the skin and glandular system.*

Beetroot should be obtained fresh and grated, or juiced for maximum benefits. A carrot 120 ml., beetroot 50 ml. and parsley juice 10 ml. is the tonic for women with menstruation or menopause problems. Try freshly grated beetroot with your next salad. Other recognized benefits of beetroot are cleansing the lymphatic system thereby also helping the immune system, *anti carcinogenic,* kidney cleansing, digestive aid and restoring health in people with general weakness, sexual weakness, prostate troubles and liver disorders. Canned beetrot does not contribute all these benefits. Let the bright, bold and raw beetroot be part of your health restoration program.

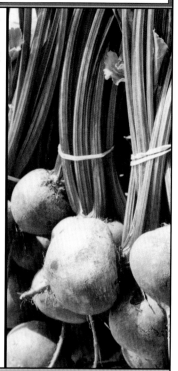

BROCCOLI *Brassica oleracea*

CALORIES - total: 34 kcal. per 100 gram
Calories from: Carb:24 **Protein:7** Fat:3

Broccoli is a good source of both vitamin A 1500 I.U. and vitamin C 94 mg. Vitamin C is heat sensitive. Prolonged cooking of broccoli is not advised, as it will 'stink-out' the kitchen, due to the loss of nutrients such as sulphur and reduce the benefits. To prepare the broccoli, place the stems only, in water and lightly steam the vegetable for two minutes, with the lid on. Add small heads of fresh broccoli in a fresh garden salad for maximum benefits. Broccoli is a good source of calcium 103 mg and phosphorus 78 mg, valuable for building and maintenance of strong bones. It also provides magnesium and vitamins: A and C; all work together to promote efficient metabolism of the minerals calcium and phosphorus. Broccoli also supplies good amounts of magnesium 24 mg and iron 1.1 mg. The iron content of broccoli is enhanced due to the addition of vitamin C. Research has shown that broccoli has anti cancer properties due to the abundance of nutrients: vitamin A & C, plus selenium 3 mg which has anticancer and antiviral properties.

Broccoli also contains *indole-3-carbinol* which the body converts into an *anti-androgen* that can inhibit the growth of prostrate cancer cells. Broccoli also contains a potent compound: *sulforaphane* which is able to destroy the 'helicobacter pylori' bacterium, the cause of most stomach ulcers and cancers. Common antibiotics do not destroy the bacteria. Broccoli is a very good source of chromium, protects against adult-onset diabetes as chromium boosts the activity of insulin in glucose intolerant people. Broccoli may also lower blood cholesterol due to the supply of *calcium pectate.*

Broccoli gives a beneficial anti bacterial boost.

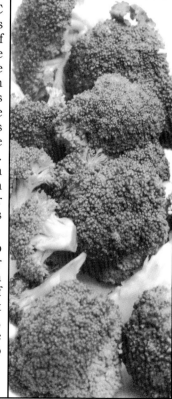

BRUSSELS SPROUTS *Brassica oleracea*

CALORIES - total: 43 kcal. per 100 gram
Calories from: Carb:32 Protein:8 Fat:3

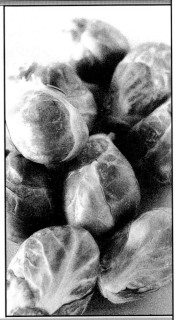

Brussels Sprouts are a very good source of the mineral sulphur and this has a cleansing and antiseptic effect on the digestive system, bloodstream and skin cells. Sulphur foods are essential for maintenance of healthy skin, nails and hair as they are a rich source of keratin, a protein substance that is also part of insulin. Brussels sprouts should not be boiled, as sulphur is heat sensitive. They can be lightly steamed or finely chopped and added to a fresh garden salad. The strong taste of raw Brussels sprouts is due to the high sulphur content. Sulphur foods also promote the digestion of protein foods. Brussels sprouts contain the nitrogen compounds termed indoles and this provides a cancer - inhibiting factor in combination with the vitamin C 85 mg and vitamin A 750 I.U. Brussels sprouts also provide selenium 2 mcg and a fair amount of potassium 386 mg, both help to protect against cancer. Brussels sprouts are also a good source of magnesium 23 mg, iron 1.3 mg and folate 61 mcg plus they provide a valuable amount of dietary fibre 4 grams with a low calorie value and a fair amount of vegetable protein. The 'small cabbage' was named after the capital of Belgium - Brussels. They also contain: *isothiocyanates* that can suppress the growth of tumours. Roll out the big brussels sprout benefits.

CABBAGE *Brassica oleracea*

CALORIES - total: 24 kcal. per 100 gram
Calories from: Carb:19 Protein:4 Fat:1

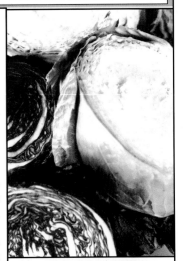

Cabbages are an excellent source of the two 'cleansing minerals': chlorine 1,045 mg and sulphur 1,710 mg. Both work as a team in expelling waste matter, cleansing of the blood and they also tend to reduce excess weight. A deficiency of chlorine foods can lead to poor liver function and various types of congestion such as sinusitis. Regular use of fresh cabbage as with coleslaw or finely chopped cabbage added to a salad will also be most beneficial for protection from the common cold and viruses. Try the taste of home made cabbage rolls and rice on a winter's night. The more the cabbage is cooked: the chlorine and sulphur benefits disperse.

There are numerous varieties of cabbage: the common, Chinese, red and savoy are the main types with the common cabbage supplying the best chlorine and sulphur content. If only for the supply of these two nutrients, cabbage would be an excellent food, but there's more!

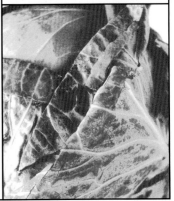

Cabbages are a good source of chlorophyll, the green magic medicine and a unique source of vitamin U. It has proved to provide healing of peptic ulcers. It is likely that the sulphur content also helps, as *sulforaphane* destroys the *helicobacter pylori* bacterium that causes the stomach ulcers.

Medicinal tonic doses of raw cabbage juice in thirteen ulcer patients, over 10 days, provided a 100% success rate, but to avoid such discomfort and bitter taste, enjoy the flavour of coleslaw regularly.

Cabbage is the main ingredient in *sauerkraut*, a product of German ingenuity. Sauerkraut is formed from fermented cabbage leaves and supplies an abundance of vital enzyme elements.

Cabbage is a good source of bromine for glandular functioning, vital during menopause plus cabbage is very low in calories and it has a very low fat content. Add the fancy dressing and hoe into it!

Carrots were used by the Greeks and Romans as medicine and they are now the most widely cultivated vegetable. The numerous varieties and colours include the white, purple, red, yellow and the 'king of carotene' the orange carrot. There are two main types of carotene both available in carrots, beta carotene 5,774 mcg and alpha carotene 2,817 mcg. There are two types of vitamin A: preformed-vitamin A (retinol) obtained from animal origin, provitamin-A (carotene) from plant origin.

Carrots are the best vegetable source of carotene which the body converts into vitamin A. Diabetics may be unable to convert carotene into vitamin A. Intake of retinol from animal origin: (cod liver oil) may be essential, especially in times of illness.

Carotene has unique protective and healing abilities, alpha carotene may be more powerful than beta carotene to inhibit tumour growths, one study showed it to be ten times more potent. Most research has been on beta carotene with benefits in the treatment of lung and pancreatic cancer. Supplements of beta carotene are not advised, it is best to obtain the natural balance from carrots with alpha and beta carotene plus active enzymes. Cooked carrots provide more useable carotene than raw carrots, apart from carrot juice, as cooking and juicing open-up the carotene starch structure.

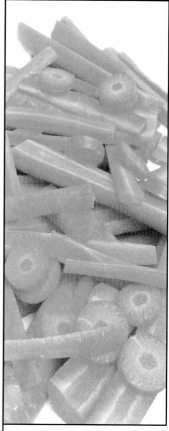

Carrots provide so much carotene, eating raw carrots will still supply ample carotene plus the benefit of numerous heat sensitive nutrients, also available in fresh carrot juice. In summary, the benefits from the exceptionally rich supply of carotene and natural phytochemicals are: boosts the immune system, improves eyesight, heals wounds, reduces high blood pressure, cleanses the liver, improves skin condition, reduces acne, reduces mucous, prevents jaundice, promotes skin protection from sunshine, protects against ulcers and generally prevents the development and reduces the duration of infections, viruses and colds.

The sulphur content 445 mg of carrots and the chlorine content 318 mg are the main reason for the remarkable liver cleansing abilities of fresh carrot juice. Cooking increases the carotene value but greatly decreases the sulphur and chlorine and potassium 341 mg content. Skin cleansing is easy with fresh carrot juice plus the supply of silicon 166 mg all promote a good complexion. The question of 'excess carrot juice', does it cause orange skin, does excess beetroot cause red skin, no, it is the elimination of toxins from the liver that can cause skin to discolour, or the inability of the body to process carotene properly. Excess of any food is a problem, limit your carrot juice intake to no more than 3 times a week, with quantities: children 120 ml. adults: 240 ml. Vitamin A (carotene) is a fat soluble vitamin, so it is not required everyday. If you need exceptional healing, have a wheatgrass juice on the other days, or mix carrot with beetroot or celery juice. Cooked carrots provide a vital balance to the meat meals, don't leave them off the plate.

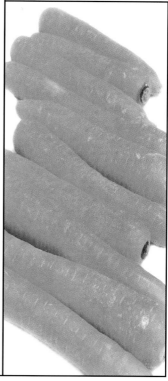

Carrots are a great food for children as carrots are the sweetest vegetable, or try honey carrots or mashed carrots for babies and for nursing mum's, carrot juice promotes lactation. Carrots provide iron 0.5 mg, copper 0.05 mg, manganese 0.15 mg, plus selenium, a natural antioxidant in combination with the abundant supply of alpha and beta carotene.

Carrots are 'the root of all natural healing power!'

CAPSICUM *Capsicum annum*

CALORIES - total: **20kcal. per 100 gram**
Calories from: Carb:37 Protein:4 Fat:1

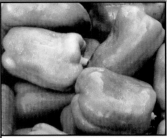

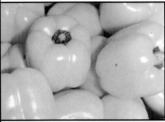

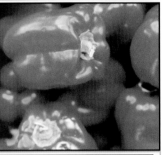

Capsicums are also known as the bell pepper or the sweet pepper. They are the best vegetable sources of precious vitamin C. The red capsicum supplies 204 mg, the green capsicum 128 mg of vitamin C. The benefits of obtaining natural vitamin C in contrast to the tablet cannot be over stated. The action of vitamin C is *dependant on a supply of bio-flavonoids,* they are contained in the white part of the associated fruit or vegetable. A vitamin C tablet may supply no bio-flavonoids and therefore the action of vitamin C is greatly retarded. The natural form of vitamin C will also supply an abundance of enzymes that will promote the numerous functions of vitamin C. The tablet is the expensive way to get what only nature can provide in correct balance for human nutrition. Remember to buy a couple of capsicums every week and prevent numerous health problems. Cooked capsicum will contain less benefits as vitamic C is heat sensitive.

Capsicums are an excellent source of vitamin P or bioflavonoids. A deficiency of vitamin P can lead to: varicose veins, arteriosclerosis, arthritis and rheumatism. Vitamin P is vital for increasing the strength of the capillaries and thereby preventing such ailments as varicose veins. Capsicums are also a very good source of vitamin A: red 4,450 I.U., green 420 I.U. Capsicum will add colour to your salads, red, orange, yellow and green slices of vitamins: 'C,A,P', children enjoy the variety of colours and a 'crisp cool capsicum' is one way to provide benefits without the 'citrus acid tang' that some children and adults cannot tolerate.

Capsicum supply low amounts of minerals, they really are a 'huge vitamin C, A, P tablet'.

CAULIFLOWER *Brassica oleracea*

CALORIES - total: **25kcal. per 100 gram**
Calories from: Carb:19 Protein:5 Fat:1

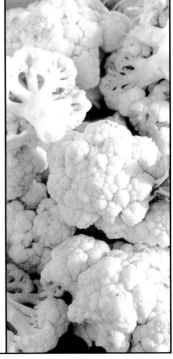

Cauliflower is the pure white vegetable and apart from the excellent supply of sulphur 1,186 mg and organic chlorine 310 mg from fresh produce, the only other nutrient benefits are vitamin C 78 mg and potassium 206 mg. If you can handle the taste of fresh cauliflower 'flowerets' in a salad, you will gain maximum cleansing benefits from cauliflower. Sulphur reduces body toxins, prevents the development of infections, cleanses the digestive system and protects against stomach ulcers. The combination of sulphur and the silicon content 337 mg gives cauliflower the power to promote hair growth, improve skin condition, promote blood haemoglobin development, plus, improve blood circulation and protect against the formation of arthritic conditions. Cooked cauliflower is common and to ensure a reasonable supply of sulphur and chlorine, lightly steam the 'head' with the stalk immersed in simmering water for 5 minutes. Cauliflower '*au gratin*'- with cheese is very common and popular. Place the steamed cauliflower heads in a baking dish, sprinkle with grated parmesan and cheddar, bake for 10 minutes - hot oven. Serve with dark coloured foods: mushrooms, spinach, carrots but avoid combining with rice, pumpkin or potatoes, too much starch, too little colour, too little flavour. Let the 'power of the cauliflower' loose once in a while and with the cheese topping, it's big in calcium and protein, ideal for growing children. Cauliflower also supply vitamins: K, C, A, folate and biotin.

Celery has a long history of therapeutic benefits and with more research, the benefits increase. In ancient Rome, celery was used to offset a possible hangover. The Greeks found it beneficial for conditions of gall stones, liver problems and constipation. During the 17th. century, Italian gardeners converted celery from a very bitter food plant to a variety which is now mass produced, blanched by covering the stems to further decrease the bitterness.

The two main active ingredients in celery that provide the unique taste and smell are: sedanolide and 3-n-butyl phthalide and they are responsible for the anti tumour qualities and cholesterol lowering properties of celery. In addition pthalides have the power to relax the muscles that line the blood vessels and thereby can decrease blood pressure. Pthalides lower the production of the hormone catacholamines, decreasing nervous stress.

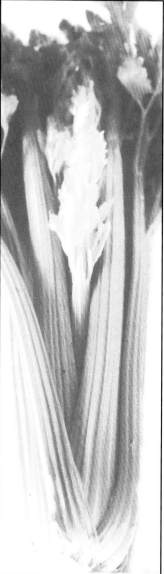

Celery is also a very good source of vitamin A in the form of beta carotene 324 mg and the relatively unknown lutein and zeaxanthin 340 mcg, members of the carotenoid family. This combination gives celery the status of being a good food for the eyes, as 'l & z' are naturally present in the human eye, to protect against phototoxic blue light and ultra violet radiation. Both 'l & z' are the only carotenoids found in the lens of the eyes and they also protect against age-related increases in lens density and cataract formation. It's nearly common knowledge now that celery is the richest vegetable source of organic sodium 96 mg -126 mg and the main benefit is that organic sodium keeps calcium soluble within the bloodstream and body cells, in fact every cell in the body is covered by a solution of saline water. Commercial salt is not completely water soluble, celery sodium is totally soluble. Refined foods, white bread in particular contain inorganic calcium elements that can accumulate, over years, leading to arthritis or the depositing of calcium around bones and moveable body joints.

Celery has the power to re-balance the problem, catch it in time, before you get stuck. Celery promotes normal blood pressure, prevents hardened arteries, oedema and it can naturally thin the blood, before that blood clot develops.

Celery also provides protection from cancer due to the ingredient acetylenic, which has been shown to stop the growth of cancer cells. In addition, the phenolic acids contained in celery block the action of the prostoglandin hormones which encourage the growth of cancerous tumours. Celery reduces the inflammatory prostoglandins that contribute to the pain of arthritis and rheumatism. Celery is a diuretic. Celery promotes virility.

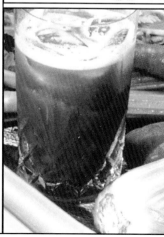

Celery eaten raw, or for maximum benefits, the fresh juice is abundant in benefits and especially during those hot summer days, celery juice will replace the lost sodium salts, protecting against cramps. Celery soup in winter can provide many of the above benefits as the nutrients in celery are mainly not heat sensitive.

Celery is a good food for diabetics as it stimulates the pancreas glands: (I. of L.) to produce insulin and carbohydrate digestion.

Celery is the weight watchers dream food, with only 17 calories per 100 gram, eat a whole bunch and fill up but not out!

Celery provides excellent amounts of chlorine 1, 780, sulphur 650 mg, silicon 430 mg and bromine 17 mg.

Celery is tops in human nutrition.

CUCUMBER *Cucumis sativus*

CALORIES - total: **15kcal. per 100 gram**
Calories from: Carb:12 Protein:2 Fat:1

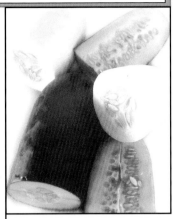

Cucumbers are a silicon food with 800 mg, very few foods contain the mineral silicon however it is a major nutrient, often forgotten in general human health but with the increasing cases of osteoporosis and osteoarthritis, silicon may eventually be recognized for it's vital role in the proper construction of bones. Cucumber supplies 16 times more silicon than wheat or wheat bran. There's a lot to be said about the 'cucumber sandwich', it will certainly provide the strength to the bones plus promote the hair growth, as hair is primarily made of silicon. Lettuce provides the ultimate silicon supply. There is no recommended dietary intake for silicon, but you can be assured it is required.

Cucumber is full of organic water (95 %), ideal for those hot days, if you peel the cucumber, most of the silicon disappears but the sulphur 690 mg and chlorine 660 mg remain. Sulphur and silicon both promote a healthy skin condition, the cucumber facial is not just for fun, it does provide the cool and beneficial qualities, both taken internally or externally.

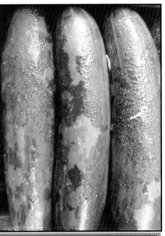

Natural chlorine in cucumber promotes rejuvenation of skin tissues and cleansing of the blood, plus chlorine promotes digestion of fats and proteins. The cucumber and yoghurt entree will be an ideal choice before the main restaurant meal.

Cucumber also contain the enzyme erepsin which is required to convert peptides into amino acids. Cucumber is an excellent diuretic and it helps to prevent kidney stone development, high blood pressure and rheumatism.

Cucumber can reduce excess uric acid in the blood, often a direct result from excess meat and chocolate consumption. Cucumbers are a good source of fibre and the seeds provide numerous nutrients such as vitamin E. Keep cool, clean and content with the cucumber qualities!

EGGPLANT *Allium sativ*

CALORIES - total: **24kcal. per 100 gram**
Calories from: Carb:20 Protein:2 Fat:2

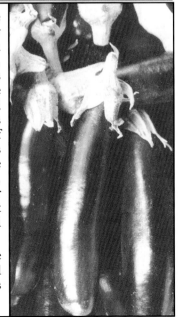

Eggplants are also called aubergine. The common colour is purple but a white eggplant is also available. The eggplant provides very little flavour on it's own so it requires French cooking or Italian ingenuity or Turkish talent to make it a delight. Herbs, lemon juice, butter and a sprinkle of cheese usually do the trick and it looks appetising, or olive oil, garlic, tomatoes and black pepper. The nutritional value of eggplant is fairly basic apart from the good chlorine 670 mg and sulphur 445 mg content. Chlorine stimulates protein digestion in the stomach. Chlorine cleanses the body of excess fats and that may be essential when the extra cheese is added on top of the eggplant. The sulphur content will promote carbohydrate digestion and cleansing of the digestive system. Eggplant will provide 3 grams of dietary fibre per 100 gram, better than none, or approx. 14% of total dietary fibre, chicken and meat supplies none. If you have never cooked eggplant before, get a good recipe, or watch your neighbour, that's the best way to begin.

Eggplants do provide the valuable phytosterols 7 mg, to boost the immune system. Eggplants soak up the oils so use a cold pressed flax or walnut oil for a big dose of the essential Omega 3. Eggplants are ready to oblige!

LEEK *Allium ampeloprasum*	CALORIES - total: **61kcal. per 100 gram**
	Calories from: Carb:54 Protein:4 Fat:3

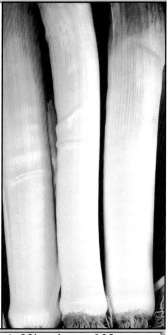

Leeks are the straight member of the onion family and the ideal winter onion with cream of leek soup and don't worry, the leek is powerful enough to offset the additional fats in cream. Leeks supply *cycloallin* which has the ability to dissolve blood clots that form on the inside of blood vessels, even cooking does not affect this special ingredient. Cycloallin also helps to dissolve fibrin from inflamed moveable joints. The carotene content 1,667 I.U. of leeks is excellent with beta carotene 1,000 mcg and lutein and zeaxanthin 1,900 mg all promote healthy eyesight and protection against some forms of cancer. Leeks contain a natural antiseptic quality due to the sulphur content and supply of allyl disulphate and cycloallin. Common onions do not supply the carotene, lutein and zeaxanthin, the leek is the unique 'onion' source and must therefore be considered most valuable. Leeks also supply good amounts of sulphur compounds which promote the secretion of bile, thereby assisting digestion of fats, 'no need to worry about the cream'. Insulin is a sulphur compound and leek are a safe foods for most diabetics. Leeks provide a fair source of organic iron 2 mg and copper, plus a fair source of folate, vitamin B6 and vitamin K.

Leeks are the sweet onion and apart from a cream soup, leeks can be added to any salad or quiche with no worries about clots.

MUSHROOMS *Agaricus campestris*	CALORIES - total: **22kcal. per 100 gram**
	Calories from: Carb:11 Protein:8 Fat:3

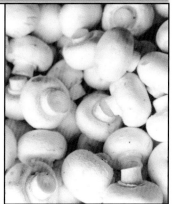

Mushrooms are in a world of their own, in the dark and full of unique nutritional benefits. The varieties are extraordinary and some are poisonous, so be sure you obtain a reputable supply. Such varieties as the Swiss brown, button, cup, flat, porcini or cap mushroom and truffles, the maitake, the shiitake, reishi and the common white, brown mushrooms have varied benefits. The Maitake mushroom contains adaptogen which helps the body adapt to stress and promote normal metabolism. It also contain polysaccharides that inhibit the growth of cancerous cells, destroy HIV and promote the activity of the T-helper cells in the immune system. They may assist in cases of hepatitis, high blood pressure and chronic fatigue syndrome. The Shiitake mushroom contains the polysaccharide - lentinan which strengthens the T cell formation of the immune system. The Reishi and Shiitake mushroom have anti tumour properties and may assist in the treatment of some cancers. In Japan the Shiitake mushroom extract is licensed as an anti cancer drug.

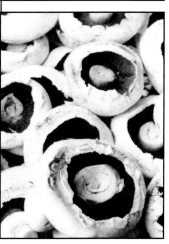

Generally speaking, mushrooms are termed probiotic, they strengthen the immune system, balance the body and provide natural resistance to disease. They contain host defence potentiators (HDP) which enhance the immune system. They also provide antiviral, analgesic, antioxidant and anti inflammatory benefits. Mushrooms are a good source of potassium 400 mg average, for healing and improved blood circulation. They contain no vitamin A, very little calcium and iron but supply fair amounts of phosphorus for the nerves and brain. Mushrooms are low in calories and supply a little 'complete protein'. Mushrooms absorb a lot of oil when fried so take it easy. Fresh mushrooms contain 90% water and are a good source of the amino acid lysine.

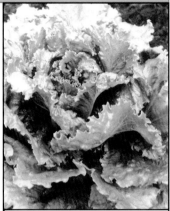

Lettuce are the lucky vegetable as they rarely get cooked and thereby they can provide an abundance of essential human nutrients. The varieties of lettuce are growing in popularity, including the iceberg, cos or Romaine, butterhead, Boston, mignonette and Great Lakes to mention a few. Generally speaking they all supply the same dominant nutrients.

The supply of chlorophyll from the green lettuce leaves provides an excellent source of healing benefits, refer to page 112. Lettuce may be the only source of living chlorophyll for some people and the simple salad sandwich, with lots of green lettuce leaves is a bonus for the blood, brain and nervous system. In addition the very good supply of vitamin K 24 - 125 mcg is essential for blood coagulation. Such factors as aspirin, x rays and radiation all deplete vitamin K from the human body, plus, frozen foods supply no vitamin K. Let the lettuce keep your blood in active defence mode, just in case!

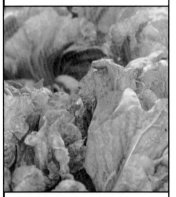

Another major benefit from lettuce is the excellent supply of the mineral silicon 500 - 2,400 mg. The iceberg lettuce is the richest source and the same goes for the supply of vitamin A 1,900 I.U. Both of these nutrients are vital for healthy skin condition and rejuvenation. Silicon is vital for skin repair and in particular for hair growth and in combination with the chlorophyll content, lettuce is possibly the only food that can positively restore hair loss. Ideally a tonic serve 120 ml. from lettuce juice mixed with carrot 50 ml., taken 3 times a week will give the body the essential elements required to 'make hair'. Meat, bread, fish and processed foods provide no silicon or chlorophyll. Keep ahead of things especially if you are likely, 'hereditary speaking' to go thin on top. A regular serve of fresh lettuce will feed the hair but the juice will absorb easier, provide greater quantity and quality.

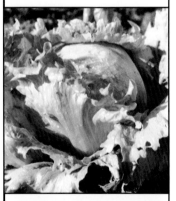

Lettuce also provide a good serve of folate 30 - 130 mcg, required for reproduction of red blood cells in the bone marrow, brain function and for a healthy nervous system. A prolonged deficiency of folate may trigger the onset of leukaemia, especially in children as they grow so fast, they need ample folate to manufacture blood cells. Remember the old saying 'if ya don't eat ya greens, your not getting any sweets'! Somehow or somewhere we need to get folate and if 'ya don't like ya greens, eat ya yellows', sweet corn is a good source for fussy children.

During pregnancy, ample folate 400 mcg is required per day for the development of the foetus. Green vegetables are a vital source of folate. The supply of chlorine 500 - 1,380 mg and sulphur 580 - 680 mg is really top quality as these are heat sensitive, but lucky for lettuce, the benefits are fully available such as purifying the blood, cleansing the body of toxins, prevention of infections plus many more. Sulphur contains keratin, a major component of hair follicles in addition to silicon. Lettuce is really ahead of the rest.

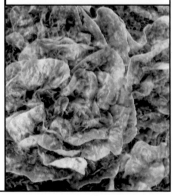

Lettuce is a fair source of organic iron .5 - 2 mg, plus trace amounts of copper 0.03 mg, manganese 0.6 mg, and vitamin C 6 - 24 mg, all required in combination for blood development. The potassium supply 247 mg exceeds the sodium supply 8 mg, vital in these days of excess salt in foods and drinks. Lettuce provides beta carotene 3,484 mcg and lutein and zeaxanthin 2,312 mcg, for protection from cancer and optic deterioration. Next time you think about lunch, crunch into a fresh 'salad!"

Onions, onions, onions! There are over 300 varieties, the common brown, red and white plus shallots and leeks, all provide similar benefits. As onions are not eaten in large quantities plus they are fairly low in the supply of the main nutrients: calcium 22 mg, iron 0.5 mg and phosphorus 27 mg, what makes onions so great! The flavour is the major benefit in cooking and as you may know you can nearly fry an onion without added oils. Onions contain natural antiseptic oils such as allyl disulphate and cycloallin. Research showed that cycloallin had the unique ability to dissolve blood clots which can form on the inside of blood vessels and in particular, the veins. The process is termed fibrinolysis and it was found that onions have this ingredient, cooked or raw. Another study suggested that cycloallin may also dissolve the fibrin formed around damaged joints or inflamed joints as with arthritis.

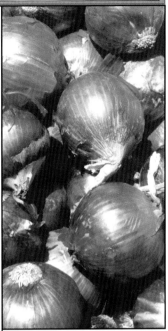

Other research has exposed the substance quercetin which is well supplied by onions, to have numerous beneficial properties. Quercetin is a water-soluble pigment, a flavonoid. It provides antihistamine and anti-inflammatory qualities. It is also classed as a phytoestrogen and was shown to inhibit breast cancer cells in test tube research. Quercetin is a potent antioxidant, protecting against heart disease. It is also valuable for diabetics as quercetin inhibits the enzyme that causes accumulation of a substance sorbitol, a cause in the deterioration of the eyes, kidneys and nerves in diabetics. Onions provide a very low glycemic index and are therefore safe and ideal for most diabetics to include with cooking. Onions also supply a fair amount of potassium 144 mg but really it is the trace substances plus the sulphur oil content that gives onion it's mighty power, not only to keep friends at a distance, but those nasty internal neighbours! Onions are also recognized to protect and relieve prostatis, reduce blood sugar, blood pressure, reduce sinusitis, colds and infections. Onion oil is often used for treatment of ear aches and catarrh.

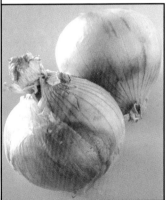

Onions also promote beneficial bacteria in the lower intestine and cleansing of the respiratory system. Onions are great but beware of the added fats, especially with the barbecue and those sausages, add heaps of onion but 'hold your horses' on all that saturated fat and cholesterol. A baked or roasted onion is really ideal and full of mild flavour. Onions will provide internal cleansing. Also try onion bread, french onion soup and if you haven't got an onion in the kitchen, it's a failure, so many recipes need it, the quiche, the pizza, the garden salad with the sweeter red onion. Chives are a great kitchen companion, you can grow them on the 21st. floor or higher and they add a charm to numerous snacks and entrees. If you have a problem with onion breath, chew some fresh parsley or mint and restore your confidence. The trace mineral molybdenum is supplied by onions, required for fat metabolism. Onions also provide trace amounts of selenium 6 mcg an antioxidant, folate 19 mcg and vitamin C 8 mg.

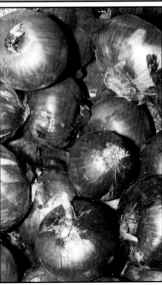

Onions provide very little vitamin A 40 I.U., and fibre 0.6 g. Last but not least, onions provide fructans as part of their carbohydrate structure. Fructan increases bifidobacteria and decrease detrimental bacteria in the intestines, reduce toxins, prevent constipation, reduce cholesterol and blood pressure.

Peel an onion for unique and unreal benefits!

PARSNIPS *Pastinaca sativa*

GLYCEMIC INDEX: 90

CALORIES - total: **75 kcal. per 100 gram**
Calories from: Carb:69 Protein:3 Fat:3

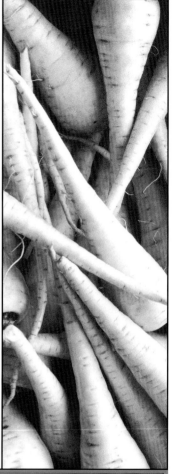

Parsnips are the essential ingredient in pasties, but very few commercial pasties contain this distinctive flavoured starch vegetable. The parsnip is one of the underestimated vegetables, it may seem pale in appearance but it can 'pack a punch' nutritionally speaking. The potassium content 541 mg of parsnips exceeds the banana 370 mg and potato 407 mg. Potassium is the foundation mineral of all muscular tissues. In addition, potassium and phosphorus 77 mg combined are vital for the transportation of oxygen into the brain. Be smart, don't forget the parsnip next shopping trip. The only problem is that potassium is fairly heat sensitive, over 30% can be destroyed by excess cooking, therefore you are 'back to bananas' for pure potassium power.

The mineral silicon 800 mg is not heat sensitive and parsnips are nearly second highest to lettuce in this essential mineral for the skin and hair, plus, if you have a problem with brittle nails, let the parsnip in before you get all cracked up. Parsnips are a rich source of organic chlorine 1,040 mg, twice that of lettuce and nearly 1,000 times that of meat, grains and cheese. The cause of numerous common ailments, especially of the respiratory and glandular system is a lack of body cleansing. Chlorine and sulphur 960 mg are both abundant in parsnips, part of the reason for their 'unique flavour'. Give your body a chance to do some spring cleaning, hoe into them in spring. The high glycemic index of parsnips (90 G.I.) is to be considered when serving them, you can roast or bake them but serve with a cream sauce, or mash them with milk and butter, or, with pasties, add a cream sauce, onions and maybe mushrooms. The rich supply of 'cleansing nutrients' can offset the added fats, as chlorine rids the body of excess fats, assists the liver and cleanses the blood. Sulphur has a cleansing and antiseptic effect on the digestive system and it also promotes fat metabolism.

Here's the last tip, don't forget the parsnip!

PEPPERS *Capsicum annuum / frutescens*

CALORIES - total: **43 kcal. per 100 gram**
Calories from: Carb:29 Protein:5 Fat:9

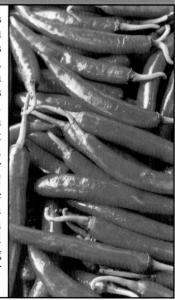

Chilli Peppers are small, bright and potent. They range in colours from green, yellow, cream, purple and red with no telling, until you try, how hot? As chilli peppers are only taken in minute amounts compared to other foods, the nutritional value is minimal, however, the benefits from the supply of nutrients is remarkable. The vitamin A content of red fresh sweet chillies 4,450 I.U., hot red chillies 21,600 I.U., hot fresh green 770 I.U., sweet green 420 I.U.; approx. half of the vitamin A is in the form of betacarotene the balance in the form of lutein and zeaxanthin. The rich supply of vitamin C hot red 369 mg, hot green 235 mg, in addition to the carotene, l & z, makes chilli a great food for the eyes, taken internally. Keep your hands away from your eyes when preparing peppers, it's bad news! Both the vitamin A and C are the main nutritional benefits, the pepper is very low in most minerals except potassium 300 mg on average. The two main special substances, so far discovered, in peppers are capsaicin and resiniferatoxin, they both proved effective, in research, to kill a majority of skin cancer cells, causing them to self destruct due to oxygen starvation. A little chilli pepper goes a long way to heat up a dish, can you handle it!

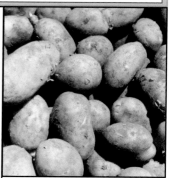

Potatoes are the greatest 'down to earth food', apart from the nutrients, they seem to put you back in place, especially after a juice fast or a hectic day in the high rise office. In context, this refers only to the full potato, not the pretty packet chips found in every store around town. The oversupply and consumption of packet chips and take - away fries needs to be mentioned first, as they are a detrimental food. They provide no health benefit, plus, they rob the pockets of parents and children plus it robs the body of the 'chance' to eat proper food. Apart from those problems, the 'free radicals', in the cooking oil, with fried chips is a major factor in the development of cancer and the added salt also contributes to heart disease. Chips and french fries supply 500 calories compared to baked potatoes, no oil, 1 calorie, that's a huge difference. The reason why they are popular is the fat content, plus additives, it tastes good, provides quick, crunchy energy and is a 'cheap as chips' when dad buys them. Children like the energy, but get ahead of them, before the next store and hand out some honey cashews or a sesame bar and get real food value.

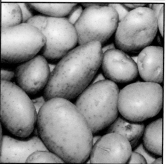

Back to the original topic, potatoes are a fair carbohydrate food 17 grams and depending on their preparation, they can be good or bad. The fact that baked potatoes have a very high glycemic index of (93 G.I), on their own, is cause for concern. The way to decrease this problem is to serve baked potatoes with mushrooms, onions, broccoli, cabbage and a dab of butter, sour cream or a cheese sauce. As meat supplies no carbohydrate content and potatoes supply a fair deal, plus the other vegetables, it is ok to have a serve of lean meat and vegies with the baked potatoes. To lower the G.I of potatoes also try mashed potatoes but they are still moderately high so it is best to add the vegies mentioned, for a balanced meal and G.I. level. Potatoes absorb fat, so it's best to have the chips or wedges as big as possible and to use the oil only once. Use safflower, sunflower or olive oil for frying, to reduce the free radical problem. The thin french fries absorb the most oil and have a 75 G.I., potato chips have a moderate 54 G.I. due to the abundance of oil. Potatoes supply low amounts of complete protein but it adds up considerably when fish or cheese is added to make a fulfilling meal. The fish and chip meal is ideal on holidays, as long as the children eat a good serve of fish, before filling up on fizzy and chips.

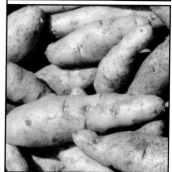

The potato has very few nutrient benefits apart from a good supply of potassium 400 - 500 mg, fair amounts of sulphur 289 mg, chlorine 155 mg, silicon 88 mg, phosphorus 53 mg, iron 0.06 mg. and that's all folks, but it was enough to keep a generation of people from starving in the early nineteenth century, in Ireland. The numerous varieties of potatoes are worth discovering for their unique variations in flavour and texture and use in specific recipes. From all over the world, the potato is used in local recipes, it's the food of nations. It supplies a little of this, a little of that and great quantities can be consumed to provide a storehouse of energy. In Ireland, an average 3.5 kilos a day were eaten 'alone' for years! Potatoes supply no vitamin A, so if you can find a carrot, we'll all be better off. A small amount of vitamin C 10-20 mg so add a slice of capsicum and not many B vitamins, so add a yeast extract gravy and you're nearly home. Enjoy the 'apple of the earth!'

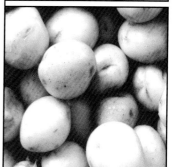

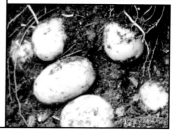

PUMPKINS *Cucurbitaceae*

GLYCEMIC INDEX: 75	CALORIES - total: **26 kcal. per 100 gram**
	Calories from: Carb:23 Protein:2 Fat:1

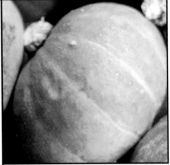

Pumpkins are related to the melon and marrow family, the Cucurbitacea, all of which seem to spread themselves out throughout home gardens and entire paddocks. For full flavour, the pumpkin flesh needs to be a bright orange and this also indicates a maximum supply of vitamin A - carotenoids 1,600 - 7,000 I.U. Over 50% of the carotene is in the form of beta carotene 3,100 mcg with beta cryptoxanthin a close second at 2,145 mcg and third, lutein and zeaxanthin 1,500 mcg.

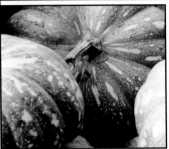

Pumpkins are the ultimate food source of beta cryptoxanthin, and research has shown a direct benefit to the respiratory system, in particular, the lungs. A decreased lung cancer risk and for smokers, a decreased blood serum level of beta-cryptoxanthin was found, plus for the 'passive smoker', the same result. Generally speaking, carotenoids are of vital value for the respiratory system, the lungs and the well known antioxidant properties of beta carotene, as mentioned with carrots, however, carrots only supply 78 mcg of beta cryptoxanthin and most vegetables contain none, a few tropical fruits supply moderate amounts.

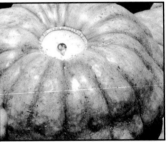

Pumpkin can be considered the 'king of cryptoxanthin' and if you know a smoker, or work in a smoky place let them know that the 'king' is inviting all of you to dinner, what a nice gesture! Pumpkin scones for afternoon tea, in the royal gardens, pumpkin soup entree, pumpkin pie for the royal gala dinner and for dessert, you guessed it, pumpkin meringue in the library with the Queen and Earl Grey. Back to business, the addition of cream with the soup or scones, or butter with the pie will improve the absorption of the beta cryptoxanthin, as with all carotenoids, they are fat soluble vitamins and the addition of dietary fat increases their absorption via the digestive tract.

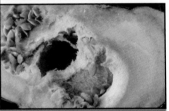

Pumpkins are low in calcium 21 mg and nearly all minerals except potassium 340 mg, silicon, iron 1mg and chlorine. Pumpkins are a great food for the eyes, skin, hair and through winter they will provide plenty of energy with a moderately high G.I. (75) but with a dab of butter in the mash, or cream soup, it's smoother on the sugar levels. Unfortunately, the smoking habit has spread the world, the 'king' is also ready to overtake the world to provide some golden royal health benefits but remember, get in before midnight!

Radishes take little room in this book and that's all they need on your plate, or pre-dinner salad appetiser. They are a great promoter of digestive juices, as they are a very good source of organic chlorine 1,000 mg, ideal for stimulating the supply of protein digestive enzymes in the stomach: *pepsinogen*. Chlorine is heat sensitive, it is great for reducing mucous and in addition, radishes supply a volatile ether oil that increases mucous elimination and has proved beneficial in cases of tuberculosis, coughs and bronchitis. Radishes also supply sulphur 715 mg, ideal for people with weak bile secretion, to assist fat digestion. The strong taste is due to the chlorine and sulphur. Don't be scared of the radish, it is not as powerful as 'big brother', the horseradish, over twice the power!

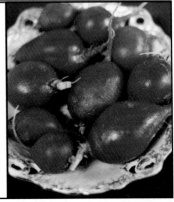

SPINACH *Spinacea oleracea*	GLYCEMIC INDEX:<20	CALORIES - total: **23 kcal. per 100 gram**
		Calories from: Carb:13 Protein:7 Fat:3

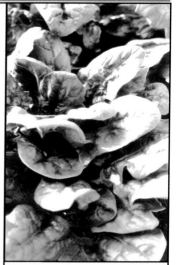

Spinach always gets a mention in health books but what about *silverbeet* (Beta vulgaris), also known as *seakale beet,* or *Swiss chard*, they are distant cousins, same with *New Zealand spinach* (Tetragonia expansa) and then there's *spinach beet* a close cousin to silverbeet, it has green stalks compared to the white stalks of silverbeet.

'Get off the garden', back to the house, in the kitchen and they all provide a valuable supply of chlorophyll, when eaten raw and 'true spinach' - spinacea oleracea is the easiest to eat raw.

They all supply fair amounts of oxalic acid 0.97 grams per 100 gram. and this is often considered a problem. Firstly, oxalic acid is a necessary part of blood 288 mcg/ 100 ml, it is produced by the body. The immune system requires oxalic acid to protect against disease. Such factors as: citric acid additives and alcohol, increase the blood oxalic acid levels. A prolonged deficiency of vitamin B6 can increase oxalic buildup in the kidneys. Magnesium 79 mg increases the solubility of oxalic acid. Eaten raw, the oxalic acid content is of no concern, it remains organic and assists the absorption of calcium and it is required for *peristalsis*, the involuntary movement of food via the oesophagus. When cooked, the oxalic acid in foods can 'lock calcium' and be one cause of kidney stones. Inadequate water intake is another cause. If you eat cooked spinach once a week, no worries, but if you eat chocolate regularly, hardly drink water, mainly alcoholic drinks and eat a lot of meat, with salt, you increase the risk of 'stone formation' and poor calcium absorption.

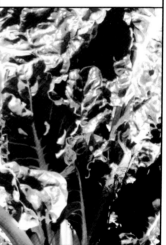

True spinach and silverbeet are an excellent source of lutein and zeaxanthin 11,000 mcg, vital for the eyes of adults, plus beta carotene for anti cancer action. True spinach is an excellent source of potassium 558 mg, the 'muscle mineral' and 'Popeye' was right, plus, the fair iron content 3 mg and a very rich folate content of 194 mg and the abundant vitamin K content 483 mg, but, remember freezing destroys vitamin K, so fresh is best or very lightly steamed is ok. Spinach is a great health restoring food!

SWEET POTATO *Ipomoea batatas*	GLYCEMIC INDEX: 54	CALORIES - total: **76 kcal. per 100 gram**
		Calories from: Carb:95 Protein:4 Fat:0

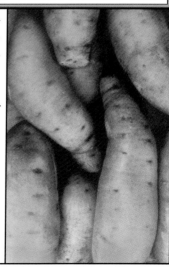

Sweet potatoes are not a yam or related to the potato family, they grow from a vine but do grow underground, like the potato. The sweet potato has a much lower glycemic index 54 G.I. and that's a great start, especially as it is packed with carbohydrate value 95% with no fat content, a good food for anyone overweight or athletic, plus it provides dietary fibre.

Sweet potatoes are a pure beta carotene 8,728 mg food, with a bit of vitamin C 38 mg, less when cooked and a fair supply of potassium 337 mg. Apart from that, a dash of iron 1 mg, magnesium 25 mg, phosphorus 47 mg, folate 14 mcg and vitamin E 0. 4mg. There's no doubt that sweet potatoes are one of the sweetest vegetables, they contain the full range of plant sugars: sucrose 2,170 mg, glucose 1,010 mg and fructose 710 mg but they are 'safe sugars' with a moderate G.I. for a stable increase in blood sugars and energy.

The beta carotene value gives sweet potato a special title, 'the sweetest anti cancer vegetable', put in on your plate and palate!

TURNIPS *Brassica rapa*

GLYCEMIC INDEX: 75

CALORIES - total: 28 kcal. per 100 gram
Calories from: Carb:25 Protein:3 Fat:1

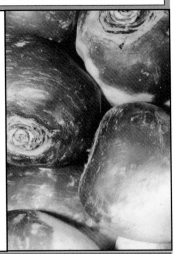

Turnips belong to the 'wallflower family', they rarely get up to dance and their closest new partner is the swede (Brassica napus) a hybrid from broccoli and the turnip. Compared to the 'amazing broccoli', turnips and swedes have no carotene character, not even a bit of beta. Neither have any significant nutritional features, they always look chubby even though they carry no fat content, they hardly contain calcium, 30 mg and have very little sign of muscle tone or potassium 191 mg. They are often a dash salty with organic sodium 67 mg and that's a good thing, because their blood count is really down in the dumps in iron 0 mg and their nerves are shaky at the knees with magnesium 11 mg and phosphorus 27 mg. Surprising the turnip even shows up at parties, maybe it's that small vitamin C of 21 mg that gives them a tiny spark of life. You can eat as many as you like, with very few calories, but anyway, best of luck if you like them, hope that didn't turn you off them!

ZUCCHINI *Spinacea oleracea*

CALORIES - total: 43 kcal. per 100 gram
Calories from: Carb:33 Protein:5 Fat:2

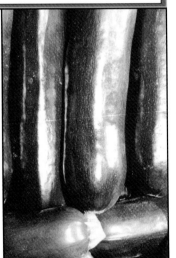

Zucchini are a vegetable marrow, often called *courgettes*. They provide similar nutritional benefits and flavour to the same family member *squash*, but compared to the pumpkin, also a marrow, they are fairly basic in their supply of nutrients.

The small zucchini, or French courgette or Italian zucchini are occasionally served at the best restaurants, with their delicate water based flavour. They are best eaten when served as a lightly steamed whole vegetable, or quickly fried, to retain the delicate moisture and flavour. The zucchini supplies a small vitamin A 323 I.U plus a good supply of potassium 200 - 400 mg, phosphorus 29 mg, calcium 27 mg, iron 0.3 mg and vitamin C 19 mg.

Zucchini are a carbohydrate food with a low starch content and a trace of fibre, 1 g, thereby they need only a slight amount of heat-steam, baking, frying to soften them. Serve lightly steamed, topped with cheese, on rice, with cashew nuts for a simple complete protein meal. The zucchini also supply a small amount of complete protein 3 g. If you are on a weight reducing program, steamed zucchini with rice and a few raw cashews: lowest nut in fat content with 47 grams per 100 gram, can provide a large meal with very few calories, a low fat content with a fair supply of complete protein.

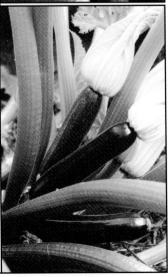

Zucchini grated, make an excellent addition to burgers, or try zucchini on the barbecue, it's full of flavour due to the added fats. Zucchini supply folate 61 mcg. Most green leafy vegetables are also an excellent source so add a little fresh lettuce or coleslaw to the next barbecue list with grilled zucchini and 'Bob's your uncle!' He says, "we'll fight those nasty free radicals!"

The zucchini is the fastest growing garden vegetable so you may have to get out at midnight to check that the courgettes do not get 'out of hand'. That's what happens, especially after a couple of night's and days of rain and thunderstorms, you will be happy with the rain, but, the zucchini get so big, your neighbour will not even accept them. He might say "I've got them growing out of my ears!" Poor thing, does he need an examination!

VEGETABLE SUMMARY CHARTS

VEGETABLES	MAIN NUTRIENTS, ANTIOXIDANTS & PHYTONUTRIENTS	MAIN BODY SYSTEM
Artichoke	fibre, stabilize the metabolism, beneficial for the liver, potassium.	digestive
Asparagus	asparagine , fluoride, bromine, glutathione, rutin, folate, sulphur, chlorine.	urinary, glandular.
Beetroot	chlorine,sulphur, manganese sodium, potassium, copper, iron.	blood, glandular.
Broccoli	vitamin a, vitamin c, calcium, indole-3-carbinol, sulphorane, chromium.	immune, glandular.
Brussel sprouts	sulphur, indoles, vitamin c, vitamin a, selenium, potassium, folate, fibre.	digestive
Cabbage	vitamin a, vitamin c, potassium, bromine, folate.	skin
Carrots	anthocyanins, isoqueritrin, queritrin, ellagic acid, perrillyl alcohol melatonin, vitamin a, potassium.	immune
Capsicum	vitamin c, anthocyanin, vitamin a, potassium,	immune
Cauliflower	fibre, potassium, iron, magnesium, calcium, phosphorus, copper	muscular
Celery	calcium, potassium, fibre, iron, manganese, copper, magnesium phosphorus, silicon, chlorine, sulphur	blood
Cucumber	liminoids, lycopene, salicyclic acid, vitamin c, biotin, b5,	joint
Egg plant	manganese, saponin, trans-resveratrol, phenolic compounds,	blood
Leek	vitamin c, lutein, zeaxanthin,	immune
Mushrooms	vitamin c, vitamin a, copper, iron, potassium, phytponutrients.	respiratory
Lettuce	citric acid, sulphur, vitamin c, antioxidants.	immune
Onions	beta carotene, chlorine, vitamin c, potassium.	respiratory
Parsnips	alkaline, bromine, vitamin c, potassium, vitamin a, enzymes.	glandular
Peppers	potassium, beta cryptoxanthin, beta carotene, lutein, zeaxanthin.	respiratory
Potato	added sodium, calcium, potassium, iron, vitamin a, oleic acid.	nil.
Pumpkin	papain, carpain, chymopapain, vitamin c, beta cryptoxanthin, beta carotene, lutein, zeaxanthin,	immune repair, skin
Radish	vitamin p, vitamin c, citric acid, calcium, phosphorus, magnesium, phytonutrients, fibre,	immune respiratory
Soinach	beta carotene, beta cryptoxanthin, lutein, zeaxanthin, sulphur.	skin, elimination
Sweet potato	fibre, copper, potassium, silicon, folate.	elimination
Turnips	chlorine, sulphur, manganese, bromelain, vit. c, copper, selenium, zinc.	respiratory, blood
Zucchini	phytonutrients, phenols, vitamin a, copper, manganese, carotene.	immune, brain

VEGETABLES - BALANCED DIET - DAILY CARBOHYDRATE INTAKE

	TOTAL DAILY (R.D.I.) CARBOHYDRATE INTAKE	ADULT MALE	ADULT FEMALE	TEENAGER	CHILDREN
		340 grams	280 grams	400 grams	270 grams
	VEGETABLES 15% OF TOTAL CARBOHYDRATE INTAKE LAUGH WITH HEALTH DIET GUIDE	51 grams	42 grams	60 grams	40 grams
65%	100 g STARCH VEGETABLES = 14 grams of carbohydrate approx.	236 grams	195 grams	278 grams	185 grams
10%	100 g LEAFY SALAD VEGETABLES = 3 grams of carbohydrate approx.	170 grams	140 grams	200 grams	133 grams
25%	100 g BRASSICA VEGETABLES = 5 grams of carbohydrate approx.	255 grams	210 grams	300 grams	200 grams
100%					

100 grams is equivalent to any one of the following: 1 medium potato, or 1 medium bowl of salad vegetables or 1 full cup of cooked brassica vegetables,, half cup raw cauliflower, or 1 small carrot, half cup raw spinach, 2 scoops mashed pumpkin, 3 cups shredded lettuce, 3 pieces celery - 15cm long, or 4 florettes broccoli or half a large parsnip.

5%	VEGETABLE JUICES 5% OF TOTAL CARB. INTAKE	17 grams	14	20 grams	13 grams
	100 gram of veg. juice = 9 grams of carbohydrate	188 grams	155 grams	222 grams	144 grams

100 grams vegetable juice = half a glass fresh juice or 100 ml. approx.

U.S. FOOD PYRAMID DAILY DIET GUIDE	Abundance of vegetables			
AUSTRALIAN HEALTHY EATING GUIDE	5 serves	5 serves	3 - 4 serves	2 serves

1 SERVE is equivalent to: half cup cooked vegetables (75 g), or, 1 cup salad vegetables or 1 small potato.

Herbs are a specialized field and only fully trained practitioners may provide accurate advice and diagnosis. The information in the following pages and charts, on herbs, is provided as a basic guide to some common herbs and their association with healing. This herb guide is not intended to be used for any treatment, diagnosis or dosage measure. Both medical and naturopathic advice is always recommended.

By maintaining a natural food diet and healthy lifestyle you can be sure of obtaining the maximum health potential. Many herbs are part of the common diet and provide well recognized benefits, but under some conditions they may be unsuitable for consumption, such as during pregnancy and for this reason proper advice is required to ensure their safety and potential.

Herbs have a long history of providing benefits and with the 'time-tested' benefits of herbs such as garlic, parsley, ginger and mint, it is safe to use them on a regular basis during most times in life. Herbs are often used just to add flavour to meals, at the same time they may provide numerous benefits. By checking through the pages 78-80, the common herbs are described with more detail. When considering the intake of a new herb, always check with a medical practitioner, as some herbs may react with common medications. Herbs are for healing and when properly diagnosed, a health condition may gain great improvement from the addition of properly prepared tonics or infusions. Give the herb kingdom a chance to add spice to your life and promote maximum healing power.

ANISE *Pimpinella anisum*

Anise produces seeds that contain a special oil; anethole provides the main benefits, either as a tea infusion or as oil. Commonly used in cough medicines and lozenges. The tiny seeds combined in cooking promote the digestion of fatty foods as they also provide the B vitamin choline. For babies with colic, regular use of anise tea, by the mother may relieve the condition. Anise oil may also be used in formula milk to relieve colic. Anise tea promotes lactation and purifies the digestive system. For a week digestive system, anise tea is beneficial and it also helps to balance acidity and relieve stomach cramps. Anise oil in a vaporiser helps in cases of bronchitis, emphysema, laryngitis and for a persistent cough. Anise oil mixed with milk may promote sleep and relieve cases of insomnia. Anise seeds are ideal to add to fish meals, pork or veal dishes and in sauces. The oil is also used in liqueurs, such as anisette. Anise oil and seeds are a valuable digestive aid.

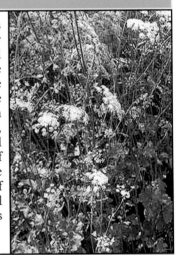

BASIL *Ocimum basilicum*

Basil provides the flavonoids: vicenin and orientin that protect cells from the effects of free radicals and radiation. Basil is a delightfully flavoured herb. The variety of oils in basil provide the main benefits, they are extracted from the leaves and contain : cineole, eugenol, estragole, limonene, myrcene and sabinene. These oils provide a powerful antibacterial effect and have proved effective against some bacteria that are resistant to the action of antibiotics. Basil oil provides anti-inflammatory action, as eugenol blocks the activity of an enzyme that causes inflammation. Basil promotes appetite, relieves headaches, stomach cramps and constipation.
Basil, the chef's best man!

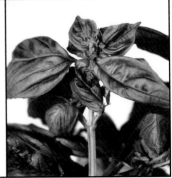

ECHINACEA *Echinacea angustifolia*

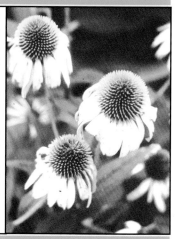

Echinacea increases the body's ability to produce white blood cells which are required especially during times of infections, viruses and colds. It is an excellent blood cleanser, removing toxins from the blood and also improving filtration and drainage of the lymphatic system, which collects toxins before they enter the blood system. Echinacea is a natural antibiotic and it may provide relief from tonsillitis and respiratory and bladder infections. It is also used to reduce fever. Externally, echinacea may relieve psoriasis, eczema, arthritis and burns. In cases of an enlarged prostate gland or weak prostate, echinacea may help. Extracts of the echinacea root may provide relief from chemotherapy and yeast infections. Echinacea is not recommended for children under two years, or during pregnancy or lactation. Also diabetics and people with auto-immune disease, tuberculosis, leukaemia, multiple sclerosis or collagen disease are not to use echinacea.

GARLIC *Allium sativum*

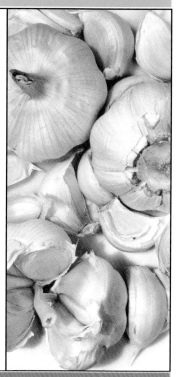

Garlic is the champion of herbs and it has broken every record since the beginning of time. The Egyptian slaves refused to work when garlic was not provided. Garlic is the best source of sulphur compounds such as allicin which provide the powerful antibacterial, antibiotic, antiviral and anti-infection action. Garlic reduces the activity of inflammations that cause common colds and viruses to spread. Allicin compounds protect against colon cancer and may stop the growth of bacteria that cause stomach cancer. The substance ajoene, a sulphur compound in garlic may help reduce skin cancer. Regular use of garlic may provide protective benefits for diabetics due to increased antioxidant levels and reduced triglyceride, insulin and blood pressure levels. Garlic also contains ally disulphate which provides the antiseptic power and antivirus activity. Fresh garlic will provide the best source of these sulphur oils, as excess cooking destroys sulphur compounds. Regular use of garlic will cleanse the body of toxins. Garlic is the ideal herb for relief of respiratory disorders, bronchitis, dysentery, cholera, typhoid fever and intestinal worms. It can also help to reduce blood pressure and improve circulation and heart action. Odourless garlic capsules taken regularly may provide a fair amount of protection. Garlic is the one essential herb in any kitchen, a clove every few days is the ideal way to stay healthy, fit and active and to protect against any nasties that want a free ride. Give garlic a go for any ailment, it provides pure white healing power.

GINGER *Zingiber officinale*

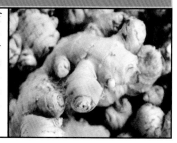

Ginger may provide relief from inflammation due to the supply of compounds termed: gingerols. Such conditions as osteo and rheumatoid arthritis and swollen joints may all be relieved with regular use of the ginger root. Gingerol reduces the production of nitric acid that causes free radical damage. Ginger may provide protection from motion sickness, sea sickness and nausea during pregnancy. Ginger boosts the immune system, relaxes digestion, provides antioxidant power and promotes sweat.

GINSENG *Panax ginseng / P. quinque folius*

Ginseng is obtained from two main varieties: Oriental and American, however true ginseng is obtained from the Chinese or Korean plant. Chinese ginseng contains the active ingredient: panax, it stimulates the entire body, relieves fatigue, improves circulation, nourishes the blood, reduces blood sugar levels and promotes normal blood pressure. It is not recommended for ailments with inflammation, during menstruation or times of fever.

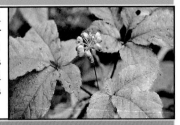

MINT *Mentha piperita*

Peppermint contains a phytonutrient termed perillyl alcohol, it may help retard tumours of the pancreas, liver and mammary glands. Peppermint oil in a vaporiser may protect against various bacteria and fungus. Peppermint also contains rosmarinic acid for improved respiration and to relieve asthma. Peppermint leaves in tea promotes digestion and helps to relieve conditions of indigestion, irritable bowel syndrome, nervousness, insomnia, migraine, headaches, coughs and heartburn.

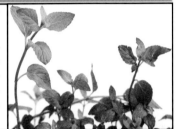

PARSLEY *Petroselinum crispum*

Parsley is rich in vitamin A 8,500 I.U. and vitamin C 172 mg, both these factors give it the power to prevent colds and viruses due to the supply of both water soluble vit. C, antioxidants and fat soluble vit. A plus antioxidants. In addition the rich supply of iron 6.2 mg provides protection from colds. Dishes such as tabouli salad provide maximum parsley power, or try a few sprigs with the carrot or celery juice for a real head rush of benefits. Parsley contains special oils such as myristicin that may retard tumour development, especially in the lungs. Parsley provides protection against carcinogens in cigarette smoke and other environmental pollutants. Another benefit of parsley is due to the supply of flavonoids such as apiin that promotes digestion and especially luteolin, protects against the effects of free radical damage, or oxygen damage to cells often due to cooked oils. Try a tabouli salad and feel at ease about the free radicals. Parsley is food for blood building due to the iron content plus folate, magnesium, manganese and copper. Parsley may help to relieve bladder infections, improve digestion, promote lactation and alleviate menstruation. Parsley when infused and applied to eyes relieves conjuctivitis. Avoid using parsley in cases of kidney inflammation and avoid the seeds and large quantities of parsley leaves during pregnancy. Parsley is a potent herb.

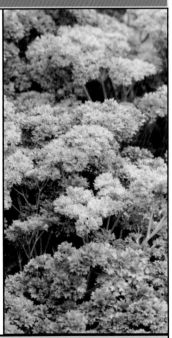

PEPPER *Piper nigrum*

Black, green and white pepper are derived from the same plant, they are varying stages of the pepper berry ripening. Black pepper is fully ripe and promotes maximum benefits such as: activates digestion and stimulation of protein digestive enzymes and fat breakdown. Pepper also provides antioxidant and antibacterial action and protects against flatulence. Pepper promotes sweating and diuretic functions. Pepper is a great spice to add.

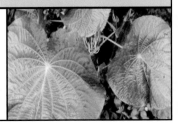

HERBS REFERENCE GUIDE

The following chart and herb glossary is provided as a basic guide to the most common herbs and their association with healing, effect on the body and mind with the basic use and preparation of the herb described.

This guide is not intended to be used for any dosage or personal application. Medical and naturopathic advice is always recommended. The benefit of the chart is to provide a view to the additional benefits for healing that Nature has provided, apart from the wide range of natural foods and a wonderful environment.

Naturopaths are trained to recognise the illness and proper dosage of herbs and often a combination of herbs is provided as a tonic, drop or emollient. Some herbs may cause problems with prescription medications. Check with a reputable naturopath and always remember that natural foods provide all the nutrients to keep healthy. It is interesting to note the effects of herbs and spices that you may use regularly. Some herbs have been used successfully for thousands of years for healing and today most herbs have well recognised functions.

ACACIA Acacia senegal	Coughs, colds, sore throat, catarrh, diarrhoea, dysentery. Dissolved in water.
ADDER'S TONGUE Ezythronium americanum	Emetic, anti-scrofulous, emollient. Fresh leaves crushed into poultice with cider.
AGAVE Agave americana	Disinfectant, laxative, diuretic, diseased liver, jaundice. Boil plant.
ALFALFA Medicego sativa	Appetiser, diuretic, tonic, bowel problems, peptic ulcers. Prepare leaves into tea.
ALOE Aloe vera	Sunburn, wrinkles, insect bikes, cuts, wounds. Break leaves to extract juice, use direct from plant.
ALPINE CRANBERRY Vaccinium sitis idaea	Gout, rheumatism, diarrhoea, disinfectant. Boil leaves into tonic or eat berries.
ALTHEA Aithea officinalis	Demulcent, emollient, diuretic, burns, carbuncles, wounds, gargle, coughs, whooping cough, bronchitis, catarrh. Place leaves, flowers or root into boiled water.
AMARANTH Amaranthus hypochondriacus	Astringent, gargle, throat irritations, dysentery, diarrhoea. Infuse leaves in water, drink the infusion.
AMERICAN CENTAURY Sabatia angularis	Indigestion, dyspepsia, tonic. Steep in boiling water, using herb leaves.
AMERICAN IVY Parthenocissus quinquefolio	Astringent, coughs, colds, tonic. Use bark and twigs chopped in cold water.
ANGELICA Angelica archangelica	Tonic, appetiser, carminative, diuretic, flatulence, headaches, colic, fever, stomach and intestinal problems. Infuse crushed seeds in boiling water.
ANISE Pimpinella anisum	Digestion, flatulence, colic, eye wash, cramps and spasms, insomnia, purifier, lactation. Crush seeds and steep in boiling water, strain, drink hot.
ARNICA Arnica montana	Wounds, bruises. Diluted infusion from dried flowers.
ARUM Arum maculatum	Bronchitis, asthma, catarrh, flatulence rheumatism, gargle. Dried rootstock only, boiled, cooked, diluted, syrup with honey.
ASARUM Asarum europaeum	Diuretic, catarrh, emetic, mucus, eliminative. Use only with medical direction.
BALM Melissa officinalis	Nervous disorders, cramps, colic, bronchial, catarrh, asthma, migraine, toothache, dizziness, melancholy, hysteria, insomnia, insect bites. Use fresh leaves, make tea.
BARBERRY Berberis rulgans	Liver ailments, high blood pressure, gargle, pyorrhea. Ripe berries or boil bark of the root into tea.
BASIL Ocimum basilicum	Appetiser, stomachic, cramps, vomiting, constipation, whooping cough. Use with meals or make into tea.
BEARBERRY Arctostaphylos uva-ursi	Gall stones, cystitis, bronchitis, kidney stones. Make tea from leaves, use small quantities only.
BEARS GARLIC Allium ursinum	Arteriosclerosis, liver problems, diarrhoea, emphysema, bronchitis, high blood pressure. Use as a salad green, soup.
BEDSTRAW Gallium (aparine, verum)	Catarrh, diaphoretic, diuretic, epilepsy, dropsy, calmative. Use herb, steep in warm water. Use fresh leaves.
BENNETT Geum urbanum	Diarrhoea, gargle, tonic, halitosis. Make decoction with herb or rootstock in water.
BETONY Stachys officinalis	Heartburn, sweating, varicose veins, worms, neurasthenia, sores, cuts. Infuse the flowering herb in water.
BILBERRY Vaccinium myrtillus	Fever, antiseptic, astringent, gargle, coughs, vomiting, eyesight. Use berries or dry and make infusion.
BIRCH Betula alba & alta	Astringent, worms, rheumatism, boils, diuretic, anthelmintic. Make decoction with inner bark or leaves in water.

HERBS REFERENCE GUIDE

BIRTHROOT
Trillium
pendulum

Antiseptic, tonic, coughs, colds, insect bites and stings. Use rootstock in a decoction with hot water or milk.

BIRTHWORT
Aristolochia
clematitus

Snakebite, abdominal and menstrual problems, childbirth. Boil rootstock or fresh plant in water.

BISTORT
Polygonum

Diarrhoea, dysentery, astringent, diuretic. Use rootstock, boil in water.

BLACK, RED & SMOOTH ALDER
Alms glutinosa, alum mbra, serrulata

Lice, scabies, scabs, astringent. Boil inner bark, apply diluted.

BLACK COHOSH
Cimicifuga
racemosa

Hysteria, whooping cough, chorea, sedative, cardiac stimulant, rheumatism, bronchitis. Use rootstock at the time berries form. Boil in water.

BLACK ROOT
Varonicastrum

Emetic, cathartic, hepatic. Use root under medical supervision only.

BLAZING STAR
Uatris-spicata/
squarrosa

Gonorrhea, snakebite. Use root extracts directly or boil root in water.

BLIND NETFLE
Lamium album

Menstrual irregularities, astringent, varicose veins and gout. Use plant or flowers infuse in water.

BLOODROOT
Sanguinaria
canadensis

Sedative, tonic, stimulant, eczema, sores. Rootstock used only under medical supervision.

BLUE COHOSH
Caulophylum
thaliclroides

Colic, childbirth, regulate menstruation, cramps. Rootstock used only with medical supervision

BLUE FLAG
Iris versicolor

Heartburn, gastritis, enteritis, migraine, dropsy. Use boiled rootstock. For bums and sores use crushed fresh leaves.

BLUE VERVAIN
Verbena
hastata

Tranquilliser, emetic, tonic, fevers and colds, insomnia, worms. Use rootstock, boil in water. Use leaves to make tea.

BORAGE
Borago
officinalts

Fever, antidote for poisons, pleurisy, lactation. Dried flowers or leaves, steep in cold water.

BOXWOOD
Buxas
sempervirens

Purgative, diaphoretic. Use under medical supervision.

BRIER HIP
Rosa canina

Diuretic, kidney stones, gout, rheumatism, eliminates uric acid. Use fruit without seeds, boil in water.

BROOKLIME
Veroiica
beccabunga

Anemia, febrifuge. Use fresh juice diluted with water or milk.

BYRONY
Byronia alba/
dioica

Purgative, constipation, whooping cough. Extracts from root, use under medical supervision only.

BUCHU
Barrosma
betulina

Aromatic, stimulant, urinary disorders, stomachic, tonic. Use leaves, steep in water.

BUCK BEAN
Barosma
serratifloia

Fever, migraine, indigestion. Use dried leaves, steep in water.

BUCKTHORN
Rhamnus-
frangula/
carthartica

Constipation, obesity, dropsy, use bark from R.frangula, use dried bark only.

BURDOCK
Arctium lappa

Neutralise poisons, stimulates bile, acne. Use leaves/root, boil in water.

BUTFERCUP
Ranunculus
acris

Rheumatism, sciatica, rhinitis. Use fresh plant only with medical supervision.

CALENDULA
Calendula
officinalis

Bruises, sprains, pulled muscles, burns and sores. Use boiled dried flowers or leaves with lard.

CAMOMILE
Anthemis nobilis

Aromatic, flatulence, colic, fever, restlessness, sores and wounds, stomach cramps. Use flowers, make tea.

CANNABIS
Cannabis saliva

Analgesic-hypnotic, antiasthmatic, antibiotic, anti-epileptic, anti-depressant, anti glaucoma, tranquilliser, euphorigenic, alcohol withdrawal. Flowering top and leaves ingested, inhaled. Note: prohibited plant in most countries.

CARAWAY
Carum caM

Stomachic, expectorant, appetiser, menagogue, carminative. Use seeds in cooking, salads, bread.

CARDAMON
Eletlaria
cardamomum

Flatulence, spice, appetiser, stimulant, stomachic. Use as flavour or spice in cooking.

CATNIP
Nepeta catana

Stomach upsets, enema, bronchitis, colic, aromatic. Use herb in boiled water, steep quickly, do not boil.

CAYENNE
Capsicum
frutescens

Appetiser, digestive, cramps, bowel pains. Use pepper with meals.

CHERVIL
Anthriscus
cerefolium

Eczema, gout stones, abscesses, dropsy, high blood pressure. Use fresh or dried herb with meals.

CHICKWEED
Stellana media

Laxative, expectorant, use herb, boil in water, use as tea/tonic. Can be eaten with salads or vegetable meals.

CHICKORY
Cichorium
inlybus

Jaundice, spleen problems, bile production, gallstones, mucus. Make tea from leaves.

CHIVE
Allium
schoenoprasum

Appetiser, digestive, anemia. Use fresh leaves.

CLOVE
Caryophyllus
aromaticus

Antiseptic, anodyne, toothache, vomiting, nausea, aphrodisiac. Use buds or oil tincture.

COLTSFOOT
Tussilago farfara

Respiratory problems, coughs, colds, bronchitis, steep in warm water. For insect bites, inflammations, bums. Use the crushed leaves decoction.

COMFREY
Symphytum off
icinale

Digestive problems, excess menstruation, use as tea. The rootstock powdered for coughs, dysentery and diarrhoea. Use leaves as a poultice for wounds, insect bites and sores.

CORIANDER
Coriandruni
satisium

Appetiser, aromatic, antispasmodic, used as spice with seeds. Externally use for relief of rheumatism and pain in the joints, make into poultice.

DANDELION
Taraxacum
officinale

Edema, stimulates bile formation, liver problems. Tonic, stimulant, constipation, gallstones, jaundice, anemia, fever, insomnia, hypochondria. Use plant direct, or steep in boiled water. Also available in herbal drinks.

DILL
Anethum
graveolens

Upset stomach, insomnia, flatulence, lactation, use fruit seeds, steep in boiled water, serve as tea or tonic.

EUCALYPTUS
Eucalyptus obulus

Antiseptic, deodorant, colds, lung disease, sore throat, asthma, bronchitis, pyorrhea, burns, infection, fever. Boil leaves and condense water to get oil. Use diluted as directed.

FENNEL
Foeniculum milgare

Aromatic, stomach and intestinal disorders, appetite stimulant, colic, abdominal cramps, flatulence, mucous, lactation. Use seeds fresh crushed, steep in boiled water. Use as a spice for any fish meal or fatty meal.

FIGWORT
Scrophularia nodosa

Scabies, tumours, eczema, rashes, skin problems, bruises. Use plant directly, steep in water.

FLAX
IJnum usitatissimum

Coughs, catarrh, chest and lung problems, make decoction with seeds in boiled water. The oil (Linseed) is used for gallstones elimination.

GARDEN VIOLET
Viola odorata

Respiratory problems, gargle, headaches, whooping cough. Use boiled rootstock solution.

GINGER
Zingiber off icinale

Stimulant, appetiser, carminative, menstruation relief, colic, digestive. Use root in meals.

GINSENG
Panax schin-seng/P. quinquelolius

Panacea, stimulant, fever, blood disease, childbirth, vogor, digestive, aphrodisiac, nerves, glands, coughs, colds, chest problems, use as a tea, oil extract or dried root only.

GOLDENSEAL
-lydrastis canadensis

Antiseptic, laxative, diuretic, catarrh, pryrrhea. Use powdered rootstock in boiled water, cool.

HAWTHORN
Crastagus oxyacacantha

Sedative, high blood pressure, cardiac, arteriosclerosis, nervous heart problems, insomnia. Use flowers, steep in water or make tea from the fruit, boil and strain.

HIBISCUS
(MUSK-MELLOW)
Hibiscus abelmoschus

Antispasmodic, itchy skin, nervine, stomachic. Emulsion made from seeds.

HOLLY
hex aquilolium/ l.opa

Gout, gall stones, bronchitis, arthritis, rheumatism, diuretic. Boil leaves in water. Berries are mildly poisonous.

HOPS
Humuhis lupalus

Sedative, hypnotic, calmative, insomnia, flatulence, intestinal cramps. Steep hop fruit in water, use freshly.

HORSERADISH
Arrnoracia ilaapthifohia

Gout, rheumatism, colitis, coughs, asthma, congestion. Use root extracts, chopped finely in salads.

IRISH MOSS
Chondrus crispus

Coughs, colds, tuberculosis, mucilaginous. The plant is generally used as a decoction, also in cough lozengers.

JASMINE
Jasminum officinale

Calming, snake bite, use flowers, steep in water. The scent is sensual when the plant is in full flower.

JUNIPER
Juniperus communis

Tonic, antis diuretic, make tea from berries. Also use spice to stimulate appetite. Juniper oil is used for bone-joint pains and as a vapour for bronchitis and lung infections.

KNOTWEED
Polygonum

Dysentery, bronchitis, enteritis, lung problems, coagulant, peptic ulcers, kidney and gall stones. Use flowering herb, steep in water.

LAVENDER
Lavandula Vera.

Sedative, tonic, migraine, stimulant, flatulence, antiseptic, cleansing, nausea. Use leaves prior to flowering, steep in water - infusion.

LICORICE
Glgcyrrhiza

Diuretic, laxative, bronchitis, congestion, peptic ulcers, fever. Use rootstock infused in water.

LINDEN
Convallana

Stomachic, colds, coughs, sore throat, flowers and leaves in tea.

LOVAGE
Levislicum

Stimulant, diuretic, stomachic. Should not be used by pregnant women. Rootstock infusion in water.

MAGNOLIA
Magnolia glauca

Dysentery, dyspepsia, tonic, tobacca cure, astringent, use bark decoction.

MALLOW
Malva-sylvestris/ rotundifolia

Expectorant, demulcent, emollient, bronchitis, respiratory ailments, use fresh plant only, make infusion or decoction in water.

MARJORAM
Origanum vulgare/ horfensis

Carminative, stomachic, tonic, coughs, colic, cramps, menstruation, regulation, seasickness, calmative, use herb and flowers, infuse in water or take as a spice with foods.

MINT
Mentha piperita/spicata Peppermint, Spearmint and Curled mint)

Stomachic, tonic, antispasmodic, nervousness, coughs, migraine, digestion, heartburn, nausea, cramps, aphrodisiac. Use as tea, leaves only before flowering, pick on a hot sunny day.

MUSTARD
Brassica nigra/ hirta

Digestive, appetiser, bronchitis, pleurisy, antiseptic. Use with foods.

NASTURTIUM
Tropaeolum majus

Disinfectant, antiseptic, congestion, colds, flood formation, expectorant. Use leaves and flowers to make juice as tonic.

NETTLE
Urtica dioica

Digestive, lactation, astringent, tonic haemorrhoids, rheumatism, diarrhoea. Cook plant, or infusion, or juice tonic.

NUTMEG
Myristica fragrans

Aromatic, hallucinogenic, flatulence, carminative, use seed ground into powder. Do not eat seeds whole as they are fairly poisonous.

PASSION FLOWER
Passiflora incamata

Sedative, nerves, diaphoretic, use as prescribed.

PENNYROYAL
Hedeoma pulegloides

Colds, nausea, diaphoretic, carminative, menstruation, headache, rashes. Not to be used during pregnancy. Make infusion.

PERIWINKLE
Vinca major/ minor

Sedative, toothache, nerves, hysteria, fits, astringent, menstruation. Use the herb as tea or chew for toothaches.

PLANTAIN
Plantago

Coughs, gastritis, respiratory, blood coagulation, worms, sores, cuts, bites, hemorrhoids, toothache, use and chew root. Make infusion or decoction.

HERBS REFERENCE GUIDE

POMEGRANATE Punica granatum	Diarrhoea, astringent, gargle, tapeworm, use as fruit in moderation.
PRIMROSE PTimula off icinalis	Insomnia, bronchitis, coughs, lung problems, blood cleanser, rheumatism, gout, skin blemishes, use flowers as infusion, or decoction with rootstock.
RAGWORT Senecio aureus	Menstruation, diuretic. Contains toxic alkaloids.
RED EYEBRIGHT Euphrasia officinalis	Eye inflammations, eyewash, coughs, colds, congestion, hay fever. Use fresh herb as infusion.
RHUBARB Rheum palmatum	Appetiser, purgative, tonic, laxative. Use in small doses as food, not for pregnancy or lactation periods. Use stem only, leaves contain high oxalic acid content.
ROSE Rosa spp.	Headaches, nerve and heart tonic, blood purifier, sores, toothache, use red rose petals. The fruit-hip is a very rich source of vitamin C, use as in tea.
ROSEMARY Rosmannus officinalis	Stimulant, liver functioning, digestion and bile production, improves circulation, raises blood pressure, use as dried herb sparingly, use oil for bruises, eczema, sores and wounds.
SAGE Salva off icinalis	Reduces perspiration, stops flow of mothers milk, nerves, depression, diarrhoea, stomach disorders, sore throat, use as infusion. Fresh leaves for insect bites and warts, crush leaves to extract juice.
SARSAPARILLA Smilax officinalis	Tonic, rheumatism, colds, fever, flatulence, blood purifier. Use rootstock infusion or as a drink.
SASSAFRAS Sassafras albidum	Rheumatism, gout, arthritis, antiseptic, diuretic, pain relief, fever, tonic. Use as infusion of bark.
SAVORY Satereja hortensis	Stomach disorders, cramps, nausea, poor appetite, gargle, aphrodisiac, use as infusion of herb.
SKULLCAP Scutellaria lateriflora	Sedative, nerves, diuretic, tonic, insomnia, rheumatism, neuralgia, menstruation, use plant as infusion.
TARRAGON Artemisia dracunculus	Digestion, kidneys, menstruation, insomnia, hypnotic. Use flowering plant as infusion.
THYME Thyrnus vulgans/ serpyllum	Sedative, bronchitis, diarrhoea, coughs, colic, antispasmodic, use fresh herb as infusion, use oil for antiseptic, toothpaste, mouthwash, warts, rheumatism, bruises, sprains, use a salve for shingles. Use as a herb in food sparingly.
WILD DAISY Beflis perennis	Laxative, tonic, purgative, burns, colds, congestion, stomach problems, liver, kidney, use as tea or use external for injuries, stiffness.

GLOSSARY

ACRID	-having a hot or biting taste.
ALTERNATIVE	-a substance which gradually restores body functions.
ANODYNE	-a substance that relieves pain.
ANTHELMINTIC	-a substance that removes worms.
ANTIOBIOTIC	-agent that fights micro-organisms
ANTIEMETIC	-relieves nausea and vomiting.
APERIENT	-laxative, stimulates bowel.
APHRODISIAC	-an agent that increases or stimulates sexual desire or potency.
APPETISER	-promotes the appetite.
AROMATIC	-a spicy fragrant herb or extract with pleasant smell.
ASTRINGENT	-a substance that contracts skin tissue or reduces discharges and secretions.
ANTISEPTIC	-a substance that destroys harmful germs or bacteria.
ANTITUSSIVE	-a substance that provides relief to coughing.
APERIENT	-provides a stimulant to bowel movement.
BALSAM	-extract of certain trees that is a healing or soothing agent.
CALMATIVE	-provides a relaxing, calming effect on the body and mind.
CARDIAC	-a substance that affects the heart either by stimulating or restoring other functions.
CARMINATIVE	-an extract that helps to relieve digestive gas
CATARRH	-inflammation of the respiratory tract, congestion.
CATHARTIC	-laxative, relieves bowel.
CHOLAGOGUE	-a substance that promotes bile flow.
COAGULANT	-promotes clotting of the blood.
DECOCTION	-a herbal preparation by simmering in water.
DEMULCENT	-soothes inflamed membranes, tissues, mainly mucous membrane.
DEPRESSANT	a substance that decreases nervous function,
DEPURATIVE	an agent that purifies the blood.
DIAPHORETIC	-promotes perspiration.
DIGESTIVE	-an ingredient that promotes or enhances digestion.
DIURETIC	-causes an increase in the secretion of urine.
EMETIC	-promotes vomiting.
EMMENAGOGUE	-increases menstrual flow.
EMOLLIENT	-a substance, lotion that often or soothes skin.
ERRHINE	-a substance that promotes or causes sneezing.
EXPECTORANT	-a substance that promotes mucus discharge.
HEMOSTATIC	-an ingredient that helps stop bleeding.
HEPATIC	-a substance that has an effect on the liver
NEPHRITIC	-a substance or tonic that heals the kidneys.
NERVINE	-an agent that produces a calming effect on the nerves.
OXYTOCIC	-a substance, potion that stimulates uterine contraction.
PECTORAL	-used for heart or chest disorders.
PURGATIVE	-a substance that has a strong laxative effect.
SIALOGOGUE	-a substance that promotes saliva secretion.
STOMACHIC	-an agent that stimulates, heals the stomach.
STRYPTIC	-a substance that contracts blood vessels, stops bleeding.
VERMIFUGE	-a substance that destroys or expels worms in the intestine.
VULNERARY	-an agent that assists in the healing of wounds.

PROTEIN INTRODUCTION

QUESTION 25	What is Protein?	Protein is made from organic compounds of carbon, hydrogen, oxygen and nitrogen; termed amino acids.
QUESTION 26	What are amino acids?	Amino acids are the individual units that make up complete protein.
QUESTION 27	What is complete protein?	The human body needs a total of 20 amino acids for growth and life. 9 amino acids are termed the 'essential amino acids' or 'complete protein'.
QUESTION 28	What foods supply complete protein?	1 - Grains 2 - Legumes 3 - Nuts 4 - Seeds 5 - Sprouts 6 - Fish 7 - Seafood 8 - Meat 9 - Poultry 10 - Eggs 11 - Dairy produce
QUESTION 29	What is the function of amino acids?	Amino acids have numerous functions. refer to chart 1 page 86

NOTE: All amounts in this book are measured in milligrams (mg) per 100 grams, unless stated otherwise.

85

What is the main function of amino acids?

1 ESSENTIAL AMINO ACIDS	MAIN BODY FUNCTION	INFANTS 3 - 6 months	CHILD 10-12 years	ADULT
HISTIDINE	- *essential for growth of children* - required in the formation of glycogen - a vital component in blood - controls mucus levels - non essential for adults	33 mg	20 mg	non essential
ISOLEUCINE	- required for blood development - assists digestion and metabolism - maintains correct nitrogen levels - regulates glandular functions - essential for growth	80 mg	28 mg	12 mg
LEUCINE	- assists the functions of isoleucine - required for blood development - regulates digestion and metabolism - assists the glandular system	128 mg	42 mg	16 mg
LYSINE	- assists digestion and storage of fats - regulates pineal and mammary glands - controls acid alkaline blood levels - essential for amino acid assimilation - regulates the gall bladder	97 mg	44 mg	12 mg
METHIONINE	- the first amino acid used in the construction of any protein. - controls fat levels of the blood - blood haemoglobin development - promotes metabolism of fats - the main limiting amino acid	45 mg	22 mg	10 mg
PHENYLALANINE	- essential for adrenalin production - promotes vitamin c absorption - assists secretion of thyroxine-hormone - gall bladder and waste elimination - formation of skin and hair pigment - assists functions of the kidneys	132 mg	22 mg	10 mg
THREONINE	- assists the functions of all amino acids - improves nutrient absorption - required for new cell development	63 mg	28 mg	8 mg
TRYPTOPHAN	- required for healthy skin and hair - promotes growth of cells and tissues - assists production of gastric juices - regulates sleep and mood patterns - transfer of mesages via seratonin - nourishes the optic system - assists in blood clotting	19 mg	4 mg	3 mg
VALINE	- required for glandular functions - essential for the nervous system - required for growth of cells	89 mg	25 mg	14 mg

Multiply the amounts in mg above by your body weigt in kilograms to obtain the total mg per day required for the individual essential amino acids.

What type of protein does the body require?

There are a number of factors when evaluating the type of protein the human body requires.

1. For adults, eight essential amino acids are required,

2. Children need the eight essential amino acids plus one extra amino acid, histidine.

3. Amino acids are used by the body in a specific ratio, as presented in chart 2. No food provides the exact same ratio but many foods provide a reasonable balance of amino acids.

4. Any food that supplies the eight essential amino acids is termed a complete protein food.

5. The supply of the eight essential amino acids must occur at the same meal.

6. The best protein foods are low in saturated fats and require the least cooking.

7. Foods that provide their 'amino acid balance' similar to the ratio in chart 2, are termed 'high quality protein foods'.

8. The term 'net protein utilization', or (n.p.u.) is used as a measure of protein foods and their supply of amino acids, compared to the 'ideal proportion' refer to chart 2. Refer to page 89.

9. There are three main 'protein variables' when evaluating protein foods. The charts on page 93 provide all three 'protein variables' in order to determine the best protein foods.

PROPORTION OF HOW THE BODY REQUIRES THE 8 ESSENTIAL AMINO ACIDS

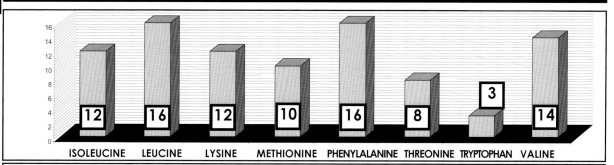

ISOLEUCINE	LEUCINE	LYSINE	METHIONINE	PHENYLALANINE	THREONINE	TRYPTOPHAN	VALINE
12	16	12	10	16	8	3	14

To calculate your approx. daily individual amino acid requirements, multiply the value above (chart 2) x your body weight in kilograms. Example: isoleucine (12 x your body weight) = (70kg) = 840 mg. of isoleucine required per day, or refer to chart, page (88) for a guide .

As presented in the chart above, the body requires a supply of the 8 essential amino acids in a specific proportion. One of the ways to assess protein is termed the net protein utilization. The (n.p.u.) refers to the supply of 8 essential amino acids from individual foods, compared to the amount required by the body in the proportion as shown above in chart 2.

For example: refer to chart 3, page 88: (MET.) methionine and you will see that for a 60 kg. person, refer to chart 3, page 88, the only foods that supply adequate methionine: 600 mg per 100 gram portion are brazil nuts, sesame seeds, tuna, cheese and turkey. The other foods and food groups do not supply adequate methionine to provide the recommended dietary intake, per 100 grams. This is termed a limiting amino acid. Obviously this can be overcome by eating larger quantities of the food.

The other factor, to gain better quality protein is to combine foods to provide a proportion with a better balance of amino acids. Refer to chart 8, page 92 for the *limiting amino acids* from a variety of food groups.

When combining foods to increase protein value, it is important that foods are properly combined at the same meal, to obtain the full benefits. For a guide to food combination, refer to pages 208 - 210.

Body weight, age and physical activity are the main factors. A person with a very active lifestyle requires additional calories and protein.

Chart 3, provides a guide to the amount of the individual amino acids required for an 'average activity level'. The *activity exercise chart* on page 11 shows an increased requirement for calories, with extra physical activity.

The balanced diet requires 30 - 40% of all calories to be obtained from protein. You can add approx. 10 - 30% protein intake per day to the figures below if you have a very active, physical lifestyle.

Basically, the figures below provide the approx. daily amino acid requirements. This chart shows body weight in kilograms and amino acid requirements in mg per day. To compare the amount of individual amino acids required, with the supply of amino acids from a variety of protein foods, refer to chart 5, page 89 and charts 11 & 12 on pages 94 - 95.

3 ESSENTIAL AMINO ACID DAILY REQUIREMENTS FOR ADULTS

measured in mg required per day, approx.	40 kg.	50 kg.	55 kg.	60 kg.	65 kg.	70 kg.	75 kg.	80 kg.	90 kg.	100 kg.	110 kg.
ISOLEUCINE	480	600	660	720	780	840	900	960	1080	1200	1320
LEUCINE	640	800	880	960	1040	1120	1200	1280	1440	1660	1760
LYSINE	480	600	660	720	780	840	900	960	1080	1200	1440
METHIONINE	400	500	550	600	650	700	750	800	900	1000	1100
PHENYLALINE	640	800	880	960	1040	1120	1200	1280	1440	1600	1760
THREONINE	320	400	440	480	520	560	600	640	720	800	880
TRYPTOPHAN	120	150	165	180	195	210	225	240	270	300	330
VALINE	560	700	770	840	910	980	1050	1120	1260	1400	1540

Chart 4 shows the average amount of protein required per day for a variety of age groups and other stages and activities. It is clear that an active person requires increased protein, compared to the average man or woman.

By referring to pages 94 - 95, more details are provided on numerous foods and their protein supply, and, the approx. amounts of those foods required in grams per day, to obtain the R.D.I., recommended dietary intake, USDA.

For men, chart 4 shows 50 grams of complete protein. On page 94, chart 11, oats, the R.D.I. requires 357 grams of oats per day to supply the R.D.I.

Example: Men need approx. 50 grams of protein per day, oats supply 14 grams per 100 gram
= 50 grams, divided by 14 grams = 3.57 grams x 100 grams per day = 357 grams of oats.

4 Recommended Dietary Intake (R.D.I.) of PROTEIN per day

INFANTS to 1 year	CHILDREN 1 -2 years	YOUTH 13 - 19 years	MEN	WOMEN	MANUAL WORKER	SPORTS PERSON	PREGNANCY LACTATION	RETIRED CONVAL-ESCENT
5-10 g	20 - 30 g	40 - 60 g	50 g	40 g	60 g	80 g	50 g	35 g

QUESTION 33

The chart below lists a variety of natural foods and their individual amino acid content. All the foods listed supply complete protein, as they supply the essential 8 amino acids for adults and the extra essential amino acid (histidine) for children. The amino acid values from this chart will be used in other charts to explain the way complete protein from different food groups compares and the way to improve protein values by combining foods. The amino acid values below are all based on 100 gram portions.

Charts 6 & 7 on pages 90 - 91 are a compilation of the information from this chart. The food groups listed on the left hand column of chart 5 are used as the average for the charts 6 & 7 on pages 90 - 91, to provide a visual guide for comparison. On charts 6 & 7, amino acid are represented individually with the approx. value required for persons from 50 kg to 80 kg, plus, the amount of the amino acid obtained from 8 different food groups.

FOOD GROUPS	NATURAL FOODS	HIS.	ISL.	LEU	LYS.	MET	PHA.	THR.	TRY.	VAL.
WHOLE GRAINS	BARLEY	239	545	889	433	184	661	433	160	643
	CORN	206	462	1296	288	186	454	389	61	510
	MILLET	240	635	1746	383	270	506	456	248	682
	OATS	261	733	1065	521	209	758	470	183	845
	RICE	126	352	646	296	135	377	294	82	524
	RYE	276	515	813	494	191	571	448	137	631
	WHEAT	286	607	939	384	214	691	403	173	648
	WHEAT GERM	687	1177	1708	1534	404	908	1343	265	1364
LEGUMES (beans & peas)	CHICK PEAS	559	1195	1538	1434	276	1012	739	170	1025
	KIDNEY BEANS	658	1312	1985	1715	233	1275	1002	214	1401
	LENTILS	548	1316	1760	1528	180	1104	896	216	1360
	LIMA BEANS	669	1199	1722	1378	331	1222	980	195	1298
	PEANUT	749	1266	1872	1099	271	1557	828	340	1532
	SOY BEANS	911	2054	2946	2414	513	1889	1504	526	2005
NUTS	ALMONDS	517	873	1454	582	259	1146	610	176	1124
	BRAZIL NUTS	367	593	1129	443	941	617	422	187	823
	CASHEW NUTS	415	1222	1522	792	353	946	737	471	1592
	COCONUT	69	180	269	152	71	174	129	33	212
	HAZEL NUTS	288	853	939	417	139	537	415	211	934
	PECAN NUTS	273	553	773	435	153	564	389	138	525
	PISTACHIO NUTS	507	880	1520	1080	370	1090	610	273	1340
	WALNUTS	405	767	1228	441	306	767	589	175	974
SEEDS	PEPITAS	711	1737	2437	1411	577	1749	933	560	1679
	SESAME SEEDS	441	951	1679	583	637	1457	707	331	885
	SUNFLOWER SEEDS	586	1276	1736	868	443	1220	911	343	1354
EGG	WHOLE EGG	1123	850	1126	819	401	739	637	211	950
DAIRY FOODS	MILK (COWS)	92	233	344	272	86	170	162	49	240
	YOGHURT	146	214	336	282	78	180	160	37	255
	CHEDDAR CHEESE	815	1685	2437	1834	650	1340	929	341	1794
TUNA	TUNA	880	1481	2178	2556	842	1074	1249	290	1554
BEEF	BEEF PORTERHOUSE	569	858	1343	1433	407	674	724	192	911
POULTRY	CHICKEN	593	1088	1490	1810	537	811	877	250	1012
	LAMB	501	933	1394	1457	432	732	824	233	887
	TURKEY	649	1260	1836	2173	664	960	1014	238	1187

6

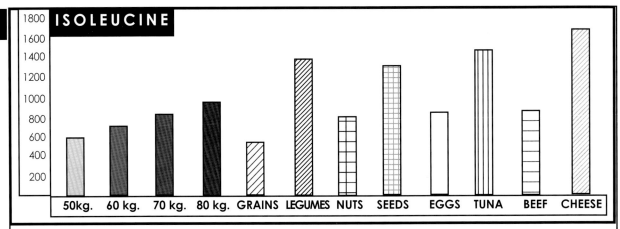

ISOLEUCINE

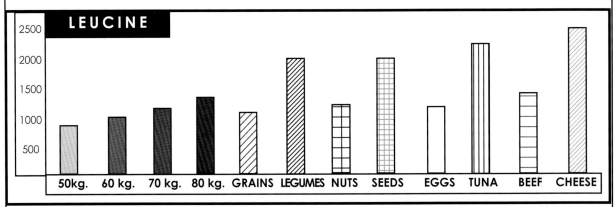

LEUCINE

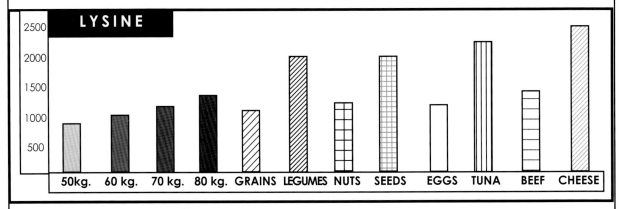

LYSINE

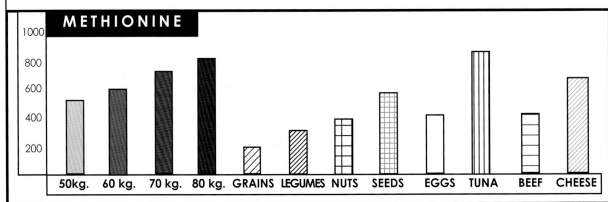

METHIONINE

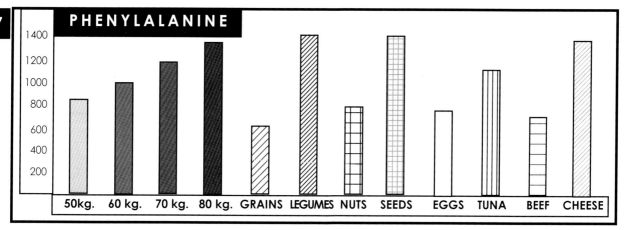

PHENYLALANINE

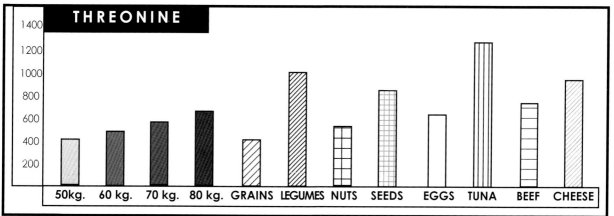

THREONINE

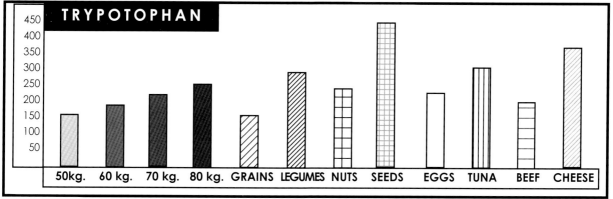

TRYPOTOPHAN

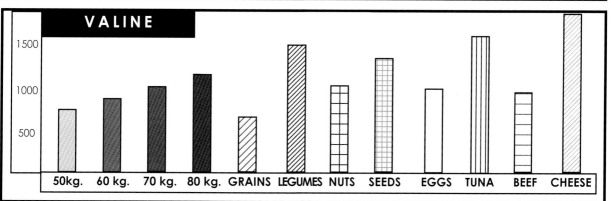

VALINE

How do I increase the protein value of a meal?

Apart from eating more food, the chart below gives a list of foods to combine, to increase the protein value, or net protein utilization (n.p.u.) of a meal.

For whole grains: wheat being the most common, the simple combination of a cheese sandwich, or pasta with cheese, or cereal with milk. For rice, legume such as kidney beans will improve the protein value of the meal and also be a good combination providing complete protein.

With the legumes, the only limiting amino acid is methionine and the best food source is brazil nuts or tahini, so you can combine a small portion and gain considerable increase in protein as with hummous; a combination of chick peas and tahini (lemon juice, garlic etc.).

The chart below displays the 'main limiting amino acids' with the protein food groups. The most common limiting amino acid with nearly all foods (except brazil nuts, tahini, tuna and cheese) is methionine. Generally speaking, by adding any of the methionine rich foods to a meal it will greatly increase the (n.p.u.). Such combinations as tahini on toast are ideal, or almonds with brazil and cashews.

Numerous traditional recipes utilize combinations that improve the protein value of a meal such as kidney beans and corn as with tacos, nachos, or spaghetti and parmesan or other cheese, or oats and milk with porridge. All these simple combinations and many more have been used for centuries and have provided good quality protein meals.

Fish, especially tuna has an excellent protein value and it does not need other foods to gain a better protein balance. Cheese is a great protein food, but, due to the rich saturated fat content, combine cheese with low fat foods, such as legumes, grains and vegetables to obtain a well balanced diet. Both meat and poultry have 2 limiting amino acids (MET. & PHA.), for the 60 kg person, from a 100 gram serve. Nearly all vegetables supply (MET) methionine and (PHA) phenylalanine and they are the ideal food to combine, especially leafy vegetables.

In summary, vary your diet, combine suitable foods and choose from the legumes group more often. Use ground seeds in pastries, breakfast cereals, pancakes, soups and cookies.

MAIN PROTEIN FOOD GROUPS	MAIN LIMITING AMINO ACIDS based on *100 gram portions* for a 60 Kg. person.								FOODS TO COMBINE TO IMPROVE NET PROTEIN UTILIZATION (N. P. U.)
	ISL.	LEU.	LYS.	MET.	PHA.	THR.	TRY.	VAL.	
GRAINS	549		399	198	574	413	149	640	add milk, cheese, legumes, egg.
LEGUMES				300					add tahini, or whole grains
NUTS			518	385	762				combine almonds, brazil and cashews
SEEDS			470	552					eat extra 30%
EGGS				401	739				milk
TUNA									complete
BEEF				407	674				vegetables for best digestion
CHEESE									complete
POULTRY				537	811				vegetables for best digestion
50 kg.	600	800	600	500	800	400	150	700	100 g is equivalent to one of the following:
60 kg.	720	960	720	600	960	480	180	840	- 2 medium boiled eggs.
70 kg.	840	1120	840	700	1120	560	210	980	- 5 slices whole wheat toast. - 1 cup of cashew nuts.
80 kg.	960	1280	960	800	1280	640	240	1120	- 1 cup of legume sprouts.

8

	What are the best protein foods?

As a summary of the protein information provided in the previous pages, chart 9 shows the; three main protein values: (1) protein percentage of original food, (2) (n.p.u.) net protein utilization and (3) the grams of useable protein per 100 gram serve.

Chart 10 provides the three protein variables and the total protein value in %. This is calculated by adding the three values of a natural food and obtaining an average in percentage. The best protein food is tuna with a 43.3% total protein value. Chart 10 also provides a list of fats, cholesterol and carbohydrate content.

On pages 94 - 95, charts 11 & 12 provide a guide to the approx. grams required per day to obtain the (R.D.I.) for protein, from a wide variety of natural foods and meals.

9

	PROTEIN % of uncooked NATURAL FOOD	PROTEIN %		N.P.U. % net protein utilization.	N.P.U. %		GRAMS of USEABLE PROTEIN	GRAMS g
1	SOY BEANS	34	1	EGGS	94	1	TUNA	22
2	PEPITAS	29	2	MILK & YOGHURT	92	2	SOY BEANS	20.7
3	TUNA	28	3	FISH & TUNA	80	3	CHEESE	18
4	CHEDDAR CHEESE	26	4	RICE	70	4	PEPITAS	17.4
5	PEANUT	26	5	WHEAT GERM	67	5	FISH	17
6	LENTILS	25	6	BEEF	67	6	WHEAT GERM	16.7
7	WHEAT GERM	25	7	OATS	66	7	BEEF	16
8	BEEF	24	8	SOY BEANS	61	8	SUNFLOWER SEEDS	13.3
9	SUNFLOWER SEEDS	23	9	PEPITAS	60	9	CHICKEN	13
10	FISH	22	10	SUNFLOWER SEEDS	58	10	PEANUT	11.1

0

	NATURAL PROTEIN FOODS ALL AMOUNTS MEASURED IN 100 GRAM PORTIONS	1 PROTEIN of natural food %	2 N.P.U. net protein useable %	3 PROTEIN content grams	1+2+3 = TOTAL PROTEIN VALUE %	TOTAL FAT CONTENT grams	SATURATED FAT CONTENT grams	CHOLESTEROL CONTENT mg	CALORIES	CARBOHYDRATE CONTENT grams
	THE BEST PROTEIN FOODS - COMBINED PROTEIN VALUES CHART									
1	TUNA	28	80	22	43.3	5	2	37	145	0
2	FISH	22	80	17	39.6	6	2	50	200	0
3	EGGS	12	94	17	39	11	11	550	160	1
4	SOY BEANS	34	61	21	38.6	5	1	0	403	33
5	CHEESE	26	70	18	38	33	18	100	402	0
6	WHEAT GERM	25	67	17	36.3	8	1	0	380	50
7	BEEF	24	67	16	35.6	18	9	70	258	0
8	PEPITAS	29	60	17	35.3	46	8	0	553	15
9	CHICKEN	21	65	13	33	13	3	60	253	3
10	SUNFLOWER SEEDS	23	58	13	31.3	47	6	0	560	20
11	OATS	14	66	9	29.6	8	2	0	388	70
12	MILK / YOGHURT	3	82	3	22.3	4	2	11	67	0
13	CASHEWS	18	58	10	28.6	43	8	0	561	29
14	SESAME / TAHINI	19	55	10	28	53	7	0	582	18
15	RICE	7	70	5	27.3	2	1	0	359	78
16	PEANUT	26	43	11	26.6	47	10	0	567	17
17	ALMONDS	18	50	9	25.6	54	4	0	598	19
18	CHICK PEAS	20	43	9	24	5	2	0	360	61
19	BRAZIL NUTS	14	50	7	23.6	67	13	0	654	11
20	WALNUTS	14	50	7	23.6	64	4	0	648	15

ORIGINAL NATURAL FOOD	COMMON daily RECIPE IDEAS	PROTEIN % NATURAL FOOD	N.P.U. % net protein utiliz.	grams useable protein	R.D.A. average man & youth 50 grams	R.D.A. average women & youth 40 grams	R.D.A. average child 10 - 14 Y. 40 grams	TOTAL FAT mg	SATURATED FAT mg	CHOLES-TEROL mg
CORN	sweet corn	3 %	72 %	5.7	625 grams day	500 grams day	312 grams day	2	2	0
	corn chips corn bread	8 %	53 %	4.2						
OATS	rolled oats porridge corn bread oat cookies	14 %	66 %	9.2	357 grams per day	285 grams per day	178 grams per day	7.8	2	0
RICE	white rice	7 %	70 %	4.9	714 grams per day	571 grams per day	357 grams per day	2	1	0
	brown rice									
	rice crackers									
	rice pudding									
	rice stir fry									
WHEAT	white flour / bread	14 %	45 %	6.3	357 grams per day	285 grams per day	178 grams per day	2	2	0
	wholemeal flour / bread									
	pasta									
	cakes									
	biscuits / crackers									
	pizza /									
WHEAT GERM	whole grain bread	25 %	67 %	16.7	200 grams per day	160 grams per day	100 grams per day	8	1	0
	added to meals									
CHICK PEAS	cooked with vegetables	20 %	43 %	8.6	250 grams per day	200 grams per day	125 grams per day	5	2	0
	hummous									
	cooked with rice									
KIDNEY / LIMA BEANS	beans with tacos	22 %	38 %	8.3	227 grams per day	181 grams per day	113 grams per day	2	0	0
	baked beans/ burgers									
	beans, rice, vegetables									
LENTILS	lentils, rice, vegetables	25%	30 %	7.5	200 grams per day	160 grams per day	100 grams per day	1	0	0
	lentil patties / soup									
PEANUT	peanuts / raw / roasted	26 %	43 %	11.1	192 g. / day	153 g. / day	96 g. / day	47	10	0
	peanut butter / sauce									
SOY BEANS	soy flour/ bread	34 %	61 %	20.7	147 grams per day	117 grams per day	73 grams per day	5	1	0
	soy with vegetables/soup									
	soy milk / cheese									
PEPITAS	pepita natural raw	29 %	60 %	17.4	172 grams per day	137 grams per day	86 grams per day	46	8	0
	pepita burgers									
	pepitas & pasta / soup									
SESAME (TAHINI)	tahini on bread / toast	19 %	55 %	10.4	263 grams per day	210 grams per day	131 grams per day	53	7	0
	tahini with salads									
	tahini in cakes									
SUN-FLOWER SEEDS	sunflower pancakes	23 %	58 %	13.3	217 grams per day	173 grams per day	108 grams per day	47	6	0
	sunflower seed snack									
	sunflower meal in bread									

ORIGINAL NATURAL FOOD	COMMON daily RECIPE IDEAS	PROTEIN % NATURAL FOOD	N.P.U. % net protein utiliz.	grams useable protein	R.D.A. average man & youth 50 grams	R.D.A. average women & youth 40 grams	R.D.A. average child 10 - 14 Y. 40 grams	TOTAL FAT mg	SATURATED FAT mg	CHOLES-TEROL mg
ALMONDS	raw almonds / apple blanched almonds / cake almond meal / pancakes	18 %	50 %	9	277 grams per day	222 grams per day	138 grams per day	53	4	0
BRAZIL NUTS	brazil nuts raw snack brazil, almonds, cashew brazil nuts / apple	14 %	50 %	7	357 grams per day	285 grams per day	178 grams per day	67	13	0
CASHEW NUT	cashews raw / snack cashews / stir fry rice cashew butter cashews / almonds	18 %	58 %	10	277 grams per day	222 grams per day	138 grams per day	43	8	0
HAZEL NUTS	hazelnuts raw / snack hazel nuts / mixed nuts hazel nuts / cakes	12 %	?	?	416 grams per day	333 grams per day	208 grams per day	62 %	3	0
PECAN NUTS	pecan nuts raw pecan nut pie / cakes pecan nut cookies	9 %	?	?	555 grams per day	444 grams per day	277 grams per day	71 %	5	0
PISTACHIO NUT	pistachio snack pistachio fettuchine	19 %	0	0	263 grams per day	210 grams per day	131 grams per day	53 %	3	0
WALNUTS	walnuts raw / with fruit walnuts in cakes walnuts in salads	14 %	50 %	7	357 grams per day	285 grams per day	178 grams per day	64%	4	0
BEEF	cooked/ stir fry beef steak barbecue	24 %	67%	16	208 g. / day	166 g. / day	104 g. / day	21%	9	78
CHEESE	cheese natural / bread cheese/ pizza / sauce cheese in cooking	26 %	70 %	18	192 grams per day	153 grams per day	96 grams per day	33%	22	107
CHICKEN	roast chicken chicken stir fry chicken casserole / soup	21 %	65 %	13	238 grams per day	190 grams per day	119 grams per day	13%	3	60
EGGS	boilled eggs / fried scrambled eggs eggs in cooking / cakes	12 %	94 %	17	416 grams per day	333 grams per day	208 grams per day	12%	4	420
FISH (average)	fish / baked/ fried / fish / chips / salad fish / burgers / patties	22 %	80 %	17	222 grams per day	181 grams per day	113 grams per day	6 %	2	50
MILK(cows) YOGHURT	milk fresh/ milk shakes milk / pancakes / cooking	3 %	82 %	3	1,200 grams per day	1,300 grams per day	833 grams per day	4 %	2	11
TUNA	tuna / salad / toast tuna mornay	28 %	80 %	22	178 grams per day	142 grams per day	89 grams per day	5%	2%	38

RECOMMENDED DIETARY ALLOWANCE CHARTS

The chart below is based on figures from the USDA, National Academy of Sciences, Food & Nutrition Board. The food sources mentioned are not from the USDA, plus, various figures in the chart are only provided as a guide. Basically the chart is provided to show the approx. amount of nutrients required per day.

There are a number of factors that may require an increase in specific nutrients, compared to this chart. Such factors as chronic illness, and various ailments, plus, smoking, alcohol, stress and physical activity levels can increase the need for numerous nutrients. Ideally, obtain a variety of the foods listed over a period of one week to obtain an excellent supply of the essential nutrients. Refer to minerals pages 147-160 and vitamins pages 161-176 for details on the functions of the individual nutrients and other food sources.

ESSENTIAL NUTRIENTS - DAILY RECOMMENDED DIETARY INTAKE CHART

TOTAL NUTRIENTS	MALE 19 - 64	MALE OVER 64	WOMEN 19 - 54	WOMEN OVER 64	PREGNANCY	LACTATION	DAILY DIET RECOMMENDED FOOD SOURCE
CARBOHYDRATES	280 - 400 grams.		230 grams. - 340 grams				grains, legumes, fruits, vegetables
PROTEIN	58 - 63 grams.		44 grams. - 50 grams.				grains, legumes, nuts, seeds, animal produce
FATS	51 grams - 65 grams.		40 grams. - 60 grams.				nuts, olive oil, veg. oils, avocado, dairy.
CALCIUM	800 mg.	800 mg.	800	1000	1100 mg.	1200 mg.	tahini, nuts, yoghurt, cheese,
PHOSPHORUS	1000 mg.				1200 mg.		pepitas, sunflower seeds, tahini, nuts.
POTASSIUM	1,950 mg.	-	5,460 mg.				wheat germ, sultanas, almonds, nuts, banana.
IRON	7 mg.		12 - 16	5 - 7	22 - 36 mg.	12 - 16 mg.	pepitas, wheat germ, parsley, mussels, tofu.
CHLORIDE	No R.D.I. Safe level approx. 1,700 -5,100 mg.						oatmeal, cheese, olives, fish in oil, peanuts
SODIUM	920mg. - 2,300 mg.						olives, salmon, cheese, rye bread, tuna
FLUORIDE	No R.D.I. Safe level approx. 3mg. - 4 mg.						oats, asparagus, apples, beetroot, corn, garlic.
SILICON	No R.D.I. No recognized level.						lettuce, sunflower seeds, vegetables, berries.
MAGNESIUM	320 mg		270 mg.		300 mg.	340 mg.	sunflower seeds, almonds, brazil, pepitas, nuts.
MANGANESE	No R.D. I. Safe level 2 mg. - 5 mg.						wheat germ, pecan nuts, walnuts, seeds, nuts.
SULPHUR	No R.D.I. No recognized level.						seafood, brazil nuts, carrot juice, vegetables,
COPPER	No R.D.I. Safe level approx. 1.5 mg. - 3 mg.						tahini, cashews, sunflower seeds, nuts, pepitas.
IODINE	150 mcg.		120 mcg.		150 mcg.	170 mcg.	capsicum, lettuce, fish, vegetables, cheese.
ZINC	12 mg.		16 mg.		18 mg.		oysters, sunflower seeds, wheat germ, nuts,
COBALT	N R.D. I. No recognized level.						fish, seafood,
CHROMIUM	No R.D.I. Safe level approx. 50 mcg. - 200 mcg.						egg yolk, cheese, rye bread , apples, wine,
SELENIUM	85 mcg.		70 mcg.		80 mcg.	85 mcg.	brazil nuts, tuna, sunflower seeds.
MOLYBDENUM	No R.D.I. Safe level approx. 75 mcg. - 250 mcg.						legumes, apricots, rye bread, vegetables, corn.
VANADIUM	No R.D.I. No recognized level.						seafood, fish, vegetables.
VITAMIN A	750 mcg. RE (retinol equivalents)					1200 mcg.	carrots, pumpkin, fruits, cheese, spinach,
VITAMIN C	40 mg.		30 mg.		60 mg.	75 mg.	guava, currants, capsicum, kiwi fruit, citrus,
VITAMIN D	No R.D.I. Safe level approx. 5 - 10 mcg. per day.						(sunlight) cod liver oil, salmon, eggs, sardines.
VITAMIN E	10 mg. alpha/TE		7 mg. alpha/TE			9.5 mg.	wheat germ oil, sunflower seeds, almonds.
VITAMIN F	No R.D.I. preferably at least 1% total calorie intake.						pepitas, walnuts, linseeds, salmon, oily fish,
VITAMIN K	No R.D.I. suggested approx. 2mcg. per kilo of body weight.						spinach, lettuce, cabbage, cauliflower.
VITAMIN P	No R.D.I. No recognized level.						capsicum, mandarins, citrus, apricots, berries.
VITAMIN B1	1.1 mg.	0.9 mg.	0.7 - 0.8 mg.		1.0 mg.	1.2 mg.	sunflower seeds, yeast extracts, tahini, nuts,
VITAMIN B2	1.7 mg.	1.3 mg.	1.2 mg.		1.5 mg.	1.7 mg.	almonds, yeast extracts, cheese, wheat germ,
VITAMIN B3	19mg. NE	16 mg. NE	13 mg. NE		15 mg. NE	18 mg. NE	peanuts, yeast extracts, bran, seeds, nuts, tuna,
VITAMIN B5	No R.D.I. No recognized level						sunflower seeds, almonds, yeast extracts, bran,
VITAMIN B6	1.3 - 1.9	1.0-1.5 mg.	0.9 - 1.4 mg.		1.0-1.5 mg.	1.6-2.2 mg.	oats, walnuts, wheat germ, seeds, garlic,
VITAMIN B12	2 mcg.				3 mcg.	2.5 mcg.	yoghurt, eggs, fish, cheese, seafood, beef,
BIOTIN	No R.D.I. acceptable level of 30 mcg.						almonds, walnuts, oats, pecan, salmon.
CHOLINE	No R.D.I. suggested : males: 550 mcg. ,females: 425 mcg.						lecithin, oats, legumes, lettuce, spinach, corn.
FOLATE	200 mcg.				400 mcg.	350 mcg.	wheat germ, sunflower seeds, vegetables.
INOSITOL	No R.D.I. No recognized level.						citrus, whole grain bread, legumes, peas, rice.

CHAPTER THREE

NUTS INTRODUCTION

Nuts provide numerous nutritional benefits and throughout the following pages there is a descriptive evaluation with the most common varieties; almond, brazil, cashew, chestnut, coconut, hazel, macadamia, pecan, pine, pistachio and walnut.

Generally speaking, nuts are a very good source of complete protein, all the essential life supporting amino acids are generously supplied by the nut kingdom, refer to page 89. Nuts can easily replace all other foods for protein value and requirements.

We are fortunate these days to have a variety of nuts from around the world to choose from and to include them with the daily balanced diet.

Many people consider nuts to be an expensive food item and unfortunately for that reason they are avoided.

Nut protein is better value than meat or poultry. Refer to the chart below.

Nuts provide an abundance of minerals and vitamins compared to meat and poultry, plus they need no cooking and that saves on fuel bills.

In addition, nuts provide numerous other benefits due to their good supply of fibre, trace minerals and antioxidants.

Nuts provide pure value per gram.

PROTEIN FOOD COMPARISON	PRICE 100 g	70 kg male	CHOLE-STEROL	IRON
ALMONDS	$ 1.40	180 g	0	4.6
BRAZIL	$ 1.19	210 g	0	3.4
CASHEW	$ 2.00	200 g	0	3.7
A.B,C NUT MIX	$ 1.50	150 g	0	3.9
PEPITAS	$ 1.95	130 g	0	11.3
SOY BEANS	$ 0.35	150 g	0	5.1
BEEF STEAK	$ 1.80	180 g	81	1.9
CHEDDAR	$ 2.50	120 g	107	0.6
CHICKEN	$ 2.00	140 g	90	0.7
LAMB	$ 3.10	160 g	75	1.0
TUNA	$ 2.50	100 g	38	1.5

Another main benefit from nuts is when they are eaten raw, as the valuable unsaturated oil content provides an excellent source of energy and health benefits, as presented in the following pages.

Animal protein foods such as meat are mainly composed of saturated fats. Once meat is cooked, a decrease in the protein value occurs plus the nasty addition of free radicals results which is really detrimental to health.

For a simple protein snack, try a handful of almonds with a ripe peach or crisp apple.

Nuts supply generous amounts of easily assimilated complete protein, minerals, vitamins and no free radicals from the abundant variety of raw nuts.

Nuts supply all the essential nutrients for the utilisation of their fat content and because most of the fats are in the form of unsaturated, they can be readily used by the body. Over half the food value in nuts is composed of unsaturated fats and these provide a very satisfying effect on the appetite with no health risk problems.

One serving of 150 grams of mixed nuts will provide an average of 900 calories or one third of the daily calorie allowance for men between the ages of 20 - 50. With such a serving, all daily protein requirements are obtained.

Nuts provide an abundance of the minerals: calcium, phosphorus, iron potassium, copper, selenium and magnesium. Each variety of nut has certain dominant nutrients, as explained in the following pages.

Research studies have shown that the unsaturated fats in nuts can actually reduce weight when they replace the saturated fats of other animal produce foods and meals.

Nuts are the answer to the big appetite and demand for calories and energy.

ALMONDS *Prunus dulcis*	C.	P.	L.	CALORIES - total: **578 kcal. per 100 gram**
	14	**13**	**73**	Calories from: Carb:80 Protein:74 Fat:424

Almonds are alkaline and for this reason alone, the almond nut in the raw state is a great food, ideal for obtaining the 75% alkaline daily food balance. All foods except fruits, vegetables and rice are acid forming, the almond is a great exception. An alkaline body balance promotes natural healing

Almonds are also a great provider of lipids especially mono unsaturated 32 g with polyunsaturated 12 g and saturated 4 g. In one study, comparing two weight loss diets, the 'almond diet' proved to reduce weight and blood pressure 30% better than the standard low calorie, low fat diet. It was found that not all the fat in almonds is absorbed, as the cell walls in the almond nut acts as a partial barrier to fat absorption. Furthermore, the abundance of mono unsaturated fats, in almonds, is ideal for energy requirements and is readily used by the body, plus, it reduces cholesterol levels in the blood.

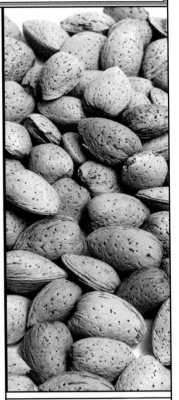

Almonds provide nearly 70% mono unsaturated lipids, 20% polyunsaturated and 10% saturated lipids. Almonds provide only a trace amount of Omega 3, but they supply 10 g of Omega 6, the other essential fatty acid. Almonds are an excellent source of vitamin E 26 mg or 90% of the daily value (d.v.) requirement. Vitamin E is a major antioxidant, it reduces the risk of heart disease as it protects against oxidation of the ldl cholesterol, or the bad cholesterol that leads to heart disease. Vitamin E also promotes blood circulation, heart muscle function and the life of body cells. One study showed a 45% decrease risk of heart disease by substituting the fats in almonds for the saturated fats in meat. In summary, lipids in almonds are safe and beneficial. For more information on almond oil, refer to page140.

In regards to the protein value of raw almonds, they provide complete protein, as they supply the eight essential amino acids, refer to chart on page 89. Almonds supply 20% protein with 21 g, or nearly 40% of the (d.v.) daily value requirement for the average adult and in regards to calories, only 20 % of daily calories, that's a very impressive figure! Almonds are an excellent magnesium food 275 mg, or 100% d.v. and this promotes blood flow and reduced risk of heart attacks, plus it is essential for the health of the nervous system and brain, as it nourishes the white nerve fibres and helps the nerves to relax. In addition, the excellent phosphorus content 474 mg is vital for the repair of the nervous system, improved blood circulation, memory and concentration. If you are writing a thesis, without almonds, it's a brain drain, almonds promote creativity, plus the good manganese content 3 mg promotes memory abilities. The calcium content in almonds is excellent 248 mg and for dairy intolerant persons, almonds are ideal. They are the best nut source of calcium and apart from tahini and tofu, only dairy is higher and it supplies considerable saturated fats and cholesterol, almonds provide safe calcium. Almonds are a great source of dietary fibre 12 g and when eaten as a snack with apples, their protein digestion is enhanced. Almonds are also full of copper 56% d.v., iron 24% d.v., zinc 22% d.v., potassium 21% d.v., B2 48% d.v., B3 20% d.v. and biotin 100% d.v., essential for fat metabolism.

Almonds are so great you could 'literally' write a book on them. Almonds can be ground and added to cereal. Almonds are perfect alkaline protein.

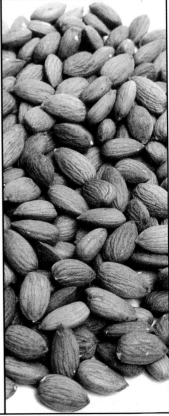

NOTE: d.v. refers to daily value for woman 25 - 50 years, refer to RDA chart page 69 for adult male and children values.

BRAZIL NUTS	Bertholletia excelsa	C.	P.	L.	CALORIES - total: 656 kcal. per 100 gram
		7	8	85	Calories from: Carb:50 Protein:50 Fat:556

Brazil nuts are exceptionally rich in the mineral selenium 1,900 - 2,960 mcg, the daily RDA is 55 mcg. with the upper level intake of 400 mcg. from supplements. Brazil nuts are so rich in selenium, it would be a big waste of money to buy a selenium supplement. One brazil nut a day will provide all the daily selenium requirements, unless you can eat a 100 gram serve of liver or 500 g of wheat germ, or 600 g sunflower seeds or a kilo of tuna.

Brazil nuts are really an essential food item. A prolonged selenium deficiency can increase the risk of asthma, heart disease, HIV infections, arthritis, senility, Alzheimer's disease, epilepsy, mental fatigue, anxiety and atherosclerosis. Selenium is vital for diabetics, as it stimulates glucose absorption. In a ten year study, an optimum selenium intake decreased cancer mortality by 50%, especially lung (46%) prostrate (63%) and colon cancer (38%). Selenium acts as an antioxidant in combination with vitamin E, against free radicals, especially from cooked oils. Selenium and the vitamin E, 6 mg in brazil nuts could be considered a life saver.

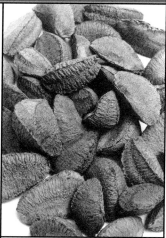

Another great benefit of brazil nuts is the remarkable supply of the amino acid - methionine 1008 mg. Brazil nuts are the best natural source of this precious *limiting* amino acid. Nearly all protein foods are deficient in the amino acid methionine and that considerably lowers the real protein potential of many foods.

Brazil nuts supply over 90% of the required methionine amounts. Most foods supply around 30% and that greatly reduces protein value. A small sprinkle of ground brazil nuts will add protein power to vegetable burgers and any meal.

Brazil nuts supply complete protein 14 g, plus an excellent source of phosphorus 725 mg, potassium 650 mg and magnesium 376 mg, plus, a good supply of calcium 160 mg. Brazil nuts supply 66 g lipids with 28 g mono unsaturated, 21 g polyunsaturated and 17 g saturated.

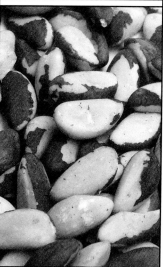

Most soils and foods are deficient in selenium. For the ultimate selenium antioxidant benefits, crack into the incredible brazil nut.

CASHEW NUTS	Anacardium occidentale	C.	P.	L.	CALORIES - total: 566 kcal. per 100 gram
		20	11	69	Calories from: Carb:110 Protein:11 Fat:69

Cashew nuts also originated from Brazil. Raw cashews have less fat than most nuts. Cashews supply 65% unsaturated fats, with 90% in the form of oleic acid, ideal for energy and reduced cholesterol. Cashews supply Omega 6, 8 g with a trace of omega 3. Roasted cashews are nice but the increase in free radicals is a problem, however, the rich supply of the trace mineral copper 2.2 mg will help protect against such problems. One handful of cashews will supply a full daily dose of copper, essential for the heart muscles, iron and fat metabolism, plus enzymes that provide flexibility to moveable joints, blood vessels and bones. Cashews are a complete protein food, but low in phenylalanine and methionine. To gain protein balance, add a few almonds and one brazil nut, with an apple for a perfect protein snack. Nearly 40% of the daily protein from one handful. Cashews are rich in magnesium 70% d.v. phosphorus 60% d.v. Cashews are soft and great for children and everybody. Cashews are worth their weight in organic copper and brain minerals, plus their pure energy value is wonderful.

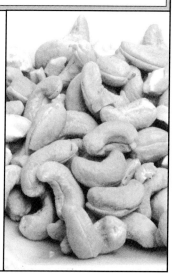

CHESTNUT	Castanea sativa	C. 89	P. 7	L. 4	CALORIES - total: **224 kcal. per 100 gram** Calories from: Carb:200 Protein:15 Fat:9

Chestnuts grow on trees and in water, the sweet chestnut *(Castanea sativa)* grows on trees and belongs to the oak family. The water chestnuts include caltrops *(Trapa natans)* and the Chinese water chestnut (Eleocharis tuberosa).

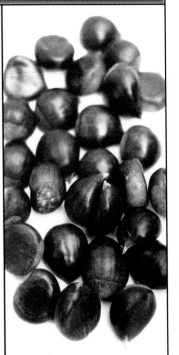

Chestnuts have the lowest calorie and fat content of any nut, 1 g and even when roasted in their shell, as traditional in Switzerland and France, there are no problems with free radicals, as the chestnut is nearly a pure carbohydrate nut 49 g. On a freezing cold day, a bag of roasted chestnuts is better than an ice cream on a boiling hot day. Chestnuts have a soft texture when roasted or boiled and children love the experience of roasting them by the fire place. It is best to slit the soft shell, to avoid explosions, but the 'boys' think that's a blast, but be careful.

Chestnuts supply good amounts of potassium 447 mg, magnesium 21% d.v., the second best nut source of vitamin A 200 I.U. and the best nut source of vitamin C 36 mg.

Chestnuts need cooking to eliminate the *tannic acid* content. In France the chestnut is a delicacy. The Maroon chestnut is top quality and in Italy the chestnut is a staple food and often ground into flour to make *farina dolce,* a specialist bread.

Chestnuts are a good source of folic acid 68 mcg, more than peas. Roasted chestnuts are the ideal food for anybody, they are the least 'fattening' of all nuts. Chestnuts are the 'look alike heart nuts'!

COCONUT	Cocos nucifera	C. 11	P. 8	L. 81	CALORIES - total: **628 kcal. per 100 gram** Calories from: Carb:68 Protein:52 Fat:508

Coconut are the biggest nut and it has been named the 'tree that sustains life' from the Sanskrit *'kalpha vrisha',* as it provides food, shelter and a delicious milk drink, also used for numerous recipes. The coconut 'meat' is termed *copra,* available as shredded or desiccated, it is great in numerous recipes and coconut cream makes a dream dish come true.

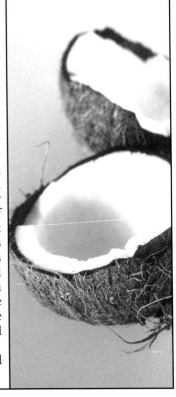

Coconut is a very satisfying food, it would be nearly impossible to eat a whole coconut. The rich supply of saturated fats is the main reason. Coconut contains 32 g of fat with 30 g as saturated fats, with no polyunsaturated fats and 2 g mono fats. Ideally, saturated fats are best avoided as they raise blood cholesterol levels, The only saving grace is that coconut is eaten raw and therefore the 'free radical' problem is eliminated. If you were marooned on a tropical island and coconut was the only food, for two weeks, you may actually get less saturated fats than the average city dweller reliant on take away foods. Coconut also provides a great supply of very beneficial fibre 9 g, stacks more than take away foods. Coconut fibre can destroy tapeworms from ingested, infected meat and it is an ideal snack for protection against constipation. Coconut milk is used for relief from stomach ulcers and sore throats in traditional tropical treatments. Half the battle in the city, is to find a fresh coconut, one that has not been allowed to ferment, but, is ripe. The taste from a quality coconut is so great, 'lucky' it's hard to eat large quantities. Coconut supply a fair amount of potassium 356 mg and a good supply of beneficial organic sodium 20 mg.

Crack open a coconut next time you need a completely cool and super satisfying snack.

HAZEL NUTS	*Corylus avellana*	C.	P.	L.	CALORIES - total: **628 kcal. per 100 gram**
		11	8	81	Calories from: Carb:68 Protein:52 Fat:508

Hazel nuts are a member of the Corylus family of trees and depending on their country of cultivation, hazel nuts may also be termed as Filberts or Cob nut. Hazel nuts are the second best nut sources of vitamin E 15 -20 mg, with the almond nut supplying 26 mg of vitamin E. A handful of hazel nuts is a most beneficial substitute for any vitamin E capsule. Hazel nuts are a fair source of Omega 6, 4 g, which in combination with vitamin E is vital for healthy arteries, regulation of cholesterol levels and prevention of heart disease.

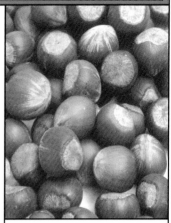

Hazel nuts are also a good source of zinc 2 mg, the mineral that is required for the breakdown of alcohol and also used as a vital component of insulin. Hazel nuts supply a fair amounts of calcium 110 mg, potassium 680 mg, phosphorus 290 mg and a very good supply of magnesium 160 mg. The supply of copper from hazel nuts is excellent 90% d.v. and in combination with the very good iron content 5 mg or 26% d.v. plus manganese 6 mg, the hazel nut is a blood builder, complete with all the tools required. All of the basic B group vitamins are supplied especially B1 43% d.v. and b6 28% d.v. The protein value 21 g of hazel nuts is complete in all essential amino acids and in order to obtain very good protein value, combine hazel nuts with cashews and brazil nuts and a few almonds. Hazel nuts are used in spreads, try the pure spread, it's fantastic.

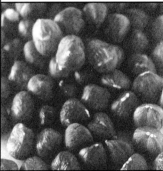

Hazel nuts are often roasted, they taste nice but may contain free radicals and by the time you buy them, they can be of minimum value. For maximum benefits, raw hazel nuts are 'ridgey didgey' in Australian terms, or authentic!

MACADAMIA	*Macadamia ternifolia*	C.	P.	L.	CALORIES - total: **718 kcal. per 100 gram**
		8	4	88	Calories from: Carb:56 Protein:27 Fat:634

Macadamia nuts are also called the Queensland nut, native to north eastern Australia. Macadamia nuts are the hardest nut to crack and thanks to some inventors, it can now be easily achieved and well worth the effort. Macadamia nuts are soft inside, full of monounsaturated lipids 60 g from a total 76 g with polyunsaturated 3 g and saturated 13 g, but, no cholesterol and no risk of free radicals, unless they are really roasted.

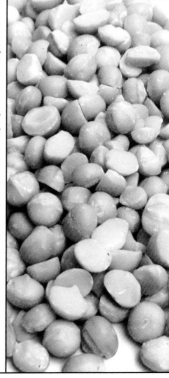

Macadamia nuts raw, are the richest nut source of monounsaturated lipids. They are nearly a unique source of *palmitoleic acid*, a monounsaturated fatty acid that assists in fat metabolism. This will help the body to use the fat efficiently as an energy source. Macadamia nuts supply 6% more oleic acid than olive oil. Macadamia nuts contain vitamin E 1 mg plus flavonoids that provide antioxidant benefits and combined with the good supply of copper 38% d.v., the antioxidant power is increased.

Macadamia nuts provide a fair supply of fibre 9 g or 36% d.v. or 136% more than meat or fish. Macadamia nuts make a perfect addition to a fruit salad, or a garden salad, no need for an oil dressing, unless it's a splash of delightful macadamia oil. Macadamia are a complete protein food 8 g or 16% d.v. and when combined with a breakfast cereal, the protein value increases to match the common meat meal. A few macadamia's go a long way to satisfy the appetite, unsalted are best, nutritionally. When you need a big energy boost, macadamia nuts are cracked up for the job.

PECAN NUTS	*Carya illinoensis*	C.	P.	L.	CALORIES - total: **691 kcal. per 100 gram**
		8	5	87	**Calories from:** Carb:57 Protein:32 Fat:602

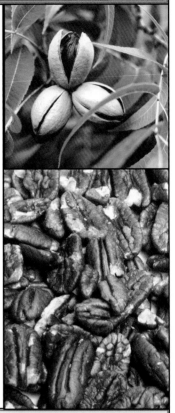

Pecan nuts are similar to hickory nuts. Pecan nuts are the second best nut source of lipids 72 g, macadamia's 76 g and pecans have half the saturated fat 6 g and ten times the polyunsaturated content 22 g of the macadamia

In a four week study, when the pecan nut diet replaced a controlled low fat diet, it lowered cholesterol by 6.7%, low density lipoproteins by 10% and triglycerides by 11% compared to the low fat diet, both with the same calorie intake.

When pecan nuts replace potato chips as a common snack food, the benefits would be even greater, as the free radicals from cooked chips is enormous. Try a handful of pecan nuts with an apple, or try a slice of pecan nut pie for that full stomach feeling, instead of chips, the benefits are enormous.

Pecan nuts are a good source of phosphorus 277 mg or 28% d.v., plus, the magnesium content 121 mg or 30%d.v. gives the pecan nut the right to claim itself as a brain food, as the magnesium content is four times that of perch - fish 30 mg, however there are 11 grams less of protein 9 g but 4% more potassium 410 mg.

Pecan nuts are a good source of dietary fibre 10 g or 31% d.v, vitamin B1 44% d.v, plus an excellent source of copper 60% d.v. and a small amount of vitamin E 1 mg, all these factors provide antioxidant benefits. Pecan nuts supply a fair portion of complete protein 9 g. Pecan nuts are not big in protein but they are great in recipes.

Pecan nuts are a most popular nut in the USA. Try a piece of pecan pie with a scoop of ice cream, it's delightful!

PINE NUTS	*Pinus pinea*	C.	P.	L.	CALORIES - total: **673 kcal. per 100 gram**
		8	7	85	**Calories from:** Carb:53 Protein:48 Fat:572

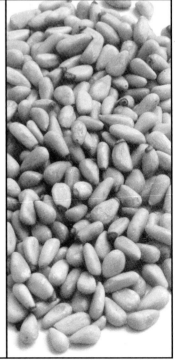

Pine nuts are also termed pignolia, they grow inside a large pine cone, from a native tree of Italy. They are used in the famous *pesto* recipe and often used in stuffings and tossed onto salads, including fruit salads such as the *strawberry pignolia* recipe. Pine nuts are best used in cooking to reduce the turpentine flavour from the supply of lipids 68 g or 105% d.v., with 50% in the form of polyunsaturated 34 g, one gram of Omega 3 and 25 grams of Omega 6. The mono unsaturated is 19 g and saturated 5 g. Pine nuts provide complete protein 14 g or 27% d.v and their protein is 50% useable.

Pine nuts are full of phosphorus 575 mg or 60% d.v. and this will promote utilization of the high calorie and fat content and benefit the nervous system, improve memory abilities and stimulate blood circulation. The magnesium content is excellent 250 mg. or 63% d.v., more than almonds and a real treat for the nervous system. Magnesium nourishes the white nerve fibres of the brain and spinal cord and 70% of magnesium is contained in the bone structure. Pine nuts are a fair source of folate, for the nervous system and brain. If you think you're going nuts up top, pine nuts are tops in brain nutrition. The iron 6 mg, copper 1mg, and manganese 4.3 mg are all very well supplied and for the blood system, pine nuts are full of power, with 3 times the iron of beef, 4,000 times the manganese and 150 times the copper. Pine nuts are waiting to beef up the blood building and brain benefits of the standard diet.

PISTACHIO NUTS	*Pistachia vera*	C.	P.	L.	CALORIES - total: **557 kcal. per 100 gram**
		20	13	67	Calories from: Carb:114 Protein:72 Fat:372

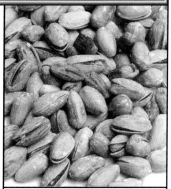

Pistachio nuts are the best nut-source of phytosterols, more specifically beta-sitoserol 198 mcg which provides protection from some forms of cancer and it also assists in blood cholesterol reduction, in combination with the good supply of monounsaturated lipids 23 g. Pistachio nuts have a low saturated fat content 5 g and a fair polyunsaturated fat content 13 g.

Pistachio are the richest nut source of the mineral potassium 1,025 mg and combined with the supply of mono unsaturated lipids, the pistachio nut is a bonus for blood circulation, if they are not salted. Potassium is destroyed by excess coffee and alcohol consumption. A handful of pistachio's after a 'hard day's night' will really help and with the good supply of B vitamins, especially B1 and B6, the pistachio benefits will boost the heart and calm the nerves. In addition, the magnesium content 125 mg or 30 d.v. will also relax the nerves and replace the loss from those extra drinks after work and protect against heart attacks. Pistachio nuts are tiny in size but huge in potassium and heart pumping benefits. They also contain calcium 107 mg, vitamin A 553 I.U. and lots of copper 65% d.v. and vitamin E 2 mg, also of benefit for the heart muscles. The supply of zinc 2 mg is vital especially for people who drink alcohol regularly. Pistachio nuts are ready to protect you!

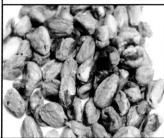

WALNUTS	*Juglans regia - nigra*	C.	P.	L.	CALORIES - total: **654 kcal. per 100 gram**
		9	8	83	Calories from: Carb:55 Protein:53 Fat:546

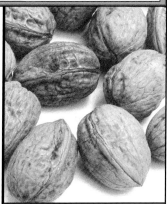

Walnuts are a valuable food for many reasons, the excellent supply of omega 3, 5.5 g is unique, as most nuts and foods supply none or only a trace amount of Omega 3. Walnuts are the richest nut source of both the 'essential fatty acids', refer to page 134. Walnuts are an Omega 3 treat as they need no cooking and therefore the oils, refer page 145, are at their maximum effectiveness especially with their good supply of biotin 1.3 mcg which assists fat metabolism.

Walnuts are a good source of folate 98 mcg, more than spinach and as folate is heat sensitive, the walnut wins the race, especially during pregnancy, as folate is essential for development of babies, plus the good iron content 3 mg and protein supply 15 g or 30% d.v. all promote healthy growth of babies.

The rich supply of polyunsaturated lipids 47 g helps to lower cholesterol. Walnuts are a good source of phosphorus 346 mg or 35%d.v. plus magnesium 158 mg or 40% d.v., both required for the brain and in addition, the great supply of Omega 3, as brain cells or neurons need omega 3. It promotes a flexible and fluid transfer of nutrients within brain cells and is vital for the development of the infants brain.

Walnuts are the best look-alike brain food on the planet. The human brain is composed of 60% fat and ideally, for maximum brain power, it is best made up from Omega 3 fats. Give your brain a regular top up with walnut oil. The iron content plus manganese 3 mg, plus copper 2 mg is great for blood building and the zinc 3 mg is vital for hormone production and development of children's bones. Walnuts on toast with honey is simple, sweet, inexpensive and full of Omega 3's plus mother and baby benefits. Walnuts are one of the first steps you can take for your baby. Walnuts are the best balanced nut. Refer to page 218 for walnut recipes.

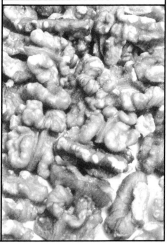

NUTS, SEEDS & SPROUTS SUMMARY CHARTS

NUTS	MAIN NUTRIENTS, ANTIOXIDANTS & PHYTONUTRIENTS	BODY SYSTEMS TO BENEFIT.
Almonds	vitamin e, protein, magnesium, phosphorus, manganese, calcium, biotin, lipids.	skeletal, nervous, brain.
Brazil	selenium, methionine, phosphorus, protein, potassium, magnesium, lipids.	immune, growth, repair
Cashew	oleic acid, copper, protein, magnesium, phosphorus, lipids.	brain, joint, circulatory
Chestnut	carbohydrate, potassium, magnesium, vitamin c, folate, lipids	muscular, blood, nervous.
Coconut	fibre, sodium, potassium.	elimination.
Hazel nuts	vitamin e, magnesium, copper, iron, manganese, b vitamins, protein, lipids.	blood, nervous, circulatory.
Macadamia	copper, fibre, lipids, protein.	muscular
Pecan	copper, phosphorus, magnesium, potassium, fibre, protein, lipids.	brain, blood.
Pine	protein, phosphorus, magnesium, folate, iron, copper, manganese, lipids.	nervous, brain, blood.
Pistachio	phytosterols, potassium, magnesium, vitamin a, copper, zinc, lipids, protein.	immune, circulatory, muscular.
Walnut	omega 3, folate, iron, phosphorus, magnesium, manganese, copper, zinc, lipids.	brain, growth, cellular, blood.
SEEDS		
Pepitas	iron, protein, omega 3, phosphorus, magnesium, cucurbitacins, zinc, copper.	blood, brain, nervous, repair.
Sunflower	vitamin e, protein, magnesium, copper, phosphorus, silicon, potassium, selenium, zinc, iron, lipids, b vitamins.	circulatory, growth, nervous, brain, joint, skin, muscular.
Sesame	protein, methionine, calcium, fibre, copper, iron, magnesium, phosphorus, zinc, lecithin, phytosterols, manganese, folate.	blood, nervous, brain, digestive, joint, skeletal, growth.
SPROUTS		
Alfalfa	phytoestrogens, iron, vitamin a, copper, selenium, cobalt, vitamin k & p.	blood, urinary, immune.
Buckwheat	rutin, magnesium, phosphorus, copper, zinc, iron.	circulatory, brain.
Wheat grass	lycopene, chlorophyll, vitamin a, vitamin k, iron, cobalt, copper, manganese, potassium, selenium, sulphur, zinc, magnesium, vitamin c, vitamin e, fibre.	immune, blood, repair, respiratory, circulatory, brain, skin, elimination.

NUTS & SEEDS -BALANCED DIET- DAILY PROTEIN & LIPID INTAKE

TOTAL DAILY (R.D.I.) PROTEIN INTAKE	ADULT MALE	ADULT FEMALE	TEENAGER	CHILDREN
	60 grams	47 grams	65 grams	45 grams
NUTS 25 % DAILY - LAUGH WITH HEALTH DIET	15 grams	12 grams	16 grams	11 grams
SEEDS 10% DAILY LAUGH WITH HEALTH	6 grams	5 grams	6.5 grams	4 .5 grams
100 g NUTS* or SEEDS* (average)* (refer below) = 23 grams of PROTEIN	65 grams	52 grams	69 grams	47 grams
U.S. FOOD PYRAMID TOTAL PROTEIN INTAKE: (includes: meat, poultry, fish, legumes, eggs , nuts and seeds).	1 - 3 serves	1 - 2 serves	1 - 3 serves	1 serve
AUSTRALIAN HEALTHY EATING GUIDE TOTAL PROTEIN FOOD DAILY INTAKE includes: meat, fish, poultry, eggs and nuts. Does not include legumes.	1 serve	1 serve	1 serve	1 serve

1 serve is equivalent to: half a cup of almonds or peanuts, or, one quarter of a cup of sunflower seeds , or, 80 - 120 grams cooked fish fillets, or 2 small eggs, or, 65-100 g cooked meat or chicken.

TOTAL DAILY (R.D.I.) LIPID INTAKE	ADULT MALE	ADULT FEMALE	TEENAGER	CHILDREN
	58 grams	50 grams	60 grams	44 grams
NUTS 25% DAILY - LAUGH WITH HEALTH DIET	14 grams	12 grams	15 grams	11 grams
SEEDS 10% DAILY - LAUGH WITH HEALTH DIET	6 grams	5 grams	6 grams	4 grams
100 g NUTS : almonds, brazil & cashew mix (average)* = 78 grams of LIPIDS	17 grams	15 grams	19 grams	14 grams
100 g SEEDS: pepitas, sesame & sunflower (average)* = 48 grams of LIPIDS	29 grams	25 grams	31 grams	23 grams
FOOD PYRAMID (TOTAL LIPID INTAKE). Includes: added lipids, not dairy or meat.	Use sparingly.			
AUSTRALIAN HEALTHY EATING GUIDE (TOTAL LIPID INTAKE) Includes added lipids. Does not include: dairy or meat.	Sometimes, or, in small amounts.			

* The average is calculated from a combination of : NUTS: almonds, brazil & cashews. SEEDS: pepitas, sesame & sunflower.

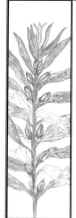

Seeds are the beginning of life. Seeds are the most compact form of life. Seeds are the universal code of nature. Seeds are latent life. Seeds are the force behind regeneration of new life, they are the most valuable asset of mankind.

From one seed we can assist nature and progressively create an infinitesimal number of the same species. The seed you plant today will need care and attention and when fully developed, that seed will return the favour and supply you with an abundance of food for enjoyment and nutrition and energy requirements.

The following pages describe the main benefits associated with the most common edible seeds: pumpkin, sesame and sunflower as well as a section on sprouting seeds.

When seeds are eaten, they provide their individual life-force and no other food-group is more compact and generous. A handful of sesame seeds may contain near five hundred individual life units, their capacity to promote your health and life are second to none. In contrast to animal products, seeds are a vital food, seeds contain no cholesterol, seeds are easy to digest, seeds are ready to sprout into life; there is no life ahead, without the seed kingdom.

A well balanced diet must include seeds, they are full of complete protein, essential oils and they provide a unique supply of essential nutrients and trace elements.

Pepitas, sesame and sunflower seeds are compatible with various fruits, nearly all vegetables, whole grains and some legume combinations.

Refer to chart page 208 for details on food combination ideas.

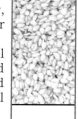

Seeds can be combined in numerous delicious ways, all depending on your imagination, range of recipes and purchase of such food.

If you have never tried any of the three basic edible seeds: pumpkin-pepitas, sesame and sunflower, you can greatly improve your health and range of recipes.

Even though seeds appear small and neglected in the packaged form, consider the colourful and abundant growth of their original source.

Numerous varieties of handy takeaway snack packs now include the seeds, they are a very good alternative to chocolate bars, the sesame bar, the pepita and honey crunch and the sunflower coated energy bars are really full of benefits. Pass me a pepita bar, please Papa!

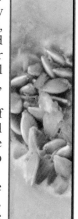

Seeds are an excellent source of numerous minerals, vitamins and the protein content is complete with an excellent supply of amino acids.

Seeds are also a source of the essential fatty acids, in particular, pepitas, or pumpkin seeds are the second richest natural source of omega 3.

For a guide to the ways to add seeds to your daily diet, refer to page 219. It is surprising how many basic meals can improve greatly with the addition of seeds, especially ground seeds sprinkled on top of the breakfast cereal, or pasta. Seeds can make a meal into a nutritional feast.

Seeds are unique providers of substances to protect against common ailments.

The following pages will describe the main benefits from pepitas, sesame and sunflower seeds.

Make the most of seeds, they are ready to multiply your nutritional intake and provide abundant benefits.

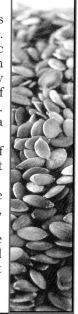

NOTE: All amounts provided in this book are measured in mg. per 100 gram serves, unless otherwise stated.

PUMPKIN SEEDS - PEPITAS *Cucurbitaceae*

CALORIES - total: **541 kcal. per 100 gram**
Calories from: Carb:72 Protein:85 Fat:384

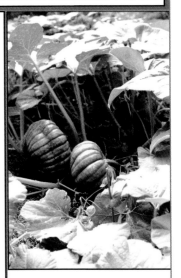

From the mighty golden pumpkin, one of the greatest natural foods is often forgotten when considering a highly nutritious diet. The seeds from the pumpkin, are often referred to as *pepitas,* a name that is derived from the Greek word *'pepon'* and translated as 'cooked in the sun'. Pepitas are available at most health stores and supermarkets. When purchasing pumpkin seeds, be sure to obtain only the inner kernel of the seed, usually a flat seed with a dark green/grey colour, as the outer white shell is gritty.

Amongst the numerous benefits of the pepitas, the organic iron content 11 -14 mg is second best in the world, apart from mussels with 14.9 mg. The small amount of vitamin C 1.9 mg will help with iron absorption. When compared to lean beef, 3.1 mg and spinach 3.2 mg, pepitas are four times the 'iron proof value' and a small 100 gram serve will provide over 80% of daily iron values. For a big iron boost, in cases of anaemia or after a big operation, or menstruation loss, pepitas provide proper recovery. For a few hints on how to use the tiny pepita seeds, place a cupful in a grinder or blender to produce a ground mixture or 'pepi-mix', add to any soups, or sprinkle over a fresh garden salad and for the best Italian pasta recipe, added to a pasta sauce, or sprinkled over the pasta and cheese, it's incredibly nourishing, with a nutty texture.

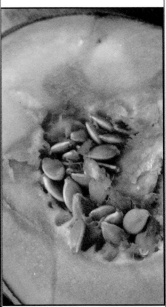

Pepitas are an excellent protein food 24.5 g or 50% of the daily protein requirement from a small 100 gram serve, now that's potent protein. Pepitas have a low saturated fat content of 9 g, a good supply of mono unsaturated 14 g and polyunsaturated lipids 21 g with an excellent supply of precious Omega 3, 7-10 g and Omega 6, 20 g. Compared to fish 0.1 - 2.2 g omega 3, pepitas are the champion omega 3 food and they really need to take prime place in every pantry. Amongst the numerous mineral benefits from pepitas, the phosphorus 1,174 mg or 117% d.v. and magnesium 535 mg or 134% d.v. is exceptional and when considering 'brain foods' pepitas get honours with distinction. Compared to fish or beef, pepitas supply over 5 times the phosphorus and with magnesium, over 17 times. The excellent supply of phosphorus promotes healing of bone fractures, concentration, growth, blood circulation and brain function.

Pepitas contain a potent source of cucurbitacins, ideal for protection and relief from enlarged prostrate glands (prostatis), as the cucurbitacins retard the conversion of the male hormone testosterone, into a more complex and potent hormone: *dihydrotestosterone* which is used by the body to produce prostrate cells. In addition, the excellent supply of zinc 7.5 mg or 50% d.v. also assists to reduce prostrate gland enlargement and it is essential for insulin conversion and protection from diabetes, ulcers, acne, dermatitis and it is vital for bone repair. The supply of the mineral copper 1.4 mg is a bonus for iron absorption, plus, pepitas supply manganese, also essential for iron absorption and as an antioxidant and for brain functioning, memory and regulating of menstrual cycles. Pepitas are a vital food for every man and woman, especially in this era of highly processed foods where the minerals zinc, copper, magnesium and phosphorus are practically swept off the factory floor. Pepitas provide anti-inflammatory power against arthritis and for a life of bliss, strength and good health, pepitas are a priority with pompous power.

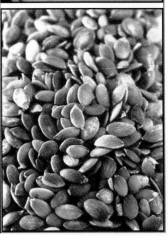

NOTE: d.v. refers to daily value for woman 25 - 50 years, refer to RDA chart page 69 for adult male and children values.

SUNFLOWER SEEDS *Helianthus annuus*

CALORIES - total: **570 kcal. per 100 gram**
Calories from: Carb:76 Protein:79 Fat:415

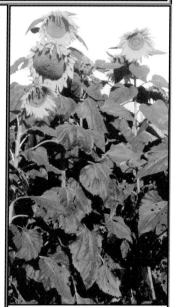

Sunflower plants attract the suns's energy all day long with a happy golden face full of amazing nutritional benefits. The name sunflower is adapted from the botanical name and Greek words helios-sun and anthos-flower. For thousands of years, originating in Mexico and Peru, the sunflower plant has provided nourishment and herbal benefits from the seeds, stems and flowers. Within the enormous sunflower, hundreds of seeds develop and for edible purposes, the inner kernel of the seed is used, unless you are a cockatoo and live for 100 years, entirely on the whole sunflower seed.

Sunflower seeds are the richest natural food source of vitamin E 31-35 mg or 115% d.v. A regular intake of sunflower seeds will promote protection from ageing, free radicals and skin cell damage, as vitamin E is a powerful antioxidant. Delicious cookies or pancakes, refer to page 219 can be made with the sunflower kernels, or grind them and sprinkle over a fruit salad, or add them to your daily breakfast cereal, they have a soft nutty texture and are grey in colour. A sunflower butter spread is also delightful on the breakfast toast.

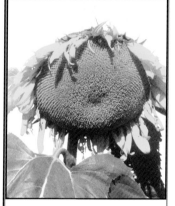

Sunflower kernels are low in saturated fat 5 g and a good source of mono unsaturated 9.5 g and polyunsaturated 33 g, mainly in the form of Omega 6, 30 g with a trace of Omega 3. The protein content of sunflower seeds is complete in all essential amino acids and they supply 23% protein and are the 10th. best protein food with 58% useable protein (n.p.u.). The supply of minerals, especially magnesium 354 mg is very good with the copper value 1.8 mg or 85% d.v. also abundant and vital for blood development, skin healing, nerve fibre protection and cartilage repair. For a big natural vitamin B1 boost, sunflower seeds provide 2.3 mg or 115% d.v. plus B2 0.3 mg and B3 4.5 mg or 23% d.v.

The price of sunflower kernels is really a big bright bonus, considering the effort involved and for added nutritional value to cookies, they are very worthwhile. The supply of phosphorus 700 mg or 70% d.v. is most beneficial for the brain, nerves, bones and in combination with the abundant supply of silicon 554 mg, also essential for the brain, nerves and bones, sunflower kernels will keep you thinking straight and walking strong. The supply of calcium 354 mg or 12% d.v. is good and the supply of potassium 700 - 900 mg or 20% daily value all add up to promote strong muscular action and proper digestion. Sunflower meal is available at most health stores, it is a rich source of protein 57% with no fat content. Sunflower meal can be added to home made bread or mixed with honey for a delicious spread, does that rhyme!

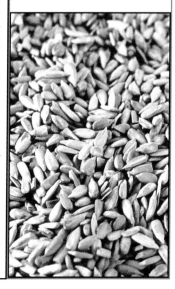

The selenium content of the kernels is very good with 59 mcg, as 70 - 80 mcg is the daily requirement, plus with the exceptional vitamin E content, the sunflower seed is a potent antioxidant. Selenium works with vitamin E to protect against free radicals and promote DNA repair and also to induce *apoptosis* or the self destruction of cancerous cells.

Sunflower kernels are an excellent source of zinc 5 mg, essential to fight infections and for body healing. Also, sunflower seeds are ideal for the reproductive system, in combination with the abundant vitamin E content. The supply of manganese 2 mg and iron 7 mg are further proof that the sunflower is the brightest supplier of surprising sun filled health benefits.

CALORIES - total: **573 kcal. per 100 gram**		
Calories from: Carb:96	Protein:61	Fat:416

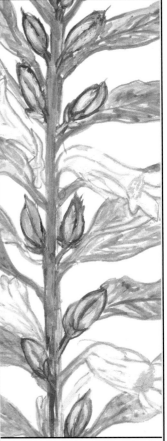

Sesame seeds have been cultivated for thousands of years, a native plant of Africa, Turkey and Arabia and a staple food in China and India. The sesame seed is referred to as the 'seed of immortality' and without doubt, some of the nutrient benefits promote long life plus the seed can last for ages after harvesting, as the substance: sesamol, unique to sesame seeds prevents the oxidation and deterioration of the precious oils. Nearly half the seed weight is made up from oils 49 g with a low saturated content 7 g, mono 19 g and polyunsaturated 23 g. Sesame seeds provide Omega 6 25 g and only a trace of Omega 3.

The protein value of sesame seeds is excellent 19 g whole and 18 g hulled. The rich supply of the amino acid methionine 637 mg promotes the metabolism of fats plus it offsets the common low supply of methionine from numerous other foods, when considering complete protein and a well balanced supply of amino acids. A small amount of ground sesame seeds added to the vegetable soup, bread or legume dish will greatly boost protein value. Sesame seeds are not easy to completely digest, unless they are ground into a paste, or tahini, halva or sesame-meal, for use in numerous recipes: cakes, biscuits, over fruit salad or mixed into vegetable burgers.

The calcium content of sesame seeds is excellent 900 - 1,100 mg or 100% d.v. Sesame seeds, ground, are the ideal non dairy calcium food and they provide more calcium than cheddar cheese 775 mg and no cholesterol. In addition, sesame seeds provide special fibres, termed *lignans* that actually lower blood cholesterol. Tahini supplies 420 mg of calcium.

The supply of the trace mineral copper is abundant 4.1 mg or 200% d.v. It provides benefits in cases of rheumatoid arthritis, as copper is part of the enzyme that reduces inflammation, plus, copper is required for the production of elastin and collagen. Apart from liver, sesame seeds are the best copper food. The supply of vitamins B1, B2, B3, B5 and B6 is very good. For an excellent supply of iron, sesame seeds provide 10 - 14 mg, or, 60 - 80% d.v. The supply of magnesium 350 mg or 80% d.v. assists sleep patterns, promotes steady nerves and may reduce migraine attacks, as magnesium reduces the *trigeminal* blood vessels from spasms which cause the pain. Sesame seeds are full of phosphorus 630 mg and zinc 7.8 mg, both values over 50% daily value. The old saying 'open sesame' originates from the fact that as soon as the sesame plant has ripened, the seeds pop out of the pods and scatter on the ground.

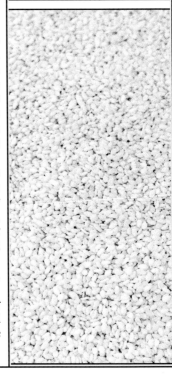

Sesame seeds are an excellent source of lecithin, required for the dissolving of fats and reduction of cholesterol. Sesame seeds contain no cholesterol and they are a rich source of phytosterols 714 mg or plant sterols that inhibit the absorption of cholesterol. In addition, phytosterols can assist with the control of blood sugar levels for diabetics, reduce prostrate enlargements and inflammation from rheumatoid arthritis.

Sesame seeds also supply manganese 2.5 mg, potassium 468 mg, selenium 5.7 mg and folate 97 mcg.

Sesame seeds decorate the daily bread rolls, but, let your imagination, some traditional sesame recipes and the super small seeds loose in your kitchen and open doors for a variety of sesame sensations.

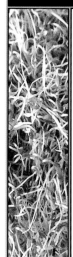

Sprouting seeds, grains and legumes is by no means a recent discovery. Over 3,000 years ago, the Chinese discovered the potential of sprouted foods and now, with modern methods of food analysis, the wisdom of their ways is revealed.

In this era, many people are still unaware of the potential of sprouted foods and unaccustomed to the ways of preparation and combination of sprouted foods with other meals. Throughout this section on sprouting, you may discover (if not already) the methods of sprouting preparation, their associated benefits and a few basic ways to include sprouted foods with other common foods.

Sprouting is a basic natural development, the original seed is transformed from a state of latent energy into a complete living form with the assistance of water, air and sunlight.

Sprouting is also termed 'seed germination'. As the seed begins to sprout, elements contained in the seed are used to provide energy, the starches contained in the seed are slowly converted into natural sugars, the protein content of the seed is transformed into available amino acids and the fat content is converted into natural sugars.

All these changes during the sprouting stage improve the nutrient quality and digestion of seeds - grains and legumes. After a few days of seed development, the most substantial contribution from that time is the 'life-rate activity' within the seed, often termed the 'enzyme activity'.

The human body requires regular supplies of various enzymes for digestion, nutrient absorption, body development and repair. Enzymes are the catalyst for all living development.

Sprouted foods are one of the best sources of living enzymes.

Apart from fruits, vegetables and sprouted foods there are very few foods that contain living enzymes. Nearly all processed and refined foods are deficient in enzyme content.

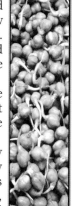

All cooked foods have very little enzyme content and without enzymes, a food cannot provide maximum nutritional benefits.

Sprouted foods are very economical. One tablespoon of raw seeds may cost about 10 cents however, when fully developed, there will be enough sprouts to fill a large salad bowl.

Sprouted foods provide a good source of vitamin C and various B group vitamins as well as a good supply of the amino acids - protein and other amino acids and such 'hard to get' vitamins as: P, K and U are all obtainable from a variety of sprouted foods.

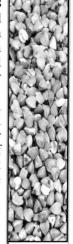

The mineral content of sprouted foods is based on the original source: whole grain, legume or seed. Sprouts are a good source of trace minerals. You can start sprouting the seed of your choice today!.

Sprouted foods are a most valuable addition to the regular diet, especially for overweight people.

A large number of overweight people have developed such a condition due to a decreasing rate of their metabolism, often due to a prolonged lack of essential living enzymes from the cooked foods eaten.

An overweight person can obtain excellent low calorie, low fat, regenerative energy from a regular supply of sprouted foods, fresh fruits and vegetables.

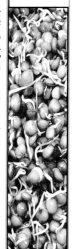

Sprout off those excess kilos. There are many recipes and ways to make sprouts taste nice. Too busy to make sprouts! Try your local sproutmarket, supermarket.

NOTE: All amounts provided in this book are measured in g. per 100 gram serves, unless otherwise stated

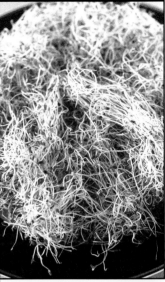

Alfalfa sprouts are one of the most popular, available at nearly every supermarket and health food store. From the tiny alfalfa seed, great health benefits can be obtained, in fact, when considered in the *dry weight*, as 90% of the sprouts weight is water, the alfalfa sprouts provides an enormous amounts of nutrients.

For example, the calcium content 1,750 mg is better than any cheese-parmesan 1,100 mg. The iron content 35 mg and vitamin A 44,000 I.U. are enormous. Ensure that your alfalfa sprouts are fresh and rinsed properly, to obtain the benefits and nice flavour. In comparison to lettuce and spinach, alfalfa sprouts provide over three times the value of calcium, iron and magnesium and for a super salad, alfalfa sprouts with tahini provides complete protein. On their own, alfalfa sprouts are not a complete protein food as they lack 4 amino acids.

In their fresh state, alfalfa sprouts provide trace minerals such as zinc 0.9 mg, copper 0.2 mg selenium 0.6 mcg and manganese 0.2 mg plus cobalt. In the dry weight, values for molybdenum 2.6 ppm have been recorded. A regular serve of alfalfa sprouts can promote blood building and cleansing; elimination of excess body acids via the urinary system.

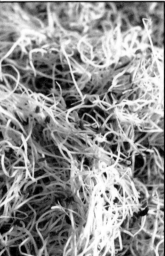

Alfalfa sprouts also provide a good supply of vitamin K 30 mcg plus vitamin P and in their dry weight, a measure of vitamin B12, 0.3 mg has also been recorded. The vitamin C content is low 8 mg but a slice of red capsicum will easily increase the supply. All the basic B vitamins are supplied in small amounts with alfalfa sprouts. A note of *caution* for persons with inflammatory or auto-immune system problems; high levels of the amino acid *canavanine*, in alfalfa sprouts, may cause such conditions to be irritated.

On a positive note, alfalfa sprouts have proven very beneficial in preventing the bacteria (helicobacter pylori) that causes stomach ulcers.

Alfalfa sprouts are a very good source of phytoestrogens, used by the body as antioxidants and for prevention of menopausal symptoms, osteoporosis, heart disease and cancer. Let the freshly prepared alfalfa sprouts add life and a beneficial bounce to your daily bread.

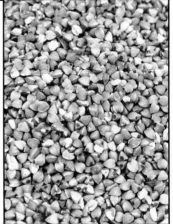

Buckwheat sprouts are hard to get and fairly easy to grow. The benefits from this relative of rhubarb are remarkable. Buckwheat and sprouts are the best natural food source of rutin, a bioflavonoid and a component of vitamin P, vital for healing of varicose veins, poor blood circulation and hardened arteries. Buckwheat sprouts promote the health of your circulatory system, plus, the good supply of potassium 350 - 460 mg will enhance the functions of rutin. Buckwheat can also be used as a breakfast cereal and obtained as buckwheat groats and cooked like rice. The magnesium content 231 mg or 58% d.v. is very good for the nervous system and combined with the phosphorus 347 mg, the brain system also benefits. The supply of copper 1.1 mg or 55% d.v. and zinc 2.4 mg will promote healing and blood development in addition to the iron content 2.2 mg. Buckwheat sprouts will help you to circulate all over!

| LENTIL SPROUTS | C. P. L.
75 21 4 | CALORIES - total: **106 kcal. per 100 gram**
Calories from: Carb:80 Protein:22 Fat:4 |

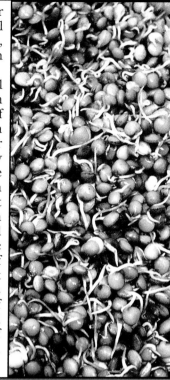

Lentil sprouts provide more iron 3.1 mg than any other sprouts, or milk, cheese, egg, lettuce or spinach. Lentil sprouts are the ideal way to obtain the maximum benefits from the lentil legume, including a very low calorie content and a fair but complete protein supply 9 g and a very low fat content 0.5 g.

Very few foods compare to the lean weight watching power of lentil sprouts. During the sprouting stage, various changes in the protein and carbohydrate content 22 g occurs to improve the digestion of the compact lentil. There are numerous recipes for lentils but often they do not include sprouted lentils, plus they may contain poor combinations. Ideally, lentils sprouts combine best with leafy vegetables and cottage cheese for a simple waist saver, or add the lentil sprouts last and make a great lentil vegetable soup, with carrots, spinach, broccoli and parmesan cheese. For the cheapest meal in town, try lentil sprouts with rice and increase the protein value by 30% for no extra charge. Fresh lentil sprouts are a good source of vitamin C 17 mg or 30% d.v plus they provide all the basic B vitamins, especially folate 100 mcg or 25% d.v. Keep a supply of lentils in your pantry for when times get tough, they can sprout new life into the kitchen and provide an abundance of energy. Lentils have been referred to as poor man's meat, but, they have none of the problems associated with meat, no saturated fat, no cholesterol and no free radicals. Let lentil sprouts into your life, add a bit of authentic flavour with spices and herbs for a lean lentil lunch and a big boost to the blood system.

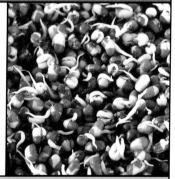

The Chinese discovered the method and preparation of mung bean sprouts, over 3,000 years ago and today, people from around the world are utilizing an important part of Chinese culture and cuisine. Mung bean sprouts provide extra benefits such as: an increase in protein availability from 23 grams up to 37 grams per 100 gram portion, complete in all the essential amino acids. The supply of B group vitamins is also improved during the sprouting process, especially vitamin B1. Mung bean sprouts are a very good source of organic iron. Refer to page 38 for more details. Take part in a little Chinese kitchen-wisdom today. Mung bean sprouts will enhance any Chinese meal or Oriental dish.

SUNFLOWER SPROUTS

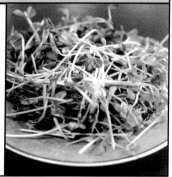

Sunflower sprouts are one of the tastiest and most delightful available. The minerals, calcium, phosphorus, iron, potassium and magnesium are well supplied, plus vitamins E and some B group vitamins. Sunflower sprouts make an ideal addition to a tossed garden salad or with a sandwich. Sunflower sprouts are easy to grow, plus they are so cheap you can really save on the shopping bill and gain a great increase in active enzymes, vitamins and chlorophyll supply. If you are too busy to sprout, buy a handy pack of sunflower sprouts next shopping day and surprise yourself with the variety of meals that can use sunflower power and presentation. Sunflower sprouts are waiting to help you shine!

Wheat is the most dominant and versatile grain in the world, however, the greatest benefits of wheat are not obtained from products such as bread and cereals. In fact, numerous health problems can be attributed to the excess consumption of refined wheat products. The ultimate value from the humble wheat grain is obtained from sprouted wheat and wheat grass shoots that are pressed into a juice, termed wheatgrass juice. Most juice bars prepare and applaud it's health and healing benefits. Dr. G.H. Earp Thomas, a soil expert calculated that 1 kg of wheat grass is equivalent to 12 kg of the choicest vegetables. For those people who are brave enough to sip or skull a dose of wheatgrass juice, it is obvious from the taste and head rush that it certainly is a potent tonic. The chlorophyll content is the major contributor of benefits, especially as it is obtained 'so fresh' and alive with enzymes and living nutrients. Usually, a small quantity 'a shot', approx. (10 tsp. or 35 g) is taken and surprisingly the nutrients from such a small serve are enormous, refer to chart. Apart from supplying over 12 minerals and 13 vitamins, wheatgrass juice provides lycopene 830 mcg, one third that of tomatoes, but, still providing proven protection from breast, lung and prostrate cancer, a powerful antioxidant and antitumour factor, able to fight against diseases caused by oxidative stress. The vitamin C content is 4 times as potent as oranges and the vitamin A (betacarotene) value is 47,700 I.U. per 100 gram, or 16,600 I.U. per 10 tsp. serve, that's potent. Both vitamin A and C protect against cancer. Back to chlorophyll, wheatgrass juice provides 185 mg per serve (10 tsp. or 35 g), the ultimate provider of chlorophyll and promoter of health and healing, as chlorophyll is loaded with oxygen. According to the Nobel prize winner, Dr. Otto Warburg, oxygen deprivation is a major contributor to cancer. Obviously, exercise is the ideal way to oxygenate the blood, but, for those people with chronic illnesses, wheatgrass juice can provide a renewed supply of oxygen, direct into the bloodstream, within 15 minutes. Smoking, alcohol, pollution, drugs, fatty foods and high protein cooked foods all deplete oxygen in the bloodstream. Chlorophyll's chemical composition is nearly identical to human blood, based on an iron atom, chlorophyll is based on a magnesium atom. This unique structure of chlorophyll was described by Dr. Birscher, a research scientist as "concentrated sun power" and stated it increases the functions of the circulatory system and the lungs, plus, neutralises toxins, cleanses and rebuilds the body. Wheatgrass juice assists in the constant requirement of the body, to manufacture healthy new red blood cells, haemoglobin. Wheatgrass juice assists the elimination of toxins such as fatty deposits, calcifications, hardened mucus, faecal matter and crystallized acids, plus it purifies the liver, cleanses the skin and can remove heavy metals from the body. One 'shot' per day will show for itself after a few days, providing renewed energy, healing of various ailments and a positive outlook, due to the remarkable supply of living nutrients, such as the rich iron 8.7 mg content. Further research will expose more about the true value of wheatgrass, especially in this era of depleted, processed and snack foods. The 'shot a day' may be the simple answer to the hectic pace of city living. Make it at home, get it from shops, buy a juice bar, whatever, just remember, wheatgrass juice is tops for healing!

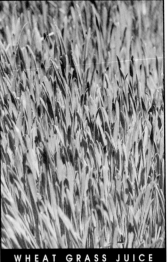

WHEAT GRASS JUICE

NUTRIENTS	3.5g.	'shot' 35g.	100g.
Calories	13	130	371
Carbohydrate	1.6g.	16g.	45.7g.
Protein	860mg.	8.6g.	24g.
Fibre	1g.	10g.	28g.
Chlorophyll	18.5mg.	185mg.	529mg.
Calcium	15mg.	150mg.	429mg
Cobalt	1.7mcg.	17mcg.	48mg.
Copper	17mcg.	170mcg.	4.8mg.
Iodine	8mcg.	80mcg.	2.2g
Iron	870mcg.	8.7mg.	24mg.
Magnesium	3.9mg.	39mg.	111mg.
Manganese	240mcg.	2.4mg.	6.8mg.
Phosphorus	14mg.	140mg.	252mg.
Potassium	137mg.	1.3mg.	3,918mg.
Selenium	3.5mcg.	35mcg.	100mcg.
Sodium	1mg.	10mg.	28.6mg.
Sulphur	10.5mg.	10.5g.	300mg.
Zinc	62mcg.	6.2mg.	1.7g.
Vitamin a	1668 I.U.	16,668 I.U.	47,704 I.U.
Vitamin c	7.5mg.	75mg.	214mg.
Vitamin e	320mcg.	3.2mg.	915mg.
Vitamin k	35mcg.	3.5mg.	100mg.

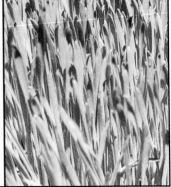

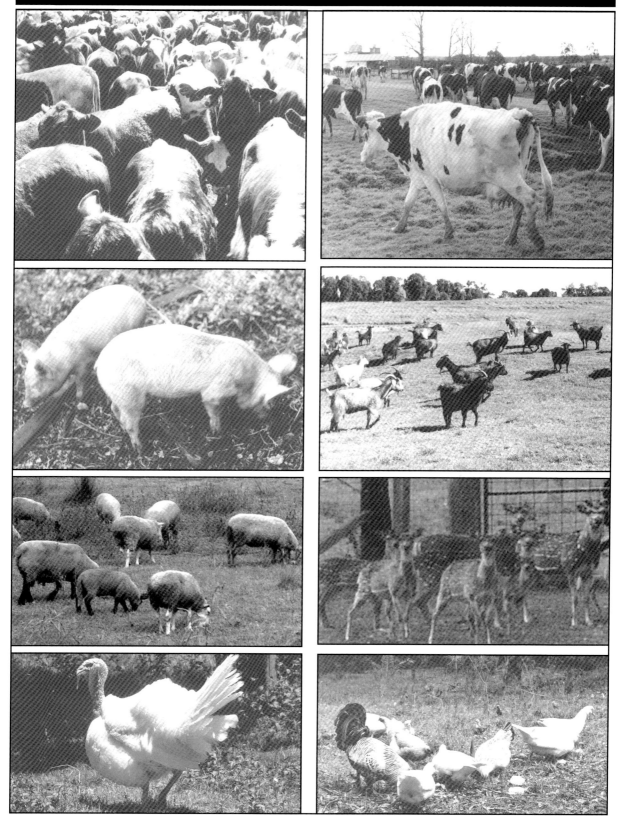

NOTE: All amounts in this book are measured in milligrams (mg) per 100 grams, unless stated otherwise.

Cheese has been made for thousands of years, the origin of cheese is thought to have developed accidentally when nomads and tribe people carried milk in containers that were made from the stomach of a milk-producing animal: cow, goat, sheep, camel or buffalo. The contact between the milk and the container, produced the earliest method of milk storage: cheese making. The special active ingredient obtained from the animal stomach is called rennet and this digestive enzyme assists the calf to digest milk from the cow. The human child up to the age of around seven also produces a milk digesting enzyme. The majority of traditional and modern methods of cheesemaking are based on the curdling effect, produced by the enzyme rennet, some cheese is curdled by the effects of lemon juice and more recently, a vegetable rennet has been developed. It is less expensive and is greatly increasing in popularity as a large variety of aged cheese and cottage cheese can be produced from this vegetable rennet.

Today there are over 400 individual types of cheese, each with a different taste, texture and appearance. From Switzerland the famous Swiss cheese, has unique characteristics nutritionally plus visually, with holes in the cheese. From Italy the famous mozzarella, from France, camembert and from England and U.S.A., the cheddar cheese. From all over the world different types of cheese are produced and available in the large urban areas, from the delicatessen or supermarket.

POSSIBLE BENEFICIAL FACTORS

1. **Low lactose content.**
2. **Protein content.**
3. **Calcium content.**
4. **Meal maker.**

1. Natural cheese made from raw milk contains the active enzymes: lipase for fat digestion and lactase: *lactose conversion*. During the natural cheesemaking process, rennet is added plus 'natural bacteria' and these will promote lactose conversion and digestion of the concentrated milk product. Natural cheese may cost more but it provides true value and easier digestion. Natural cheese is eager to please!

2. Cheese is an excellent source of *complete protein* plus it promotes the protein value of many recipes. The simple 'peasant's lunch', the cheese on bread provides the protein, the energy and other nutrients to continue a hard day's work. As cheese is a good supplier of the common 'limiting amino acid' methionine, it improves the overall protein value: net protein utilization of many meals. A small amount of cheese, 50 grams when combined with kidney beans, or rice or the salad sandwich can provide over half the daily protein requirements. It is easy too add much cheese to a meal and the pizza is a classic for excess cheese. Depending on other foods in the daily diet, over 100 grams of cheese per day is excess. Refer to protein chart page 89 for details on cheese protein.

3. The *Calcium content* of cheese is excellent, a far better choice than milk especially as it is easier to digest. Cheese supplies on average 700 mg. of calcium per 100 gram and it easily supplies over half the daily calcium in one serve: cheese and salad sandwich, grated parmesan on pasta. Up to one quarter of the weekly calcium supply can be obtained from natural cheese.

RECOMMENDED DAILY CALCIUM INTAKE					
PER 100 GRAMS	CALCIUM	CHILD 4-8	CHILD 9-18	MALE 19-50	MALE 51-70
CHEDDAR	728 mg.	800mg.	1300mg.	1000mg.	1200mg.
EDAM	738 mg.	FEMALE 9-18	FEMALE 19-30	FEMALE 31 - 50	FEMALE 51 - 70
FETA	500 mg.	1300mg.	1000mg.	1000mg.	1200mg.
MOZARELLA	653 mg.	PREGNANCY under 18 years		PREGNANCY 19 - 45 years	
PARMESAN	1200 mg.	1300mg. day		1000mg. day	
RICOTTA	208 mg.	LACTATION under 18 years		LACTATION 19 - 45 years	
SWISS	971 mg.	1300 mg. day		1000 mg.day	

4. Cheese is a *meal maker* and it adds flavour to numerous recipes due to the rich saturated fat content and the individual cheese culture. Grilled cheese is not recommended for good health as it will contain 'free radicals'. Grated cheese, sliced cheese or cubes of cheese on rye bread, salads, pasta, dry biscuits and continental breads can provide a very satisfying meal or snack, full of protein, energy and calcium. Enjoy the natural cheese 'meal making' benefits at work or play.

NOTE: d.v. refers to daily value for woman 25 - 50 years, refer to R.D.I. chart page 69 for adult male and children R.D.I. values.

CHEESE - FATS

There are two main groups of cheese: soft cheese and hard cheese and today the supermarket has huge varieties of both groups of cheese. There are also two main types of cheese: natural cheese and processed cheese.

Processed cheese is available in numerous varieties and flavours with any number of additives. Check labels for bleaching agents, preservatives, colours and ideally, avoid *processed cheese*. The packaging of individual slices in plastic adds to the price and the cheese does 'go off' fairly quickly compared to 'true natural cheese' that can last for months and just get's 'better with age'. Most 'natural' supermarket cheese provides the benefits mentioned but they may only last a week, refrigerated.

Processed cheese was invented by Mr. J.L Kraft in 1917 and since then, processed cheese has taken over in the diet of many people. All cheese may contain the following problems, if taken in excess. Natural cheese has the 'long lasting' benefits and rich, full flavour.

POSSIBLE DETRIMENTAL FACTORS

1. **Excess saturated fats / cholesterol**
2. **Processed cheese additives**
3. **Calories**
4. **Salt content**

1. Cheese is full of fats especially *saturated fats* and it also contains a fair amount of cholesterol. It is easy to obtain both excess fats and cholesterol from cheese. On average, hard cheese is 30% fat, plus 100 mg. of cholesterol.

Keep your cheese intake to a bare minimum and enjoy it to the maximum.

2. Cheese is full of *salt* and it also provides abundant *calories,* ideal for the energetic youth and sports person but for the 'not so active', cheese is best in small serves. The charts will show the comparison between the supply of nutrients and the daily allowance (R.D.I). Cheese will easily supply the daily protein, calcium, sodium and lipids, but it is best to keep cheese intake to approx. one quarter of total daily calories, as 200 grams, of cheddar cheese 'alone', or 66 g, will start to 'tilt the scales' on daily lipids, as 87 g is the adult daily R.D.I. Two cheese sandwiches will be approx. 200 grams. Add as much lettuce and other vegies and get a balance without so much cheese.

LIPIDS / SODIUM / IRON / PROTEIN RECOMMENDED DAILY INTAKE

AGE GROUP	LIPIDS (fats & oils)	SODIUM grams (approx.)	IRON	PROTEIN	CALORIES kcal.
CHILD 0-6 months	28 g.	.14 g.	6 mg.	13 g.	650
CHILD 1 -3 years	38 g.	.2 g.	10 mg.	14 - 16 grams.	1300
CHILD 4-6 years	58 g.	.2 g.	10 mg.	24 g.	1800
CHILD 7-14 years	80 g.	. 4 g.	10-12 mg.	28 - 45 grams	2000
* TEENAGERS 15 - 22	80 g.	. 4 g.	10-12 mg.	45 - 58 grams	2500
FEMALES 11- 23	78 g.	.5 g.	15 mg.	44 - 46 grams	2200
* MEN 23 and over	87 g.	. 5 g	10 mg.	63 g.	2900
* WOMEN 23 - 50 years	66 g.	.5 g.	15 mg.	50 g.	2200
*MEN & WOMEN 51 and over	59 g.	. 4 g.	10 mg.	50 - 63 grams	1900-2300

* CHOLESTEROL MAXIMUM DAILY INTAKE 300 mg (ADULT).

CHEESE SUPPLY OF LIPIDS & CHOLESTEROL

PER 100 GRAMS	TOTAL FAT	CHOLE STEROL	SATU- RATED	POLY	MONO
CHEDDAR	33 g.	107 mg.	22 g.	1 g.	9.5 g.
EDAM	27 g.	89 mg.	18 g.	.7 g	8.2 g.
FETA	28 g.	89 mg.	15 g.	.6 g	4.6 g.
MOZARELLA	21 g.	78 mg.	13.5 g	.8 g	6.7 g.
PARMESAN	26 g.	67 mg.	17 g.	.6 g	7.2 g.
RICOTTA	13 g.	50 mg.	8.3g.	.4 g	3.7 g.
SWISS	28 g.	92 mg.	18 g.	1 g.	7.5 g

CHEESE COMPARISON CHART

PER 100 GRAMS	SODIUM	IRON	PROTEIN	CALORIES
CHEDDAR	628 mg.	.67 mg.	25 g.	406
EDAM	978 mg.	.42 mg.	25 g.	360
FETA	1128 mg.	.64 mg.	14 g.	267
MOZARELLA	378 mg.	.17 mg.	19.6 g	285
PARMESAN	1620 mg.	.82 mg.	35 g.	397
RICOTTA	84 mg.	.36 mg.	11.3 g.	175
SWISS	264 mg.	.17 mg.	29 g.	382

MILK - INFANTS & CHILDREN

Milk is the first natural food. Mother's milk is the perfect food for development of content and healthy infants and depending on the duration of breast feeding and the health of the mother, a child will obtain all the essential nutrients to assist the early vital stages of growth and development.

As the mother's milk is the best food for babies, special care should be taken by the mother to ensure that she also obtains the best foods: natural foods to promote milk production: (carrot juice).

There are a few other, very important elements supplied by mother's milk, such as colostrum and bacillus bifidus, a natural bacteria that protects the child from other harmful bacteria and it also assists digestion of the milk-sugar: lactose.

As the child is weaned off mother's milk, the use of formulas, cow's milk and other milk are usually given as the next main food. For those children who obtain both a supply of mother's milk and other milk, the natural bacteria provided by the mother's milk will assist digestion of the other milk, until such time that no more mother's milk is available. From that time onwards, the 'new milk' will supply its own bacteria. The addition of acidophillus yoghurt will be the best supplier of 'friendly bacteria' to help protect and promote the infants / child's digestive system. It will also promote the digestion of milk and the breakdown of lactic acid. The addition of mashed foods, especially carrots, pumpkin and broccoli will soon provide the child with nutrients not supplied by cows milk or goats milk.

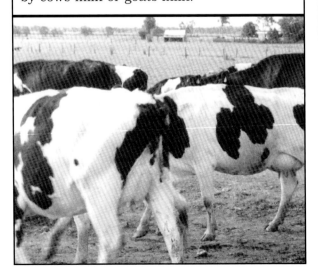

Within the developing digestive system of children a very important 'temporary digestive enzyme' is produced, called rennin. On average, this digestive enzyme will remain within the child's digestive system until the first full set of teeth commence to develop, usually around the age of seven.

Slowly, from that time onwards, the ability of a child to digest milk depends greatly on their health and their body's ability to adapt to a new system of milk digestion. The special enzyme, rennin, is required to convert the caseinogen content of milk into the form of casein. It curdles milk by converting the soluble casein into insoluble casein which combines with calcium to form calcium caseinate, the curd which is digested by the hydrochloric acid and pepsin (pepsinogen) in the stomach. Human 'mother's milk' protein provides 40% casein and 60% whey. Cows milk protein provides 80% casein and 20% whey. In comparison to human milk, cow's milk contains 200% more caseinogen. The function of caseinogen is mainly to assist in the production of the hormone: thyroxine, used by the thyroid gland to control the general metabolism, nervous system, glandular system, mental development and growth rate.

Cow's milk contains 2 times more caseinogen and is designed for calves, which have a growth rate four times that of human children. Physical and mental imbalances may occur in some children and teenagers from excessive consumption of cow's milk, more than I litre per day for teenagers, 500 ml. children (7-12 years). For most adults, cows milk is not recommended as a regular food source. In addition, for babies and children, the thymus gland provides lymphocytes to protect against disease and infection. Up to the age of seven, the thymus gland continues to grow and protect the body and by the time of puberty, it ceases to function. The thymus gland functions as a 'junior' immune system and needs more than milk to maintain it's functions. It is the fat content of milk that promotes the rapid growth in babies. Mother's milk contains 4.5 grams of fat per 100 gram, whole cows milk contains 3.3 grams of fat with both having a similar saturated fat and cholesterol value.

MILK - LACTOSE INTOLERANCE

Milk is a popular drink amongst the general public, possibly due to the powerful marketing campaigns that state benefits such as protection from osteoporosis, however there are more factors than 'meet the eye' when evaluating milk, especially for adults. One survey of adults showed that water was the most popular drink with 215 litres consumed per year, soft drinks 150 litres, coffee 106 litres, beer 94 litres, tea 28 litres, juices 23 litres wine and spirits 14 litres and milk 82 litres per year. The total of all these drinks equals approx. 2 litres per day and as 2.1 litres of *pure water* alone is required by the body for proper body functioning (kidneys, evaporation, food oxidation and during sleep), in a cold climate, it is clear that insufficient water is obtained, on average, per day, per person.

The daily 'average' milk consumption was approx. 220 ml. per day, per adult, the equivalent of the added milk to 5 cups of tea or coffee. This amount of milk is not considered excessive but the kidneys may suffer from a poor supply of 'pure' water, as tea, coffee, milk, soft drinks, beer etc. require filtration by the kidneys.

POSSIBLE DETRIMENTAL FACTORS

1. Over consumption
2. Lactose intolerance
3. Teenage acne
4. Homogenisation / Pasteurisation
6. Calcium content / iron content
7. Respiratory disorders

1. *Over consumption* of cows milk may easily occur in teenagers and the elderly due to the advertising campaigns that promote milk. Teenagers may consume over 1 litre of milk per day thinking it is necessary for their growth. Milk often takes the place of other important foods that are necessary for growth. Milk satisfies the appetite quickly and is available at every local store. For the elderly, milk is promoted for prevention of osteoporosis, brittle bones but other factors are important for strong bones. Moderate regular sunlight and exercise, plus the minerals magnesium, phosphorus and zinc, which are undersupplied by milk. Only humans drink milk after the infancy stage, animals survive on other foods.

2. *Lactose intolerance* is a very common problem with milk consumption. Lactose is the sugar portion of milk, it is a disaccharide: glucose and galactose, no other food contains lactose apart from milk. The perfect food for infants: mothers milk contains approx. 75 grams of lactose per litre, cows milk supplies 45 grams per litre.

The enzyme lactase in the small intestine is usually active in children up to the age of approx. 5 years and then progressively slows down. Without the enzyme lactase, milk will not be digested properly and the common condition of 'lactose intolerance' may develop. One survey showed that 15% of whites and 70% of blacks in the USA had lactose intolerance. Over 80% of all people from Japan, Taiwan, Philippines, Thailand and many Arab countries are 'lactose intolerant or 'lactase deficient'. People from Switzerland and Denmark have approx. 5% 'lactose intolerance'.

Undigested lactose ferments in the colon by bacterial action causing carbon dioxide 'gas' and lactic acid, possibly resulting in flatulence, cramps, and diarrhoea.

Everybody has a different lactose tolerance, decide for your own health, is it worth all that 'gas' to drink milk from a cow.

4. *Teenage acne* may result from excess milk protein (casein) as it may over stimulate the thyroid gland, general metabolism and the secretion of hormones. Also milk may contain traces of hormones as residue from the cows diet. The fat content of milk after pasteurisation is not beneficial as it does not contain the 'essential fatty acids', plus it contains saturated fats which can enter the bloodstream before filtration by the lymphatic system. Another common problem is due to the hormone progesterone contained in milk from pregnant cows. About 80% of all cows milk is derived from pregnant cows. Progesterone is broken down into androgens which promote premature sexual development and hormone production. Research showed teenage acne was reduced remarkably when milk drinking was stopped. The bacteria produced from milk digestion is also a problem. Avoid milk if you have a teenage skin problem, keep clear off milk!

5a. Homogenisation is the process that unifies the milk and cream content, it saves you the effort to 'shake the milk' but places great effort on the body later. During homogenisation, the fats in the cream and milk get pulverised and fragmented. These 'minute fats' are able to 'hide' from the lymphatic system which is designed to initially process and filter all digested fats. The milk fats are able to enter the bloodstream directly and may accumulate to cause problems with the heart and circulatory system. More fat enters the bloodstream from homogenised milk than from unprocessed cheese, cream or butter.

5b. Pasteurisation is the process where raw milk is heated to 62° Celsius for 30 minutes or 161° Celsius for 15 seconds. Pasteurization was implemented to protect the community against possibly harmful bacteria in batches of spoilt milk from the dairy farm. It is recognized that the pasteurisation process does not eliminate all bacteria and microorganisms. In addition, pasteurisation may also alter the protein structure of milk, as heating breaks and 'tangles' the protein molecules and makes them difficult to digest or break down. For better digestion, pasteurised milk can be reboiled quickly to help dismantle the 'tangled' protein molecules.

For many centuries, the practice of boiling raw milk quickly has maintained a sterile product and according to modern research, it does not destroy the nutritional value.

6a Calcium content of milk is possibly the main media marketing factor especially for prevention of osteoporosis. Calcium is required to promote strong bones. Milk does supply calcium but considering the fact that many people are 'lactose intolerant', it cannot be classed as the ideal calcium food. Such foods as natural cheese, yoghurt, carob, tahini, tofu, almonds, green vegetables and salmon are full of calcium. Refer to chart. Other associated factors with osteoporosis are just as vital as the calcium intake such as: 1 - lack of sunlight, 2 - lack of weight bearing activities, 3 - menopause and hormone action, 4 - lack of other minerals 5 - unstable supply of calcium.

The efficiency of calcium absorption can vary considerably. Ideally, maintain a regular intake of calcium foods rather than large amounts in one day. The body adapts to a pattern of calcium absorption. Ideally, a good serve of yoghurt an hour before bedtime provides maximum value, as during sleep the body will require calcium and when not available, bone 'demineralization' may occur during the long hours of sleep. Vitamin D sunlight will promote calcium absorption. Rest easy with a regular intake of yoghurt as calcium promotes a good night's sleep and yoghurt does not have the 'lactose problem'.

NUTRIENT COMPARISON CHART

PER 100 GRAMS	MILK	ALMOND	KIDNEY BEANS	PEPITAS
CALCIUM	119	232	28	51
IRON	.04	4.6	3	11.3
POTASSIUM	151	768	358	801
MAGNESIUM	13	270	45	531
PHOSPHORUS	93	502	147	1166
MANGANESE	.004	1.9	.47	2.9
ZINC	.38	2.9	1.1	7.4
VITAMIN A	126	9.8	0	72

6b. The Iron content of milk is really overestimated, it is best not to rely on milk for iron. The RDI for children from 1 - 10 years is 10 mg. For the daily iron supply, approx. 20 cups of milk is required. Also, most other minerals, vitamin A and B vitamins are undersupplied. Milk provides a basic supply of a few nutrients and a variety of possible adverse factors, as mentioned. In some children, excess milk intake has lead to anaemia and leukaemia.

7. Respiratory disorders are common from excess cows milk intake due to the production of mucus as a by-product of milk digestion. Mucus is produced by the body to eliminate toxins. It acts as a barrier against acids in the stomach. Milk contains very little vitamin A to protect the respiratory system from infection. Carrot juice contains nearly 30,000 times more 'A' than milk.

GOATS MILK / CHEESE

The benefits of goats milk when compared to cow's milk are numerous.

The composition of the fat globules in goats milk is finer than in cow's milk, thereby allowing better digestion. Goats milk is composed of more medium chain triglycerides (mct's), or fatty acids, than cows milk. These mct's are absorbed easier into the digestive system and lymphatic system. In addition the mct's lower cholesterol and provide a special form of energy that is easy to metabolise. Goats milk supplies approx. 20% more calcium and phosphorus than cows milk. One cup of goats milk supplies approx. 33% of the daily calcium for the adult female and 27% of phosphorus.

Goats milk and cheese are used throughout the world. Goats milk is often preferred to cows milk as it is less allergenic. Obviously, soy milk, or rice milk is the best choice for those with high lactose intolerance and milk allergies. The protein in goats milk and cheese is easier to digest. It contains less beta -lactoglobulins than cows milk, these are the most complex milk proteins to digest. The beta-lactoglobulins in goats milk are digested more efficiently and less protein residue remains in the digestive system after ingestion, thereby protecting against bacterial problems and mucus development that clogs the respiratory system.

Goats milk does not need to be homogenised. The fat globules are smaller than in cows milk and they remain suspended evenly in the milk. When considering to feed infants with goats milk, once breast-feeding has ceased, it is best to obtain advice. Due to the low folate content 0.40 mcg, compared to human mother's milk, 5.2 mcg, or cows milk 4.9 mcg, it is best not to give infants only goats milk. Add foods such as mashed broccoli with 64 mcg. of folate and foods with vitamin C and E. Goats milk provides complete protein with 3.6 g, human milk only supplies 1 g, cows milk supplies 3.2 g. The casein, alpha s-3 casein, in goats milk is softer and more flexible than the casein, alpha-s-1, in cows milk. Goats milk contains only small amounts of alpha s-1, compared to cows milk, thereby it is easier to digest. Over half the milk consumed in the world is from the goat. Goats milk is sweet and sometimes salty due to a very good source of organic sodium. Go the goat!

YOGHURT

Yoghurt has a long-proven health history dating back thousands of years, possibly just after the domestication of farm animals. During the early 1900's and up to this present day, research into the nutritional qualities of yoghurt has provided very encouraging results that are also backed up from generations of people throughout the world, especially: Turkey, Balkans region, Greece, Egypt, Arabia, Algeria, India & China. Today, more people throughout the world obtain the benefits that only yoghurt can provide. Yoghurt can be prepared from cow's milk, goat's milk, buffalo milk, sheep milk and soy milk.

BENEFICIAL FACTORS OF YOGHURT

1. Acidophillus bacteria
2. Easy digestion
3. Calcium content
4. B vitamins and other benefits
5. Protein value

During the process of yoghurt making the 'raw milk' is boiled to kill any 'wild bacteria' that can interfere with the added 'culture'. The culture is a natural bacteria and the two most common natural bacteria are: *lactobacilus acidophillus* and lactobacillus bulgaricus. Both are closely related however the L.B. acidophillus has proven to be the most effective in maintaining a correct and prolonged supply of natural bacteria within the digestive system, up to 48 hours.

The word 'bacteria' may concern some people and so it must be pointed out that various types of bacteria are obtained from other produce: meat, cheese, milk, eggs, poultry, fish and seafood as well as processed and take away foods.

The bacteria that is formed from those foods can produce harmful effects, if allowed to accumulate in the lower digestive system. Natural yoghurt will destroy harmful bacteria within the lower digestive system and colon and replace a 'friendly bacteria' containing valuable antibiotic qualities which provide a natural balance and cleansing for the lower digestive system. An estimated 450 different types of bacteria can live in the human digestive system. Ideally, choose the yoghurt made from non - pasteurised milk.

YOGHURT - ACIDOPHILLUS

'Lactobacillus acidophillus' bacteria is considered the most powerful yoghurt 'culture'. Other strains of bacteria used in yoghurt making and often combined with 'acidophillus' are lactobacillus bifidus, lactobacillus bulgaricus and lactobacillus thermophillus.

As a group they are termed: probiotics. It is possibly better not to obtain a yoghurt that has more than one culture as they may interfere with each other's function.

The term dysbiosis is used to describe the condition when the balance of 'bad - pathogenic' bacteria are prevalent in the intestines, compared to the 'friendly' bacteria. Such factors as antibiotics, analgesics, the contraceptive pill and steroids can cause dysbiosis.

Also, a diet low in fresh fruits, vegetables, legumes, fibre and high in animal protein and fats plus processed foods all promote dysbiosis. Acidophillus yoghurt taken regularly will 'balance the bacteria' and avoid the problems associated with dysbiosis such as flatulence, constipation, diarrhoea, bloating, chronic fatigue, skin problems and irritable bowel syndrome. Acidophillus is also available in *tablet form* for anyone who is unable to digest yoghurt.

However, the calcium content benefit is missing. Also, acidophillus bacteria secrete antibacterial and antifungal substances termed bacteriocins which stop the growth of pathogens.

Yoghurt is a *simple food to digest*. The common ingredient with all types of milk products is lactose, often called 'milk-sugar'. Most adults are unable to digest lactose properly. Lactose is converted by the digestive system into the form of glucose: energy via the enzyme lactase. As mentioned in the section on milk, there are two main factors regarding lactose. Firstly most children have the necessary digestive enzymes lactase and rennin to assist conversion of lactose. After the age of 7-14 years, these enzymes are no longer active in the human body. During the yoghurt making process, lactose is converted into simple sugars: glucose and galactose, by the bacterial action of fermentation. For adults, yoghurt is the best way to obtain the dairy product benefits.

The *calcium content* of yoghurt is ideal and one of the best natural ways to obtain the daily calcium requirement. One cup 227 grams of plain non fat yoghurt supplies 450 mg. of calcium. That is nearly half the daily requirement for men and women from 19 to 50 years. For the elderly, yoghurt is an excellent food as it requires no chewing and is simple to digest. Ideally, one cup of natural acidophillus low fat yoghurt mid morning or one cup before bedtime will ensure a very regular intake of calcium and that's exactly what the body needs, plus moderate, regular sunlight, to protect against osteoporosis.

For growing children, yoghurt is really an essential food especially from the age of 9 - 18 years, as the digestive system needs help to process the milk and cheese in their diet, plus they no longer have the 'enzymes' to assist in lactose conversion, plus they need 1,300 mg. of calcium a day. Meat supplies hardly any calcium plus meat promotes toxins in the lower digestive system.

YOGHURT & DAILY CALCIUM INTAKE				
PER 100 GRAMS & PER CUP MEASURE	CALCIUM 1 cup.	CALCIUM 100 g.	CHILD 4-8	CHILD 9-18
PLAIN LOW FAT YOGHURT	415 mg.	182 mg.	800 mg.	1300 mg.
PLAIN NON FAT YOGHURT	452 mg..	198 mg.	FEMALE 9-18	FEMALE 19-30
FRUIT LOW FAT YOGHURT	314 mg.	138 mg.	1300 mg.	1000 mg.
PLAIN WHOLE MILK YOGHURT	227 mg.	100 mg.	MALE 19-50	MALE 51-70
WHOLE MILK 3.25% FAT	291 mg.	119 mg.	1300 mg.	1200 mg.
LOW FAT MILK 2% FAT	297 mg.	121 mg.	FEMALE 31-50	FEMALE 51-70
LOW FAT MILK 1% FAT	300 mg.	123 mg.	1000 mg.	1200 mg.

The *protein content* of whole milk yoghurt by weight is only 3.5 % and for the average woman, approx. 1,600 grams would be required to satisfy the protein R.D.I. Low fat yoghurt provides approx. 5.2 grams of protein. The net protein utilization of yoghurt is very good, the same as milk at 80% n.p.u. thereby the protein value is used effectively. Yoghurt does not require other foods to increase the amino acid balance. As yoghurt is approx. 60% water content, by weight, it may not appear to supply good protein, but a cup of yoghurt a day supplies approx. 1/5 protein for women. Yoghurt has so many other benefits, the protein is just a bonus.

Eggs are a symbol of life. The chicken goes before the egg alphabetically but the egg is first in protein availability with the highest net protein utilization of any food at 93%, chicken has a n.p.u. of 65%.

One large egg contains approx. 6 grams of protein and 90% of the protein is useable by the body.

To obtain all your daily protein from eggs would be more than difficult, it would be harmful, mainly due to the cholesterol. The average adult requires from 45-55 grams (approx.) of protein per day, in egg terms that is about 8 eggs but in regards to the main problem with excess egg intake: *cholesterol,* 8 eggs supply nearly 1,700 mg.

The recommended daily maximum of cholesterol, per adult, is 300 mg. People cannot live by eggs alone. *One large egg contains approx. 200 mg. of cholesterol,* or two thirds the daily limit.

Enjoy your free range eggs and carefully manage your intake.

CHOLESTEROL & EGG FACTS

1. Only the egg yolk contains cholesterol.
2. Cholesterol is also made by the liver for the absorption of fats and utilization of fat soluble vitamins. 4. Obese people produce more cholesterol than average weight people. Weight loss diets can decrease the body's manufacture of cholesterol. 5. The average dietary intake of cholesterol from one survey showed the average man obtained approx. 330 mg. per day, women 212 mg. per day. 6. The liver can increase and decrease cholesterol manufacture according to dietary intake.

The choline (B vitamin) content of eggs is abundant with 215 mg per large egg. Choline contains a phospholipid known as lecithin which can lower blood cholesterol and remove cholesterol from tissues. A lack of choline can contribute to high blood cholesterol levels.

The high cholesterol level in eggs may be reduced by the rich choline content and to be really sure, add some *lecithin granules* supplement to your next scrambled eggs, or add it to soup and be 'confident about your cholesterol'!

The supply of other nutrients from eggs is fairly basic. The iron content is 2.8 mg. per 100 gram, kidney beans supply 3 mg, almonds 4.6 mg. beef 1.9mg. pepitas 11.3 mg and parsley 6 mg. The vitamin A content is fair at 520 I.U. per 100 gram, carrots supply near 30,000 mg, no comparison. The vitamin D content is fairly good and for those people 'stuck indoors' in hospital or unable to tolerate any sunlight, the egg may provide a small but valuable dose in addition to the best source: fish oils. Dairy products also provide a fair source. Eggs are not a calcium food, same as meat so if your diet has few other foods, add some almonds or cheese. The biotin (B vitamin) content of eggs is good but raw egg white contains avidin which can prevent biotin from reaching the blood. Raw egg white in egg nogs etc. also contains albumen protein which can pass into the blood undigested causing allergies.

The great benefit of eggs is their versatility in recipes, the omelette, cakes, pastries and pasta to mention a few. Eggs are best kept refrigerated to prevent bacterial growth. Bring eggs to room temperature before boiling. Proper cooking of eggs is essential to avoid bacteria and salmonella poisoning. Boiled eggs are simple and free of 'added fats'. Fried eggs are full of saturated fats and free radicals if butter is used, ideally use cold pressed olive oil or canola oil, or poach them, scramble or mix into the omelette with leafy green vegetables. Children enjoy dipping 'soldiers' into soft boiled eggs and it provides them with 'high density protein'.

Nutrient content (1 large egg)	Whole egg	Egg yolk	Egg white
Protein (grams)	6.25	2.78	3.25
Calories (k.cal)	75	59	17
Total lipids (g.)	5.01	5.12	0
Saturated fat (g.)	1.55	1.55	0
Polyunsaturated (g.)	.68	.68	0
Monounsaturated (g.)	1.91	1.91	0
Cholesterol (mg.)	213	213	0
Calcium (mg.)	25	23	2
Iron (mg.)	.72	.59	.01
Vitamin d (I.u.)	24.5	24.5	0
Biotin (mcg.)	9.98	7.58	2.34
Choline (mg.)	215	214	1
Vitamin a (I.u.)	317	317	0

POULTRY

Poultry includes the 'common chicken' plus duck, goose, turkey, pheasants and quail. Poultry varies in it's supply of nutrients as can be seen from the chart below. In regards to protein, chicken and turkey are 'on par' at approx. 21 grams per 100 gram with a (n.p.u.) of 65 %. A 300 gram serve of chicken will supply all the daily protein for an adult male, but, no fibre and no carbohydrate content. Without the addition of fibre rich foods, chicken is 'lost in the digestive system' and that may lead to toxins in the colon. Chicken is classed as a 'nutrient dense' food implying it supplies protein, iron and zinc, but the iron content is fairly low at 0.7 mg per 100 gram and the zinc content is 0.8 mg, neither are 'big in value' but the protein makes up the balance to be classed as a nutrient dense food.

Poultry are very low in calcium, 11 mg, even less than eggs 25 mg or beef 25 mg. With many people relying on these 3 foods for a majority of their daily protein and food supply, a calcium deficiency is likely to develop especially considering the average (r.d.i.) for adults is about 1,100 mg.

Ideally, regular intakes of natural yoghurt, cheese, tahini and almonds are required to balance the calcium deficiency. Also, acidophillus yoghurt will help reduce harmful bacteria in the lower digestive system (colon) that often result from regular chicken and meat diets. Ideally, obtain free range roast chicken and serve with generous amounts of fibre rich vegetables or a generous large serve of coleslaw salad.

POULTRY per 100 gram serve	Chicken	Duck	Goose	Turkey
Protein (grams)	20.8	11.4	16	21
Calories (k.cal)	172	403	370	158
Total lipids (g.)	9.2	48	33	7.3
Carbohydrate	0	0	0	0
Fibre	0	0	0	0
Saturated fat (g.)	2.6	23	8	2
Polyunsaturated (g.)	1.9	5	3.8	1.6
Monounsaturated (g.)	3.8	19	18	2.7
Cholesterol (mg.)	63	75	80	65
Calcium (mg.)	11	10	12	13
Iron (mg.)	.7	2.4	2.5	1.2
Sodium (mg.)	62	1.3	73	58

Poultry contain similar amounts of cholesterol but in regards to the total fat content, duck is very rich in saturated fats, with 23 g. Chicken 5 g is less than lean beef 9.6 g in total fat. Lean beef 4.2 g has about the same saturated fat content of chicken 4.5 g. In regards to cholesterol, chicken supplies 90 mg and beef 78 mg. Unless added fats are used, the cholesterol levels are fairly safe for one serve of either per day. Fried chicken is more a concern than roasted chicken due to the excess fats, free radicals and cholesterol absorbed into the bread crumb layer, especially if the cooking oil is used several times. A home roast chicken is the safest way to ensure quality control on the oils. Most fast food outlets have chicken as the number one seller and undoubtedly, it is one of the most over consumed take away foods. Limit your craving for chicken by allowing other meals such as bean tacos, fish, nuts and baked vegetables to 'get in' before the hunger rush starts!

The topic of 'free range' has been discussed for years and 'mass produced eggs' and poultry are still on dinner plates. The nutritional value of eggs is said to be the same with factory or farm eggs and the color of the yolk is determined by the feed type: wheat based produces a pale yellow yolk, corn based produces a golden yolk. Mass produced hens are given a 'well controlled diet', mainly soy and corn, antioxidant's, mould inhibitors and scraps from beef or chicken production. Hormones are not used generally speaking, but antibiotics are required to protect against disease outbreaks. Some flocks include over 1 million. The cage system is preferred for sanitation, the air is force ventilated, no sunlight and automatic feeders activated by a time clock, move food mash into troughs. Hens produce eggs for about 19 months and then moult and rest for about 6 weeks and produce again for about 8 weeks until moulting. That is usually the end of their life. A free range bird gets sunlight, fresh green feed and insects and can exercise and relax when the sun goes down. The price is often more for free range produce especially in the city but the cost is worth it's weight if the hens are given a decent outdoor life and not treated as an 'internal machine'.

Saltwater, freshwater and shellfish (including crustacea). For thousands of years fish have been obtained by humans and in the early stages, primitive hooks and nets were used to catch fish and that tradition continues in some parts of the world today. Freshly caught and then fire-baked fish is well worth the effort of a few hours fishing. Ask any fisher about the taste of fresh fish compared to canned fish, batter fish or un-frozen fish and discover for yourself the benefits of fresh fish, at least once a week. *Fresh fish*, on ice, is no more that one day since the catch.

POSSIBLE BENEFICIAL FACTORS

Fish is an excellent source of *complete protein,* on average the protein content is 24%. The *net protein utilisation* of fish is 80% whereas meat is only 67% useable protein. Therefore fish is considered a higher quality protein than meat and most other foods.
The chart below shows the individual amino acids values for a variety of fish compared to other foods. Most common fish supply similar protein. Sardines have a lower (n.p.u.) of 69%. Tuna is the best supplier of protein with a combination (n.p.u.) of 80 % and 28% complete protein.
Refer to page 93 for details.

The chart below provides the daily amino acid requirements for children, females and males. These figures are provided to compare the daily protein required with the supply from fish and other foods. A 100 gram serve is equivalent to the weight of two medium eggs (approx.). Children *need more protein than adults* and for some amino acids, more than twice the protein is required for children over 35 kilograms. To calculate your daily protein requirements for a specific weight, refer to the protein chart on page 88 and compare it to the amounts supplied below. Fish is the i*deal food* at least twice a week *for growing children* , it provides *compact protein and their stomach fills quickly!* A 140 gram serve of fish or 120 grams of tuna will supply the total daily protein for a child of 35 kilograms. For beef it would be approx. a 180 gram serve. Adults, male and female, require approx. 180 grams of fish or 140 grams of tuna to supply the *total daily protein requirements in one meal.* For beef approx. 220 grams are required. For adults, fish is recommended twice a week and whenever the *choice between meat or fish* is available, catch the fish protein and other benefits.
For *'absolutely amazing protein',* try fish crumbed with wheat germ, 2 ground brazil nuts and a whipped egg mix.

Fish is the complete protein dish.

FISH - PROTEIN (AMINO ACID) COMPARISON CHART per 100 gram portions										
NATURAL FOODS	N.P.U.	ARG.	HIS.	ISL.	LEU.	LYS.	MET.	PHA.	THR.	TRY.	VAL.
BASS	80%	1064	523	818	1451	1628	526	658	778	199	916
COD	80%	1069	525	823	1451	1640	528	697	783	199	919
MACKEREL	80%	1116	549	859	1510	1711	552	728	817	208	960
PERCH	80%	1118	549	860	1522	1711	552	729	818	210	962
SALMON	80%	1180	585	916	1616	1829	588	777	873	223	1025
SARDINES	69%	1486	730	1142	2016	2276	735	970	1087	277	1276
TUNA	80%	1416	684	1062	1888	2124	696	908	1026	259	1180
BEEF porterhouse	67%	1096	594	779	1372	1444	444	678	757	194	843
RICE - raw	70%	561	183	306	602	275	153	265	265	91	428
WHEAT- raw	60%	453	216	360	684	306	154	468	288	144	446
WHEAT GERM - raw	67%	1825	687	1177	1708	1534	404	908	1343	265	1364
KIDNEY BEANS -ckd.	40%	536	242	384	677	564	129	451	367	101	451
PEANUT - raw	43%	3509	757	1007	1946	1007	266	1483	718	314	1181
PEPITAS raw	60%	3982	672	1244	2052	1808	543	1208	893	425	1944
SOY BEANS ckd.	61%	1164	448	814	1338	1164	224	873	721	244	814
TAHINI	60%	2532	502	737	1306	549	562	897	710	375	958
EGGS	90%	776	294	760	1066	820	392	686	596	194	874
* CHILDREN (R.D.A.) 35 kg.		na.	na.	980	1470	1540	770	770	980	115	875
* FEMALE (R.D.A.) 55 kg		na.	550	550	825	660	715	770	385	192	550
* MALE (R.D.A.) 70 kg.		n.a.	700	700	980	840	910	980	490	245	700

These amounts are from the WHO (1985) and are provided as a guide for comparison purpose only.

FISH - OMEGA 3

Fish is a good provider of the 'essential fatty acid' *Omega 3*, especially tuna, salmon, mackerel, mullet, trevally, sardines, herring, anchovies and gemfish.

Omega 3 is valuable for control of cholesterol and for the brain, nervous system, skin, eyes and growth. Refer to page 166. The saturated fat content of fish on average is low compared to other animal protein foods.

Fish supplies approx. 50 - 70 mg of cholesterol per 100 gram but the Omega 3's and vanadium content will help utilize the cholesterol. It is better to use a cold pressed olive or canola oil to bake the fish, ideally steamed fish with rice and a sprinkle of cold pressed olive oil served with green beans, potatoes and carrots for a complete 'catch of benefits'.

As can be seen from the chart below, fish is a good source of omega 3, meat does not supply omega 3 but does supply Omega 6. Both Omega 3 and 6 are 'essential' in the diet. Fish does not supply omega 6 but it is available from all nuts and seeds, dairy foods, margarine and all oils

There are two types of fish: oily fish and low fat fish. Mackerel, mullet, trevally and sardines are the main oily fish, with salmon, trout and tuna supplying a fair amount of fats. These fats are of great benefit due to the supply of Omega 3. When compared to meat, fish is always lower in fat content, especially the saturated fats. For a complete low fat protein meal, baked perch, snapper or cod are an excellent choice. The low fat fish contain approx. 10% fat compared to meat and during a period of a year, by replacing 2 meat meals per week with baked fish, you can obtain 90% less fat and over 120% less saturated fats, that's a 'big' saving in kilograms, saturated fat problems and cholesterol problems. Fish is ready to reduce your weight on the scales!

FISH - SEAFOOD PROTEIN / FATS CHART

FISH & PRODUCE 100 GRAM SERVES COOKED	TOTAL % PROTEIN grams.	TOTAL % FAT grams.	SAT. FAT mg.	OMEGA 3 mg.	CHOLES TEROL m.g.
BASS	13	1.6	.5	.74	80
COD	18	.67	.67	.23	44
MACKEREL	19	13.8	3.2	3.3	71
PERCH	19	1.6	.24	.42	42
SALMON	20	6.3	.98	2.5	55
SARDINES	25	11.4	1.5	1.4	142
SHARK	21	4.5	.92	1.1	50
SNAPPER	20	1.3	.28	.46	36
TROUT	21	6.5	1.1	1.5	58
TUNA	24	4.9	1.2	1.4	38
T bone steak	17	25	11	0	71
BEEF frankfurter	11	29	12	0	50
Crab	18	2	.08	.12	41
Crayfish/ Lobster	18	2	.17	.15	96
Oysters	6	2.5	.62	.94	54
Prawns / Shrimps	20	2	.32	.65	153
Scallops	17	.75	.07	.25	30
Round steak	19	17	7	0	66
Lamb chops	15	17	8	0	58
Veal breast	14	14	6	0	56

Long before nutrition became a common term, fish oils from cod and halibut liver have provided a 'unique *food source* of vitamin D' especially for people in Artic and low sunlight areas. Vitamin D is easily obtained via sunlight but if it happens to be dark for many months, or you have to live indoors, or, work indoors during daylight hours or 'in a mine', get a supply of vitamin D and A from fish oils supplements. Also if you are in hospital for months or on the 'play station' all day instead of in the playground, your supply of vitamin D will be inadequate, especially for growing children and people with bone problems.

Fish, especially tuna is a good source of the trace mineral selenium. Fish supply all the main minerals in fair amounts plus vitamin A, E and most of the B complex including B12. Ocean fish also supply iodine. Fish is often termed a 'brain food' and the minerals magnesium, phosphorus, iodine, zinc, manganese and the trace mineral vanadium are all brain nutrients and available from fish plus the *high protein content* makes fish a 'brain food'. Fish and seafood are the best reliable source of vanadium. The supply of vanadium within the brain is required for cholesterol control and prevention of cholesterol formation within arteries. Fish, on average supplies similar cholesterol compared to meat however nearly all *'land foods'* are deficient in vanadium. Fish also supply the Omega 3's to protect against cholesterol accumulation.

'Hook onto the great fish benefits'!

SEAFOOD - CRUSTACEA

Seafood includes an incredible range of produce with a wide variety of benefits. Clams, Crab, Crayfish, Eel, Kelp, Lobster, Oysters, Prawns, Scallops, Shrimps, Snails, and Spirulina to mention the main groups. *Crustacea* includes crabs, crayfish and lobster. Clams are an excellent source of the mineral iron with 13.8 mg per 100 gram, meat supplies only 1.9 mg, pepitas supply 11.3 mg. Clams also provide the other essential blood building minerals: manganese and copper. If you feel weary and get sick often, iron may be lacking in your diet. Clams have a low fat content with only 73 calories per 100 gram. Crab meat is a good source of the mineral zinc with 6.4 mg per 100 grams, a low fat content and compared to other crustacea, the cholesterol content is low and the protein content of 18% is complete with all essential amino acids. Crab meat is also low in calories with 83 calories per 100 gram and no carbohydrate content and so it is advised to have plenty of salads, or rice with the 'crab feast'. Crayfish / Lobster are the expensive seafood, full of selenium for antioxidant benefits and it also promotes vitamin E effectiveness. Cholesterol is abundant in crayfish / lobster, if you can afford to eat them, can you afford the added cholesterol problems. Eel has a similar fat content to mackerel and sardines with 12% fat and over 60% is in the form of mono unsaturated, the cholesterol content is fairly high and fortunately the monunsaturated fats reduce blood cholesterol. In some countries, the eel is a delicacy and for some people they are too fatty. A farmer once commented about a certain person: 'slippery as a bag of eels!

Kelp is generally obtained from the botanical species: *macrocystis pyrifera, or, fucus vesiculosis* it is termed the 'first crop' in ancient Roman, Greek and Chinese history. Kelp is the richest source of natural iodine and for people living inland or whose ancestors lived by the sea and are now inland, iodine deficiencies are likely unless regular seafood is obtained. Kelp is known to contain nearly all trace elements plus main minerals and many vitamins. A kelp salt shaker is the best way to obtain the trace nutrients regularly or try the kelp crackers and 'balance your body' as that is the most formidable function of kelp, it restores a natural balance to the glands and entire body. Don't be weary, give 'kelp the chance to help'! The ocean is full of minerals washed from the earth which sediment on the ocean floor where kelp grows. Kelp is 'food for the future', it may become the 'new penicillin'. 'Forget to add the common salt'! Oysters are the richest food source of zinc. If you need to 'boost your reproductive life', zinc is essential plus it promotes healing of numerous disorders. The (R.D.I.) of zinc is 12-15 mg, one medium oyster supplies approx. 13 mg. Normal intake of zinc per day is 12 - 15 mg for adults. Zinc promotes the functions of the immune system. Excess amounts of zinc depress the immune system. One dozen oysters is definitely excessive or 152 mg of zinc. Share half a dozen or 38 mg of zinc next time you dine and share the fun and benefits 'once a fortnight' or every anniversary! Prawns are the 'over consumed seafood' mainly because they are the richest seafood in cholesterol and 'thrown on every barby' (barbecue). They are a good source of protein but the risk of high blood cholesterol needs to be 'alerted' especially if you eat a 'few snags' (sausages) the same day or eggs, chocolate, ham, or especially kidney and liver. Scallops are a safe seafood in regards to nutrients and cholesterol but as with all seafood the risk of toxins from polluted waters can be concerning. The same applies to land produce, chemicals grouped as dioxins are more prevalent in meat 81 pg. dairy 24 pg. and fish 7.8 pg. Dioxins accumulate in fat tissues of animals-humans posing a cancer hazard and reproductive problems. 'Keep our oceans clean'.

SEAFOOD - NUTRIENT COMPARISON CHART									
measured in 100 grams.	PROT-EIN %	FAT %	CHO-LESTE-ROL	IRON mg.	SELE-NIUM mcg	ZINC mg	VIT. A I.U.	VIT. B12 mcg	VIT. E I.U.
CLAMS	13	.97	71	13.8	24	1.3	300	49	1.5
CRAB	18	.60	41	.59	36	6.4	23	11	-
EEL	18	12	126	.50	6.5	1.6	3485	3	6
KELP	17	.56	0	2.8	.7	1.2	120	0	-
LOBSTER	19	.89	95	.63	41	3	70	.92	2.1
OYSTERS	7	2.5	54	6.6	52	90	332	19	1.2
PRAWNS	20	1.7	153	2.4	37	1.1	10	1.2	1.1
SCALLOPS	17	.7	33	.3	22	.95	51	1.5	1.5
SNAILS	23	.4	65	5	-	1.6	84	9	-
SPIRULINA	57	7.7	0	29	7.3	2	570	0	7.5
ALMONDS	18	54	0	4.7	7.8	2.9	10	0	39
CHEESE	25	33	107	.67	14	3.1	1071	.83	.53

Possibly the greatest nutritional debate is based on the question of meat. No other natural food obtains such 'heated' debate and the general public are pushed into meat consumption as it is always on the 'hot plate' or menu and take away display.

The over consumption of meat can cause problems. Throughout this section on meat the information will firstly provide the list of problems associated with a regular meat diet and then the benefits.

POSSIBLE DETRIMENTAL FACTORS

1. Excess consumption of meat.
2. Excess saturated fat intake.
3. Low carbohydrate content.
4. Excess cholesterol intake.
5. Uric acid, nitrates, adrenaline.
6. Antibiotics, hormones, drugs.
7. Low calcium content.
9. Excess body acids.
10. Obesity development.
11. Processed meats.
12. Bacteria, long digestion time.
13. Free radicals.
14. Lacking the supply of omega 3.
15. Low in numerous nutrients.
16. Other factors.

POSSIBLE BENEFICIAL FACTORS

1. Moderate protein content.
2. Supply of vitamin B12.
3. Long lasting 'full stomach feeling'.

1. Excess consumption of meat.

As with nearly all foods, any excess is not beneficial. The serve of meat often takes up 70% on the dinner plate and the small quantity of foods 'on the side' barely provides sufficient nutrition for a proper balanced diet.

The balanced diet requires 50% carbohydrates, 35 % protein and 15% lipids. On average, meat (steak) supplies a proportion ratio of 0% carbohydrates, 28% protein and 72% lipids. Unless the diet supplies a balance of carbohydrate foods without added fats, the common meat-meal can become a 'big' problem!

The fat from 2 lamb chops or 2 sausages or 2 slices of bacon easily exceeds the daily 'lipid limit'.

2. Excess saturated fat intake.

The average beef steak supplies the proportion of 45 g saturated fats, 1 g poly unsaturated and 9 g mono unsaturated. The essential fatty acid, omega 3 is not supplied by meat. Saturated fats can be used for energy but ideally the carbohydrate foods are the best energy foods as they require less digestive effort and generally speaking, they supply the associated nutrients to support energy production. Excess saturated fat intake can lead to heart disease.

An excess consumption of saturated fats per day is more than one main meat meal per day, or over 100 grams of cheese or one meal of bacon and eggs.

Saturated fats do provide a 'full stomach' feeling for many hours and this can be considered both a bonus and a detriment. Once consumed, the digestive system attempts to process the protein content of meat, within the stomach. Saturated fats slow down the protein conversion and can cause problems later in the small intestine and colon. Saturated fats are not processed in the stomach, they are converted into fatty acids and glycerol in the upper part of the small intestine (duodenum). This 'delaying factor' of saturated fats can seem like a satisfying meal but for the digestive system, it is in 'the too hard basket'. Saturated fats increase blood cholesterol levels in addition to those supplied by the meat.

3. Low carbohydrate content.

As mentioned previously, meat supplies hardly any carbohydrate content or more 'to the point' no roughage or fibre content. Both these factors can become a problem for the regular meat eater. Especially if their diet also includes refined foods: white bread, chips etc., as there will be insufficient natural movement in the lower digestive system.

This can lead to constipation and over the long term, colon cancer can develop due to the bacteria caused from the buildup of toxins within the large intestine.

Nearly all animal protein foods are very low in fibre and carbohydrate content.

It is essential to obtain such foods as pears, apples, rice bran, figs, coconut, legumes, bananas and other fruits and vegetables regularly in order to protect against the meat 'getting stuck in a rut'!

MEAT - CHOLESTEROL - SATURATED FATS

4. *Excess cholesterol content.*

Meat does supply cholesterol, beef 81 mg and in combination with the saturated fat content, the risk of an excess (BCL) blood cholesterol level is common for people who consume daily meat meals, plus other rich cholesterol foods and the various 'risk factors'. The factors that are vital for lowering blood cholesterol levels are the Omega 3's, such foods as walnuts, hazel nuts, pecan nuts and cold pressed flax oil in particular and fish are rich in Omega 3. Apart from lowering the (BCL), the Omega 3's can also lower blood triglycerides, or blood fat levels. The Omega 6's also help lower blood cholesterol. The mono unsaturated lipids also lower blood cholesterol and in addition they moderately reduce the bad (LDL) low density lipoproteins and maintain the good (HDL) high density lipoproteins. Olive oil is a rich source of mono unsaturated lipids and it is recommended for it's ability to reduce the 'bad fats'. Other risk factors for regular meat eaters that increase (BCL) are smoking, obesity, lack of exercise, refined foods, take away foods, chocolate, milk, cream, cheese, eggs and especially prawns, crabs, crayfish, brains, kidney, liver and sausages. Added lipids in cooking can easily 'top the scales'.

The maximum daily cholesterol intake for an adult is 300 mg. per day. One meal of 2 sausages and 1 egg will easily exceed. Many 'common meals' will exceed the maximum daily cholesterol and saturated fat intake. To be sure your cholesterol is not 'climbing up the wall', have a medical check, especially for people who have a regular meat diet with the associated risk factors.

BLOOD CHOLESTEROL LEVELS
measured in (mmol per litre)

Very high level	6.5 and above
High level	5.5 - 6.5
Average level	4.2 - 5.4
Low risk level	Less than 4.2

Cholesterol is produced by the liver at approx. 1,000 mg per day. It is required for hormone production, cell structure, vitamin D synthesis and the metabolism of fats. Excess cholesterol intake from foods can lead to the narrowing of arteries which directly affects blood flow and pressure, as the cholesterol particles, especially the (LDL) can attach to the arterial walls. In addition, saturated fats and refined carbohydrates: white bread, sugar etc., increase the (LDL) bad lipids in the bloodstream and increase blood cholesterol levels. Research has shown that 'dietary cholesterol' inhibits the anticancer action of the large white blood cells.

MEAT-CHOLESTEROL / FATS CHART

MEAT PRODUCE 100 GRAM SERVES COOKED	TOTAL FAT grams	SAT. FAT grams	CHOLES TEROL mg
Beef steak lean	22	9	81
Chicken lean	5	4.5	90
Crab	2	.5	70
Crayfish/ Lobster	2	.5	150
Ham	10	4	100
Kidney	3	1.5	550
Lamb chop	14	7	75
Liver	12	5.5	400
Oysters	2.5	1.5	53
Pork	27	11	100
Prawns	2	1	110
Rabbit	4	2	65
Salami	38	13	99
Sausages (2 med)	20	10	200
Veal roast	1	.5	100
Chocolate	30	19	100
Eggs (2 average)	12	4	420
Pate	30	13	150

RECOMMENDED LIPIDS INTAKE PER DAY

	MINIMUM	MAXIMUM
Children (5 -12)	30grams	60grams
Teenager	40grams	80 grams
Men sedentary work	30grams	40 grams
Men active physical	40 grams	80 grams
Women sedentary	30 grams	40 grams
Women active physical	40 grams	60 grams
Athletes, hard physical	80 grams	120 grams

5. Uric acid, nitrates, adrenaline

Uric acid from meat is a problem, as it builds up in the bloodstream forming sharp crystals. The white blood cells attempt to rid the blood of the uric acid crystals, however they are unable to digest the uric acid crystals and 'sadly' the white blood cells are destroyed in the process. The resulting dead white cells release a corrosive digestive juice which is known to attack the delicate lining of joints, possibly one major cause of arthritis. Coffee, chocolate, and tea also contain uric acid. In addition kidney stones are often caused by excess uric acid. Some meats such as sausages, frankfurts and some processed 'luncheon meats' contain nitrites and they can be linked to cancer causing nitrosamines in the stomach. Adrenaline is produced in animals and humans during conditions of fear, excitement and other states of heightened awareness. The abattoir is a place where animals are penned in for a few days, not fed and finally they are lined up and during this latter stage the animals sense fear. Adrenaline is pushed through their system into the blood and tissues. Adrenaline can be transferred to humans from the eating of meat and it can cause over - stimulation of the thyroid gland and general metabolism. In some cases it can promote aggressive tendencies. In India, for thousands of years, the warriors were allowed meat, the others were forbidden meat. The elephant is generally a placid plant eating animal, however the tiger, a pure carnivore, becomes aggressive quickly.

It is the adrenaline that 'triggers' the action.

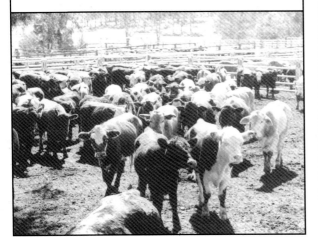

6. Antibiotics, hormones, drugs

6. *Antibiotics, hormones, drugs* are often contained in meat and meat products. The use of antibiotics in humans is already at 'peak levels'.

With meat production, ask any farmer, they also use antibiotics, hormones and drugs for the care of their herd, but it may transfer to the person who eats the meat. Hormones given to promote growth, may also transfer into the meat and other drugs required can also be transferred. Even though DDT has been banned nearly 20 years, animals can still show trace amounts which transfer to the human via a meat meal. Other chemicals that are used in meat production are: tranquillizers, toxaphene, chlordane, stibestrol, methoxychlor, dieldrin, lindane and aureomycin. Research shows that fresh fruits and vegetables help to take toxic chemicals from the body.

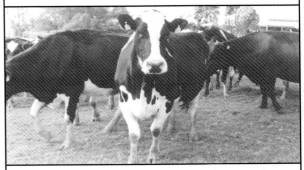

7. The *low calcium content* of meat is a concern as it is the main body mineral and the condition of osteoporosis, brittle bones and low density bones is certainly not helped by eating meat. For women after menopause, bone loss increases and calcium rich foods are essential. Excess meat will reduce the appetite for other foods and possibly add to the bone leaching, due to the low calcium supply. Cramps and high blood pressure can also be due to a calcium deficiency. Meat makes weak bones, balance your diet with calcium rich foods!

CALCIUM COMPARISON CHART per 100 gram.	
Beef steak	25 mg.
Almonds	235 mg.
Cheese cheddar	734 mg.
Tahini	422 mg.
Adult RDA approx.	1100 mg.

8. Excess body acids. The ideal balanced diet requires 75% fresh foods, 25% cooked foods. Nearly all cooked foods are acid forming. Meat is one of the most acid forming foods. When the blood is in an acid state it can lower the immune system's ability to protect and heal the body. Excess acidic foods cause the body to produce more mucus in an attempt to protect against the acids. Alkalinity in the blood is vital for the process of reproduction. For maximum healing, the blood needs an alkaline balance. Minerals are the main provider of both acid and alkaline elements. The pituitary gland controls the body's acid - alkaline balance. Nearly all fruits and vegetables, almonds and rice are alkaline foods. Most other foods, especially crustacea, meat, poultry, fish and eggs are acid forming. A constant acid diet can cause a person to be discontent as such conditions as headaches, sluggish liver, poor circulation and constipation can all be attributed to excess body acids.

Coffee, alcohol, soft drinks and tannin tea are also acid forming to the blood. The best advice for the regular meat eater is to ensure that adequate servings of fruit and vegetables are obtained regularly and to choose legume meals whenever possible.

10. Obesity is a 'growing problem' in some countries and there are a few reasons as to connection between meat and obesity. Calories do add up in the diet and with meat, over 50% of the calories are from fats, lean ham 75% fat, sirloin steak 76% and trimmed sirloin steak 35% fat. Most of the fat is saturated and often 'extra fats or oils' are added to the meat when cooking, they are 100 % lipid content. Overeating is a major cause of obesity and with meat, it is common to see large portions on the plate completely eaten with extra serves later. It is 'full of flavour', for some, with added sauce to encourage the appetite further, plus the saturated fats satisfy the appetite. Over years, a person can consume more quantity as their stomach stretches, plus the belly (intestines) and if there is no reason to stop eating, obesity increases. Obesity is often related to a slow metabolism and the excess intake of processed and take away foods, soft drinks, alcohol, chocolate and the 'hereditary' family meals.

12. Bacteria, long digestion time, for meat, digestion time is longer than any other food group, especially if added fats are combined. Meat requires 5 - 6 hours preparation in the stomach, poultry 4 - 6 hours, cheese 3 - 4 hours. The problem really occurs later in the small intestine and particularly in the large intestine, the colon. The adult human digestive system is approx. 10 meters long, most carnivorous animals digestive system is only 2 meters long. As meat putrefies easily in a warm environment, the digestive system of humans is an ideal breeding ground for bacteria as it can take up to and over 18 hours for the meat-chyme to pass out of the body. Meat provides no fibre and unless the diet includes fibre rich foods, the meat-chyme can 'hang around' the colon for days. This is a major cause of colon cancer plus the absorption of numerous toxins, leading the way to poor health due to the strain on the immune system.

13. Free radicals are abundant in cooked, fried and roast meat. The barbecue is the greatest provider of free radicals, so make sure you eat the salads with flax or olive oil to protect against the damage. Free radicals are now recognized as cancer causing elements within cooked fats and oils.

14. Supplies no Omega 3 an 'essential fatty acid' required for life, from the diet. Meat supplies Omega 6 and large quantities of saturated fats. Refer to chart page 134.

15. Low in numerous nutrients as meat is cooked, all heat sensitive nutrients are depleted. It is not a 'nutritious' food, due to the low mineral and vitamin content (refer to chart),plus the numerous detrimental factors mentioned.

NUTRIENT COMPARISON CHART				
PER 100 GRAMS	BEEF	ALMOND	KIDNEY BEANS	PEPITAS
CALCIUM	5	232	28	51
IRON	1.9	4.6	3	11.3
POTASSIUM	318	768	358	801
MAGNESIUM	20	270	45	531
PHOSPHORUS	188	502	147	1166
MANGANESE	.013	1.9	.47	2.9
ZINC	3	2.9	1.1	7.4
VITAMIN A	24	9.8	0	72

MEAT - PROTEIN EVALUATION - SUMMARY

Meat protein values are often considered to be the only source of the essential amino acids or commonly termed 'complete protein'. This is certainly not true. Apart from the main groups of seafood, poultry and dairy foods, numerous other main food groups such as nuts, seeds, grains and legumes also provide the eight essential amino acids or complete protein. By referring to page 89, a chart of numerous natural foods provides the 'facts and figures' to verify that complete protein is available from numerous foods.

On pages 90 - 91, a chart provides a guide to the average amino acid supply of the main food groups, plus the amount of each amino acid required per day for different body weights. It is obvious from the charts that meat - beef is not the best protein food and on page 93 the question of 'what are the best protein foods' is provided in the most complete evaluation of all protein factors.

Apart from *numerous* 'possible detrimental factors' detailed in the previous pages on meat, the protein from meat is complete and it provides a fair supply of the essential amino acid. The protein value of meat can be considerably less compared to the 'ideal lean beef' value on the charts.

Excess cooking of meat is common and that reduces the protein (amino acid) value plus increases the risk factors. Also many of the nutrients are 'leached out' during excess cooking, via the juices. The added fats greatly decrease the protein value as they retard and reduce proper protein digestion in the stomach resulting in poorly prepared proteoses and peptides. Animal protein foods, especially meat require considerable digestive energy to convert the food into useable protein. Primary proteins: nuts, seeds, grains and legumes require half the digestive time and energy compared to meat.

Vitamin B12 is often 'a bone of contention' when the requirement for meat is discussed. Meat is not the only source of vitamin B12, refer to page 171.

Summary of meat: the countryside is *cleared* for meat production and in some places it has become desolate due to over grazing and consequently the major problem of soil salination does occur with a huge expense (reforestation) required to rectify the problem. Meat is over consumed and that results in health problems (as mentioned). Meat takes the place of numerous other meals as people become less able to 'cook'. The basic meal of 'meat and three vegies' *everynight* is 'overkill'!

It takes just as much time to prepare any of the 'hundred's of meatless meals. The 'habit' of eating meat can be so compelling that people say 'they can't live without meat', that is because it has been the major food in their diet for years and without meat the 'plate would be empty'.

There are over 100 'complete protein meals' apart from meat and many of them have supported civilizations for centuries. See if you can get a 'piece of the action' from a properly prepared meatless meal and 'give it a go' to discover new recipes. Don't let the habit of daily meat eating take over your health, weekly food budget and life.

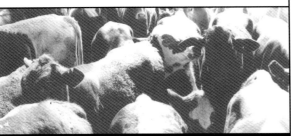

THE BEST PROTEIN FOODS					
NATURAL PROTEIN FOODS	PROTEIN % of natural food	N. P. U. net protein useable	grams of useable protein per 100 grams	TOTAL PROTEIN VALUES	TOTAL PROTEIN VALUE in %
1 TUNA	28 %	80 %	22 %	130	43.3 %
2 FISH	22 %	80 %	17 %	119	39.6 %
3 EGGS	12 %	94 %	17 %	117	39%
4 SOY BEANS	34 %	61 %	21 %	116	38.6 %
5 CHEESE	26 %	70 %	18 %	114	38 %
6 WHEAT GERM	25 %	67 %	17 %	109	36.3 %
7 BEEF	24 %	67 %	16 %	107	35.6 %
8 PEPITAS	29 %	60 %	17 %	106	35.3 %
9 CHICKEN	21 %	65 %	13 %	99	33 %
10 SUNFLOWER SEEDS	23 %	58 %	13 %	94	31.3 %
11 OATS	14 %	66%	9 %	89	29.6 %
12 MILK / YOGHURT	3 %	80 %	3 %	86	28.6 %
13 CASHEWS	18 %	58 %	10 %	86	28.6 %
14 SESAME / TAHINI	19 %	55 %	10 %	84	28 %
15 RICE	7 %	70 %	5 %	82	27.3 %
16 PEANUT	26 %	43 %	11 %	80	26.6 %
17 ALMONDS	18 %	50 %	9 %	77	25.6 %
18 BRAZIL NUTS	14 %	50 %	9 %	71	23.6 %
19 WALNUTS	14 %	50 %	7 %	71	23.6 %
20 CHICK PEAS	20 %	43 %	7 %	70	23.3 %

QUESTION 36	What are Lipids?	Lipids is the term used to describe the group of fats & oils.

QUESTION 37	What food groups supply Lipids?	There are 6 main food groups that supply lipids.

QUESTION 38	What are the 6 main food groups that supply lipids?	1 - Nuts 2 - Seeds 3 - Fish 4 - Seafood 5 - Meat 6 - Dairy produce

QUESTION 39	What other foods or food groups supply lipids?	1 - Seed, Grain, Legume and Vegetable oils 2 - Avocado, olives 3 - Margarine 4 - Fried foods 5 - Take away foods 6 - Snack foods

QUESTION 40	Are all lipids beneficial?	No. Lipids that are heated or chemically altered are not beneficial.

NOTE: All amounts in this book are measured in milligrams (mg) per 100 grams, unless stated otherwise

QUESTION 41	What effect does cooking have on Lipids?

Lipids that are heated undergo a chemical change in their molecular structure.
Oxygen which is naturally attached to the lipid structure becomes *oxidated*, during frying, cooking or intense heat. These 'oxidated molecules' release from the lipid structure and become 'free radicals'.
These *free compounds* attach to other nutrients within the blood, in search of more oxygen and nourishment, such as vitamins, causing them to become oxidised and to deteriorate. Free radicals damage skin cells and other body cells. Refer to page 138 for more details on the problems with cooked oils.

QUESTION 42	How can you protect against 'free radicals'?

The simple answer is to restrict the intake of deep fried foods and cooked oils and to use such methods of cooking as steaming, boiling and shredding to prepare most meals. Other methods such as baking and roasting can reduce the need for added lipids. Ideally, the balanced diet requires 75% fresh foods and 25% cooked foods.
Vegetables can be either steamed or baked without added fats and once the meal is served, add fresh cold pressed oils: olive, flax, canola, sunflower or walnut oil, or tahini or butter to provide that flavour enhancing benefit, without the free radical problem.
Chicken is the over-consumed food and even though it is a low fat food when roasted, deep fried chicken is full of harmful fats within the crumbed coating.
Eggs can be boiled or poached. Barbecues are another common function and the sausages especially are a real concern with their enormous supply of saturated fats and free radicals, when over consumed.
In summary, it is possible to avoid over 90% of common cooked lipids.
Such factors as an increased intake of vitamin E foods such as tahini, almonds, hazel nuts or wheat germ oil and selenium rich foods such as brazil nuts can also provide protection from the free radical problem, as they promote cell life and protect against rapid oxidation. The ideal diet must also include foods that provide the *essential fatty acids: Omega 3 and Omega 6*, as they are vital for numerous body functions.

QUESTION 43	What are the essential fatty acids?

There are 2 essential lipids required with the diet, as they cannot be produced by the body and they are required for numerous vital body functions.

The two essential lipids are: alpha linolenic acid, also referred to as Omega 3
                    and: linoleic acid,   also referred to as Omega 6
Omega 3 and Omega 6 are collectively termed the 'essential fatty acids', or vitamin F

The word Omega is the last letter in the Greek alphabet and it means 'last of series' or final development, but for those seeking the ultimate lipids, let the Omega's be first.
These 'essential fatty acids' belong to the group of *polyunsaturated* lipids.

QUESTION 44

What are the 3 main groups of Lipids?

Monounsaturated lipids have one space in the chain of carbon atoms and this allows for two carbon atoms to share two bonds with each other.

H	H	H	H	H	H	H	H	H	
C	C	C	C	C	C	C	C	C	H
H	H	H			H	H	H	H	

Polyunsaturated lipids have four or more 'free carbon atoms' forming two or more double bonds which gives them the ability to transport 'many' nutrients.

H	H	H	H	H	H	H	H	H	
C	C	C	C	C	C	C	C	C	H
H	H			H			H	H	

Saturated lipids have all their carbon atoms attached to hydrogen atoms, they are usually solid at room temperature and are mainly from animal fats.

H	H	H	H	H	H	H	H	H	
C	C	C	C	C	C	C	C	C	H
H	H	H	H	H	H	H	H	H	

QUESTION 45

What is the main function of the three groups of lipids?

Mono unsaturated lipids: such as olive oil, hazel nuts, almonds and macadamia nuts are used by the body for energy, for the breakdown of cholesterol and they are also stored as body fat in the adipose tissues. Monounsaturated oils are the best to use in cooking, if you have to cook and fry, but ideally they are consumed in the natural state, as a *cold pressed* oil.

Poly unsaturated lipids: especially Omega 3 and Omega 6 are the great carriers of nutrients such as: vitamins A, D, E and K. They also transport and breakdown cholesterol, manufacture other fatty acids, regulate the transfer of oxygen, aid in the protection of the nervous system and the cellular system and cell structure. Also, they are vital for the blood clotting process, they participate in the manufacture of body hormones, regulate healing and are required for development of the foetus and for mental development especially in infants. Poly unsaturated lipids oxidise quickly and are best taken as *cold pressed* oils with a fresh garden salad. Canola oil and walnut oil are a rich source of both Omega 3 and 6. Flax oil is the richest source of Omega 3. When used for cooking, especially frying, oils oxidise into peroxides or free radicals. They cause damage to the arteries, skin cells and may eventually cause cancer. If you have to cook and fry to enjoy a meal, restrict the quantity. Don't toil over spoilt oil!

Saturated lipids: are not essential for health or life. Most natural foods provide a portion of saturated fats in addition to mono and poly unsaturated. See chart page 135. Saturated fats are used mainly for energy. Animal produce foods are the main source of saturated fats, in the average diet. Saturated fats provide a 'full stomach feeling' and easily satisfy the appetite for lengthy periods. These two 'benefits' are often the reason for their common consumption, however, numerous problems are associated with a regular consumption of saturated fats with the animal produce foods, refer pages to pages 114 -130.

Saturated fats are the hardest to digest and they are the most likely to be stored as body fat.

QUESTION 46

What foods are the best source of Omega 3 & 6?

Omega 3 is the 'hard to get' essential fatty acid. Flax oil, nuts, seeds and fish are the best source of Omega 3. Meat supplies only a trace of Omega 3. Such foods as margarine and most cooking oils are a rich source of Omega 6. The ideal intake of the essential fatty acids is: three Omega 6 to one Omega 3. The 'average diet' ratio is 20 Omega 6 to 1 Omega 3. Due to this 'common' imbalance, it is recommended to increase the intake of 'Omega 3 foods'.

OMEGA 3 & 6 FOOD VALUES measured in grams per 100 grams		
NATURAL FOODS/OILS	OMEGA 3	OMEGA 6
Almonds	trace	10
Brazil	trace	23
Cashews	trace	8
Pine nuts	1	25
Walnuts	5.5	28
Linseeds/ flax seed	20	6
Pepitas (pumpkin seeds)	9	20
Sunflower seeds	trace	30
Sesame seeds (tahini)	trace	25
Canola oil	7	20
Soy oil	7	51
Meat	trace	6
Chicken	0.1	1
Fish (average)	2	0.1

QUESTION 47

What are the main functions of Omega 3?

The main functions of the essential Omega 3 is for the production of prostaglandins.

They are the regulators of blood pressure, kidney function, blood clotting, inflammatory responses, nerve transmission and also required for the production of hormones, cell maintenance, supple skin and various digestive functions. In addition, a regular balanced intake of Omega 3 may help prevent depression, obesity, asthma, diabetes, high blood pressure, cancer, attention deficit syndrome, rheumatoid arthritis and heart disease.

Approx. 2 - 4 g of Omega 3, per day is the recommended minimum. Omega 3 foods reduce the appetite by stabilising blood sugar levels. Omega 3 foods help to increase metabolism and thereby promote activity and weight loss. An excess of Omega 6 foods and products, such as margarine, can reduce the activity of Omega 3 and it's numerous essential functions.

Omega 3 is vital during the early stages of a babies development, especially for the brain. Numerous mental disorders can be traced to a prolonged Omega 3 deficiency. Refer to pages 123-125 and 166 for more details on the vital functions of Omega 3.

OMEGA 3 IN FISH & SEAFOOD measured in grams per 100 grams	
Bass	0.74
Cod	0.23
Mackerel	3.3
Perch	0.42
Salmon	2.5
Sardines	1.4
Shark	1.1
Snapper	0.46
Trout	1.5
Tuna	1.4
Crab	0.12
Crayfish	0.15
Prawns / shrimps	0.45
Scallops	0.25

QUESTION 48

What are the main functions of Omega 6?

The main function of Omega 6 is the transport of nutrients, oxygen and energy throughout the body. Omega 6 is also required for blood clotting, regulating body healing and the manufacture of hormones. Omega 6 is polyunsaturated, it has three double bonds within the chain of carbon atoms, the first bond located at the number 6 carbon atom, hence the name Omega 6, refer to page 133 for the polyunsaturated carbon chain diagram. Omega 3 has two double bonds, the first carbon bond positioned at number 3 carbon atom. Both Omega 3 & Omega 6 belong to the group of polyunsaturated lipids.

<table>
<tr><th colspan="4">QUESTION 49</th></tr>
</table>

QUESTION 49	What foods provide the unsaturated and saturated lipids?

As can be seen from the chart, the main *monounsaturated foods* are: almonds, cashews, hazel nuts, macadamia, pecan, pistachio. and olive oil. Olive oil supplies 76% of the lipids as mono unsaturated.

Refer to page 142 for details on the benefits of olive oil.

The main *polyunsaturated foods* are: walnuts, soy beans and fish, with the oils, corn, safflower and sunflower all providing over 50% polyunsaturated lipid content.

The main *saturated foods* are: *coconut, butter, cheese, cream, chocolate, ice cream, milk, yoghurt, beef and lamb.*

The figures in this chart do not add up to 100% as some of the minor fatty acids figures are not available in each group.

Apart from the foods in the chart, there are numerous other foods that supply both unsaturated and saturated lipids.

QUESTION 50	Is margarine a beneficial food?

Margarine is often classed as polyunsaturated, however, as can be seen from the chart, most of the lipid content (45%) is in the form of monounsaturated.

Margarine is *processed* via 'hydrogenation', which converts vegetable oils into a semi-saturated state. In addition, margarine usually contains additives such as colouring (160 A) food acid (330) antioxidant (306, 320) preservative (202) emulsifier (471) added vitamins and salt.

The oils used for margarine originate from a heat and chemical process. These oils are then *hydrogenised,* a process where hydrogen is mixed into the oils, causing saturation of the fatty acids. This converts them into *'trans fatty acids'* which increase blood cholesterol levels, deplete skin cell life and tax the immune system. So the question is 'what do I spread on my bread, sandwich or salad roll'. Ideally, cold pressed olive, flax or canola oil sprinkled and spread on the bread, or use avocado or tahini, all of which promote health.

Trans fatty acids need to be avoided. They promote heart disease, hardened arteries and may upset the delicate balance in the glandular system and also hormone functions.

Another problem with margarine is that an excess intake of Omega 6, in margarine and in processed foods, upsets and depletes the important functions of Omega 3. Keep a lid on things and balance your Omega's. Choose margarine with canola oil, mix in a tablespoon of flax oil and remember that margarine was invented for convenience, not for health.

FOOD LIPID BALANCE CHART (%)			
	MONO.	POLY.	SAT.
ALMONDS	68	19	8
BRAZIL	33	37	25
CASHEW	58	16	20
HAZEL	77	10	7
MACADAMIA	76	3	14
PECAN	60	25	8
PISTACHIO	68	13	14
WALNUTS	18	68	8
AVOCADO	43	12	18
CHICK PEAS	42	42	trace
PEANUT	47	29	30
MILLET	33	33	33
MARGARINE	45	32	19
POULTRY	45	20	30
OLIVE OIL	76	7	11
SESAME SEEDS	38	42	14
SOY BEANS	23	51	17
WHEAT GERM	27	46	18
COCONUT	6	2	88
BUTTER	34	2	57
EGGS	40	12	30
CHEESE	28	4	64
CREAM	29	4	62
CHOCOLATE	38	2	57
ICE CREAM	29	4	63
MILK	29	4	63
YOGHURT	27	3	65
FISH (average)	20	50	25
BEEF	35	2	60
LAMB	36	3	54
VEAL	40	2	40
PORK	40	2	40
CORN OIL	28	53	10
SAFFLOWER OIL	15	72	8
SUNFLOWER OIL	19	63	13

What is cholesterol and what does it do?

Cholesterol is described as a waxy fat-like substance. Cholesterol is part of every living cell in the human body, as an essential component of cell membranes.

Cholesterol is produced by the liver, approx. 1,000 mg per day. It is required for functions such as the manufacture of hormones such as oestrogen, cortisone and testosterone.

Apart from the human body producing cholesterol, animals also produce cholesterol.

When such produce as meat, chicken, seafood and dairy is eaten by humans, added cholesterol is obtained via the animal produce, as it is also an important component in animal cells.

The great increase in cholesterol levels for many people is not only due to an excess intake of animal produce foods. Processed foods and other foods with a high glycemic index, refer to page 16, such as french fries, rice cakes, baked potatoes and white bread and refined carbohydrates also increase cholesterol. Plus, soft drinks have a high glycemic index.

The conversion of such foods and drinks into energy results in *carbon fragments* which the body uses to make cholesterol. Saturated fats also supply carbon fragments after digestion and conversion into fatty acids and they also promote an increase in blood cholesterol.

Such foods as organ meats and crustacea are especially rich in cholesterol.

Cholesterol is vital for cell construction, excess cholesterol is lethal and can cause obstruction.

QUESTION
52

How do I reduce blood cholesterol naturally?

To reduce blood cholesterol naturally, it is advised to;

1. Restrict the intake of foods that contain high cholesterol.

2. Restrict the intake of foods rich in saturated fats (butter, cheese, chocolate, meat and sausages etc.)

3. Reduce the intake of foods that have a moderately high glycemic index, high glycemic index or very high glycemic index, refer to page 16.

4. Ensure that the diet includes legume meals regularly: kidney bean tacos, hummous or lentil soup.

5. Obtain a regular intake of rolled oats or barley.

6. Obtain foods rich in natural lecithin such as sweet corn and soy in the form of soya grits.

7. A natural lecithin supplement is also available at health stores, it is a concentrated source and may be helpful for promoting a reduction in blood cholesterol.

8. Limit total cholesterol intake to less than 300 mg per day.

9. Limit intake of pastries, cakes and biscuits.

10. Obtain regular moderate exercise.

NOTE: The ideal blood cholesterol level is less than 4.2 mmol. / litre. High cholesterol is 5.5 - 6.5 mmol / litre. Very high cholesterol is over 6.5 mmol / litre.

FOOD CHOLESTEROL CHART	
measured in mg. per 100 gram.	
Beef Steak	70 mg.
Brains	1800 mg.
Butter	250 mg.
Cheddar cheese	100 mg.
Chocolate	100 mg.
Cream cheese	120 mg.
Swiss cheese	85 mg.
Chicken cooked, lean.	100 mg.
Egg (whole raw)	550 mg.
Egg yolk	1,500 mg.
Fish (average)	50 mg.
Hamburger meat	80 mg.
Kidney	550 mg.
Lamb chops	70 mg.
Lard	95 mg.
Liver	400 mg.
Lobster	150 mg.
Milk (cows, full fat)	11 mg.
Oysters	250 mg.
Pate (average)	150 mg.
Prawns	110 mg.
Salmon (canned	50 mg.
Sardines	140 mg.
Sausage cooked	200 mg.
Tuna	40 mg.
Turkey (no skin)	60 mg.
Veal chops	90 mg.

Is lecithin really that important?

Lecithin is part of every living cell in the body, especially in the brain and liver. Lecithin is also part of the glandular system and required in the tissues and the muscles of the heart and kidneys.

Lecithin is made up from a mixture of substances that are collectively known as phospholipids. They consist of the essential fatty acids, phosphorus and the B complex vitamins: choline and inositol. Research has shown that with mentally impaired people, the brain-lecithin content is often as low as 19%. With mentally stable people, the brain-lecithin content is 28%. Lecithin is vital for prevention of nervous breakdowns in combination with the B complex vitamins and magnesium. During times of stress, lecithin within the body is used rapidly. If it is not replaced with the diet, fatigue, irritation and mental confusion may develop.

Lecithin is termed 'nature's tranquillizer'. The majority of processed, refined and take away foods have no lecithin content, are loaded with cholesterol and often have a high glycemic index. Protect your body, nervous system and brain for 'goodness sakes', with a little lecithin every few days. Some margarines have added lecithin, that's one positive thing about margarine but it still contains those nasty trans fatty acids, 'keep a lid on things, feed your brain with lecithin! Lecithin granules are available at most supermarkets and health stores. Lecithin can be added to soups, gravy, bread, muffins, omelettes or scrambled eggs.

Try a 'pinch' to start and then obtain a regular pinch every few days. Your brain will regain, your blood cholesterol will naturally level, your nerves will not be disturbed and your health will be better than wealth.

Is butter better than margarine?

Butter is a natural food, it contains no trans fatty acids in the natural state, margarine does contain trans fatty acids. Once heated, butter is no better than margarine as the fats will be converted into free radicals.

Butter is made from cream and milk, a rich source of saturated fats which the body can use only in moderation. Salted butter often contains 140 mg of sodium chloride (salt) per 100 grams, that is a fair amount, so best use unsalted butter for the best health value.

If your diet is well balanced with ample fruits and vegetables, legumes and oats, the addition of butter with bread or toast, or the sweet corn, rice dish or potatoes will be no concern.

If your diet is rich in animal product foods, especially bacon, sausages, meat and cheese, the extra butter will add up quickly to be a cholesterol and weight concern.

If you want a 'better butter' try the soft butter with added cold pressed oil. To make your own better butter at home, using the food processor; mix approx. one quarter cold pressed walnut oil with three quarters unsalted butter. Add 1 tsp. of wheat germ oil, 2 tsp's. flax oil, 1 tsp. of lecithin granules and with a dash of kelp salt, it becomes the 'award winning butter for the future'!

BUTTER - MARGARINE - SPREADS CHART
(all measured in 1 teaspoon or 5 gram portions)

FOOD TYPE	cholesterol	TOTAL FAT	SATURATED
Butter	10	4	2.5
Margarine	0	4	1
Margarine reduced. fat.	0	3	.5
Margarine with olive oil.	0	3	.5
Avocado	0	.7	0
Tahini	0	3	.2
Hommus	0	.8	0
Cream cheese	6	1.6	.9
Olive oil	0	5	.5

Why are cooked oils harmful?

Cooked oils are possibly the most common health risk problem, especially for people who consume regular take away foods, deep fried foods and chips cooked in oils.

Nearly half the fat that people consume is termed 'hidden fat', you can be sure it's there because it 'tastes nice'.

Any oil or fat that has been heated will go through a process where the oxygen attached to the lipid structure becomes 'oxidized' or 'lifeless' so it desperately tries to stay alive by attaching to other living nutrients within the bloodstream.

These 'lifeless oxidised particles' are termed 'free radicals' and as the name implies, they are free to roam around causing trouble.

They 'enjoy' destroying skin cells and the result is premature ageing, they 'enjoy' destroying cellular structures resulting in damage to the internal linings of arteries, they 'enjoy' breaking down DNA resulting in possible birth defects, they also attack the immune system when 'it's down', so they are nasty 'to the bone'. Why do we enjoy them! They taste good for a few seconds and provide a 'long lasting' meal.

Well, don't leave it too late to 'enjoy' the abundance of flavour from 'pure cold pressed oils': canola, flax, sunflower, soy, safflower, olive and walnut oil, plus, fresh nuts are really underestimated and often pushed to the side due to their price. As they say 'you get what you pay for'!

Rescue yourself from the increasing menace of 'radicals'!

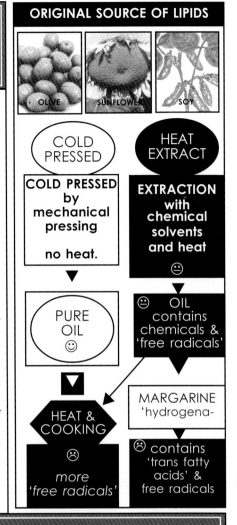

ORIGINAL SOURCE OF LIPIDS

OLIVE SUNFLOWER SOY

COLD PRESSED

HEAT EXTRACT

COLD PRESSED by mechanical pressing

no heat.

EXTRACTION with chemical solvents and heat ☺

▼

PURE OIL ☺

☺ OIL contains chemicals & 'free radicals'

HEAT & COOKING ☹

more 'free radicals'

MARGARINE 'hydrogena-

☹ contains 'trans fatty acids' & free radicals

Do lipids really add on the calories and weight?

Lipids supply 9 calories per gram, carbohydrates and proteins supply only 4 calories per gram. The balanced diet requires 50% carbohydrates, 30 - 40% proteins and 15 - 20% lipids.

If the *carbohydrate* intake is based on refined foods, they will actually increase the need for insulin and excess insulin is a cause for increased storage of body fats.

Protein foods on their own are less likely to increase body weight, unless they are taken with added fats and oils Excess protein can be stored as fat or used for energy, but it is not a clean burning energy fuel, as it produces harmful ammonia during conversion into energy.

The 15 - 20% daily intake for lipids includes all those added fats and oils in the diet with cooking, processed foods and the actual fat content in the foods consumed.

It is very easy to obtain excess fats and associated calories from the diet, especially if the diet does not include the recommended 75% fresh foods with 25% cooked food formula. Added fats make a meal, or snack food more tasty and that can easily result in excess consumption. Also, cooked foods lack numerous nutrients that control fat metabolism.

Don't let the cooked foods take over your diet, keep 'ship shape' naturally!

Regular exercise is also the key to natural weight control.

CHAPTER FOUR P

OILS INTRODUCTION

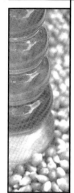

Oils can be extracted by various methods, the best method for human consumption is when the oil has been 'cold-drawn' or usually referred to as 'cold pressed'.

The cold-pressed method is usually achieved with hydraulic equipment and it does not change the chemical structure of the lipid elements, thereby providing the correct balance for human digestion, absorption and metabolism. Cold pressed or 'virgin oil' is obtained with one pressing.

The majority of oils that are available from the supermarket are extracted with chemical solvents and heat processes as that is the most economical way to produce oils. Apart from the chemical solvents and the heat processes there are further processing and bleaching techniques used to make the oil clean tasting, odourless and light coloured.

All those extra processing techniques are designed to get every drop of oil from the original source, however, the amount of chemical residue that remains in those oils is something to be avoided. The only way to be sure of obtaining top quality oil is to see the label 'cold pressed' oil.

Heat and chemical processes destroy the vital vitamin E content. One of the most noticeable effects from regular use of chemically extracted oils is poor skin condition, due to a deficiency of especially vitamin E

Very few processed foods and natural foods supply a good amount of vitamin E. A deficiency of vitamin E may be a major factor that contributes to skin cancer, as vitamin E protects against ultraviolet radiation. Whole grain bread is meant to supply a daily serve of vitamin E, white bread supplies no vitamin E. Almonds are rich in vit. E.

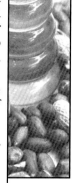

It is important to know that the more polyunsaturated oils and margarine consumed, the greater the need for vitamin E in order to prevent cellular deterioration and arterial damage.

Another vital factor is the requirement for, and the supply of the essential fatty acids, in particular Omega 3. Very few oils and foods supply the 'hard to get' Omega 3.

Canola and walnut oil are well balanced with both the essential fatty acids. Linseed or Flax oil is exceptionally rich in Omega 3, with nearly 4 times the Omega 3 content compared to Omega 6. Add Flax oil to other oils or margarine.

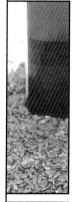

Margarine and most seed oils supply abundant Omega 6, but most oils supply either no Omega 3 or only a trace of Omega 3, refer to pages 134 - 135 for details on the unique functions of Omega 3 and the problems with margarine and excess Omega 6 intake.

The following pages will provide specific details and associated benefits for 15 individual 'cold pressed' oils. Due to the ability of oils to enhance food flavour, most processed foods, take away foods and restaurant meals will include considerable amounts of added fats and oils, but it is hard to know what type of oils they use. Ideally, when at home, make up for the restaurant meals by including cold pressed oils to salads, especially those 'well balanced oils' such as flax, canola, or walnut oil.

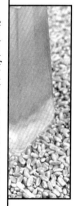

NOTE: The following chemical additives and preservatives may be found in oils that have not been extracted with the 'cold pressed' method: Propyl gallate, Methyl silicone, BHT, BHA, Polyglycerides, Polysorbate 80, Oxystearic.

A common solvent used to extract some oils is Hexane, a derivative of crude petroleum refinement.

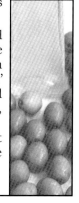

NOTE: All amounts in this book are measured in milligrams (mg) per 100 grams, unless stated otherwise.

AVOCADO OIL

VITAMIN E	CALORIES - total: 884 kcal. per 100 gram
0	Saturated:11.6g. Poly:13.5g. Mono:70.6g.

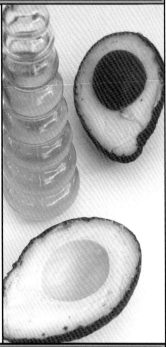

Avocado oil is second best to olive oil for the rich supply of mono unsaturated, with 70% of all lipids in the form of oleic acid. The benefits of using avocado oil on a fresh salad or as a replacement for butter or margarine are well worth discovering. Oleic acid is known to reduce low density lipoproteins and to also protect against the accumulation of arterial plaque, thereby reducing high blood pressure. The avocado fruit supplies 77% lipid content and with 70% in the form of oleic acid, the avocado-butter is without doubt, a great way to obtain a nourishing spread that can be consumed regularly as it contains no cholesterol plus it has the potential to reduce cholesterol. Avocado oil supplies a trace amount of Omega 3, 0 .1 g and a fair supply of Omega 6, 1.9 g. The avocado fruit is an excellent source of glutathione, a potent antioxidant with the power to inhibit numerous carcinogens. The common use of deep fried foods and cooked oils is the main cause of dietary carcinogens. Such foods as potato chips, french fries and barbecued meats are full of cooked oils, they contain the 'free radicals' that lead to cell destruction and the onset of cancerous tissues. The avocado and avocado oil are ready for the rescue. Mix two tsp's. of flax oil and 1 tsp. of wheat germ oil to a cup of avocado oil. The power of vitamin E and Omega 3 will provide the coalition force to knock out those oily radicals.

ALMOND OIL OIL

VITAMIN E	CALORIES - total: 884 kcal. per 100 gram
39.2 mg.	Saturated: 8.2 g. Poly:17.4g. Mono: 69.9g.

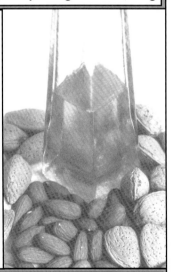

Almond oil has been used for thousands of years as a facial cosmetic. The Roman ladies cherished the rejuvenating benefits and today you can obtain the same treatment with little expense. A small bottle of pure almond oil will go a long way in providing essential nourishment for the skin and the rich supply of vitamin E, 39 mg is the main factor. Almond oil supplies 87 % unsaturated lipids, mainly in the form of mono unsaturated 70 %, with nearly 60 % being in the form of oleic acid. The oleic acid content of almond oil is completely digestible and it has the ability to improve the transfer and absorption of the fat soluble vitamins: A, D, E and K. Almond oil is a good source of Omega 6, 10 g and it supplies only a trace of Omega 3. When added to a salad dressing, the rich oleic acid content in almond oil will enhance the effectiveness of vitamin E and promote skin cell life, as vitamin E protects against oxidation. Excess use of margarine is a major cause of poor skin condition as it increases the rate of vitamin E oxidation. Almond oil is ready to liven your life internally and externally with beautiful benefits.

APRICOT KERNEL OIL

VITAMIN E	CALORIES - total:884 kcal. per 100 gram
8.7 mg.	Saturated: 7 g. Poly: 31 g. Mono: 62 g.

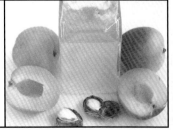

Apricot kernel oil is a rare beauty, a rich source of oleic acid 62 % and a fair supply of vitamin E, both contributing to promote healthy skin condition when used externally. Apricot oil provides an excellent supply of phytosterols 580 mg, refer to corn oil. Apricot oil is ideal for sensitive skin, premature aged skin and for babies skin, it provides a softening effect on the skin and easily penetrates the skin, it is odourless and does not feel oily. Apricot kernel oil can also be added to a fruit salad. Appreciate the benefits of apricot oil.

CANOLA OIL	VITAMIN E 17 mg.	CALORIES - total: 884 kcal. per 100 gram Saturated: 7 g Poly: 31 g Mono: 62 g

Canola oil has become a common cooking oil, but, cooked oils are of no health benefit. Canola oil is a good source of both Omega 3, 7 g and Omega 6, 20 g, plus a good supply of vitamin E. The balance between Omega 3 and Omega 6 is in the ideal proportion (1 Omega 3 to 3 Omega 6). Canola oil is nearly 70 % mono unsaturated. Canola oil also provides a good supply of vitamin K 122 mcg. Canola oil is a great choice for daily use and for a balanced supply of the essential fatty acids. Cold pressed canola is the best.

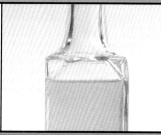

COCONUT OIL	VITAMIN E .1mg.	CALORIES - total: 862 kcal. per 100 gram Saturated: 86.5 g Poly:1.8 g Mono:5.8 g

Coconut oil is 86 % saturated fat, the richest source from any food and the minute supply of polyunsaturates means that it provides none of the essential fatty acids: Omega 3 or Omega 6. The small amount of mono unsaturates 6 g may just be sufficient to help reduce the increase in cholesterol from the saturated fat content of the coconut. Fortunately, the coconut and oil contain no cholesterol so it seems that on it's own, the oil is safe but preferably used externally only. Numerous beach style suntan lotions contain some coconut oil, it is a rich oil and can provide a unique holiday glow and scent when applied liberally. Coconut oil is extracted from the white flesh part of the nut, it is termed copra and also used for desiccated coconut, as livestock feed and as a fertilizer. In these days of increasing ultraviolet radiation, the use of coconut oil decreases due to the risk of skin cancer from excess sunlight. Nearly all calories from the coconut are derived directly from the compact saturated lipid content.

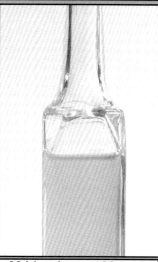

CORN OIL	VITAMIN E 14.3 mg	CALORIES - total: 884 kcal. per 100 gram Saturated:12.7 g Poly:58.7 g Mono:24.2 g

Corn oil has been used in Peru for thousands of years, it is easily extracted from the corn kernels and is a good general purpose cooking oil. Corn oil is a good source of vitamin E and it provides a small amount of vitamin K 1 . 9 mcg. Corn oil is a rich source of Omega 6, 50 mg but it does not supply Omega 3. A combination of half corn oil with half flax seed oil would provide a balance with the Omega 3's, as flax oil provides only 15 g Omega 6 and 58 g Omega 3. The corn-flax oil combo would be as good as oil gets when obtained cold pressed. Corn oil is exceptionally rich in phytosterols 968 mg, more than wheat germ oil 553 mg and olive oil 221 mg. Most other oils supply either no phytosterols or only a small amount.
Phytosterols are recognized to block cholesterol from entering the bloodstream plus they have been shown in clinical research to reduce symptoms of an enlarged prostrate, reduce inflammation in cases of rheumatoid arthritis and they help control blood sugar levels with diabetics. Ideally, make a salad dressing from cold pressed corn oil, add a dash of vinegar, flax oil and reap the benefits, including the good supply of vitamin E and Omega 6. Corn oil, on it's own, is too rich in Omega 6. An excess of Omega 6 can interfere with the functions of Omega 3, as they both compete for enzymes to manufacture other essential fatty acids. Corn oil is ready to combine for numerous benefits, cob onto them!

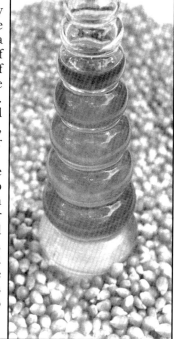

LINSEED - FLAX OIL	VITAMIN E 17.5 mg	CALORIES - total: 884 kcal. per 100 gram Saturated: 10 g Poly: 68 g Mono: 22 g

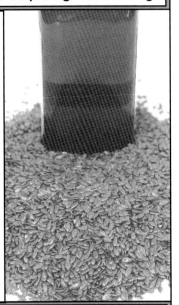

Linseed oil is obtained from the Linacea family or the common flax plant. The early Romans and Greeks used linseed oil as a food plus it is common in some European countries. Edible linseed / flax oil is available, it is deodorized and refined and can also be used externally as a poultice for boils. It makes an excellent addition to other common oils, especially to increase their Omega 3 content. Linseed oil is the richest source of the vital Omega 3's 58 g and a good source of Omega 6 15 g. No other oil or natural food, apart from fish, has an abundance of Omega 3 compared to Omega 6. With an increased use of polyunsaturated margarine in the average diet, the intake of Omega 6 is excessive plus the problem of trans fatty acids can lead to increased cholesterol, damage to cell membranes and hormone production.

The excellent supply of Omega 3 in linseed oil is vital for the nervous system, brain function, fetal development and for protection from depression, autism and learning difficulties. Just a drop of edible linseed oil in the margarine can make a bright difference, or add it to the salad dressing or add some linseed to bread or breakfast cereals. Linseeds are full of O 3.

MACADAMIA OIL	VITAMIN E 1 mg	CALORIES - total: 718 kcal. per 100 gram Saturated: 12 g Poly: 2 g Mono: 59 g

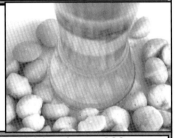

Macadamia oil is obtained from the nut tree native to Australia's north coast region of New South Wales, the trees flourish amidst the rolling hills. Macadamia oil is nearly 60% mono unsaturated, helpful for reducing cholesterol and reducing low density lipo-proteins. Macadamia oil is mainly oleic acid with a nearly unique source of paimitoleic acid. Macadamia oil is low in the essential fatty acids: Omega 3 and 6. Macadamia oil makes a marvellous addition to a salad dressing with a taste that's hard to crack!

OLIVE OIL	VITAMIN E 14.3 mg	CALORIES - total: 884 kcal. per 100 gram Saturated:13.5g Poly:10g Mono:73.9g

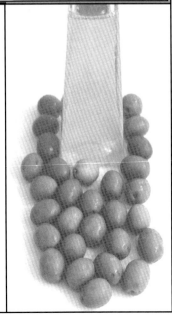

Olive oil has now become a popular addition to the Western diet, after thousands of years, the nutritional benefits of olive oil are being researched and acclaimed the world over. The exceptionally rich monounsaturated content 74 % is ideal for lowering blood cholesterol levels and especially for protection from the low density lipoproteins, as olive oil is less likely to oxidize and form into arterial plaque. The substance oleuropein, in olives, inhibits the sticking of monocyte cells to the arterial walls.

When olive oil replaces saturated animal fats in the diet, a great improvement in arterial health and cholesterol levels occurs. The polyunsaturated content of olive oil supplies a small amount of both Omega 3, 0.7 g Omega 6, 8 g. plus a good supply of vitamin E 14 mg and vitamin K 60 mcg. Olive oil can be used as a replacement for butter, in Italy, bread is dipped into olive oil and served with lunch salads and pasta. The oleic acid content of olive oil is helpful for reducing inflammation in cases of rheumatoid arthritis and may also help in cases of asthma. Olive oil has proved beneficial in reducing the risk of colon cancer and also for reduction of the high triglyceride level in some diabetics. Virgin olive oil mixed with walnut oil in salad dressings is wonderful.

PEANUT OIL

VITAMIN E 15.7 mg

CALORIES - total: 884 kcal. per 100 gram
Saturated: 16.9 g Poly:32 g Mono: 46.2

Peanut oil is obtained from the Arachis Lypogaea plant, it is a legume. Peanut oil is often referred to as 'arachis'. Cold pressed peanut oil is composed of 80 % unsaturated lipids and 20 % saturated. The valuable supply of essential unsaturated fatty acids is mainly in the form of oleic acid - 70% and polyunsaturated linoleic acid, or Omega 6, 20 %. The method of oil extraction is most important to the quality of peanut oil. The 'cold pressed oil' is the best choice. Peanut oil helps transport adrenaline throughout the body. Peanut oil is a good cooking oil as it can be used several times without breaking down. The fair supply of vitamin E with cold pressed peanut oil is a bonus for the circulatory system.

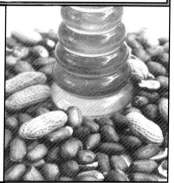

SAFFLOWER OIL

VITAMIN E 34.1 mg.

CALORIES - total: 884 kcal. per 100 gram
Saturated:6.2 g Poly:74.6 g Mono:14.4 g

Safflower oil is obtained from the safflower seed which is a member of the 'Compositae' family of plants and one that ancient civilisations cultivated near the banks of the river Nile. Safflower oil is the richest source of unsaturated lipids, with linoleic acid being the dominant 'essential fatty acid'. Nearly 90% of safflower oil is unsaturated and over 70 % or 74 g is in the form of linoleic acid (Omega 6) and 20% oleic acid. Safflower oil supplies 10 grams of linoleic acid per tablespoon. A most common result of a linoleic acid deficiency is dermatitis, that is also prompted by excess emotional stress and physical exhaustion. This high proportion of unsaturated lipids gives safflower oil the ability to protect your body against excess blood-cholesterol caused from excess consumption of animal fats and a lack of natural whole foods such as fruits, vegetables, whole grains, legumes, nuts and seeds. A high blood-cholesterol level can be most detrimental to the heart muscles and the circulatory system. Such symptoms as arteriosclerosis, heart disease, chilblains and cramps may all be due to excess blood cholesterol levels. As safflower oil does not provide Omega 3 (linolenic acid) it is best to ensure that the diet also includes such foods as salmon, fish, walnuts, pepitas and linseed oil, as there may be a link between *excess* intake of Omega 6 and heart disease. Margarine is a common source of Omega 6, so spread lightly.

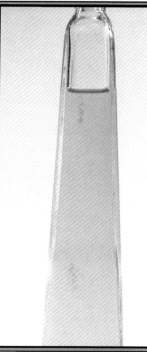

SOY OIL

VITAMIN E 9.2 mg

CALORIES - total: 884 kcal. per 100 gram
Saturated:14.4 g Poly:57.9 g Mono:23.3

Soy oil is a reliable source of the two essential unsaturated fatty acids, however the balance of Omega 6 is in excess compared to Omega 3. Over 85% of soy bean oil is made up from unsaturated lipids with Omega 6, 51 g and Omega 3, 7 g.
Over 50% of soy oil is composed of linoleic acid or Omega 6.
Soy oil also supplies approx. 25 % oleic acid, mono unsaturated lipids. To obtain a well balanced oil, mix 2 teaspoons: approx. 30 g of edible linseed oil to 5 teaspoons: approx. 70 g of soy oil and greatly increase the Omega 3 balance and value.
The combined oil of 30 g linseed oil with 70 g. soy oil provides approx. Omega 3, 22 g and Omega 6, 40 g. Just as your car needs 20 w / 50, your body needs Omega 3 w 6, a teaspoon a day equals 3 g /Omega 3 and 5 g Omega 6.

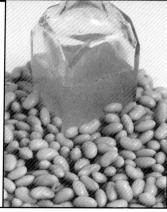

SESAME OIL

VITAMIN E
1.4 mg

CALORIES - total: 884 kcal. per 100 gram
Saturated: 14 g Poly: 41 g Mono: 39 g

Sesame seeds are termed 'the queen of the oil bearing seeds'. Sesame seeds are 45% protein and mineral content and over 50% lipid content. For every 500 grams of sesame seeds you can obtain over one cupful of top quality oil. Sesame oil is an excellent source of unsaturated lipids with over 80% being unsaturated and 14% saturated lipids. The extraction of sesame oil is a simple process that requires no chemical solvents or additives as there are no husks to be removed and a top quality oil can be obtained with one cold-pressing. Sesame seeds are grown throughout many parts of the world especially Turkey, China, Africa, South-Central America, India and the southwest parts of the USA. In some of these places, sesame oil is referred to as Gingelly oil or Benne oil. The sesame plant produces a special substance known as sesamol, an excellent natural preservative that retards sesame oil from turning rancid. In places that have very hot weather such as Turkey from where the sesame paste tahini originated, sesame oil will last longer than other cold pressed oils. Sesame oil supplies an abundance of phytosterols 865 mg and they reduce cholesterol plus they retard the absorption of cholesterol. Sesame oil has a rich and distinct flavour, for an authentic middle east recipe, use sesame oil.

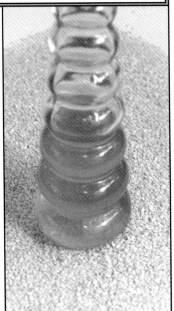

SESAME -TAHINI

VITAMIN E
40 mg

CALORIES - total: 570 kcal. per 100 gram
Saturated: 6.7 g Poly: 21 g Mono: 18.1

Tahini is made from ground sesame seeds with a similar consistency to thick honey. One of the main benefits of tahini is that it can be easily digested and within half an hour after digestion, tahini can enter the bloodstream and supply valuable nutrients such as the excellent source of vitamin E, 40 mg, thereby providing numerous health benefits. Vitamin E also promotes the functioning of linoleic acid and this is most beneficial as it retards ageing of body cells, thereby helping to preserve that youthful look and also to retain proper focusing of the eyes with the older generation.

Tahini is one of the most versatile foods as it combines well with bread or on toast, or, as an alternative to butter, as an ingredient in salad dressings, as a dip, in hummous, halvah or mix into a fruit salad or pour over a fresh garden salad, a most nourishing complete protein meal, refer to page 89. Tahini is an excellent source of calcium 420 mg and if you are allergic to dairy, tahini is the best alternative. The phosphorus content 750 mg is excellent, ideal for the nervous system and brain and as tahini is an excellent source of vitamin T (the sesame vitamin), the nourishment for the brain and memory are exceptional. The magnesium 96 mg plus copper 1.6 mg and zinc 4.6 mg are abundant and vital for the nerves, skin, strong bones, blood vessels, healing and the immune system. The B1, 2, & 3 content are very good, essential daily for the nerves, skin and digestion. There are two types of tahini: hulled and unhulled, they have similar nutrient benefits, the hulled tahini is more palatable and lighter in colour. No kitchen pantry, or breakfast or lunch setting is complete without tahini, it is one of the greatest natural foods for strength, growth, repair and health. Add a teaspoon of flax oil to your tahini for a complete supply of the essential fatty acids. Tahini also contains lecithin, choline and inositol. A regular serve of tahini will ensure your body has all it needs to heal, regenerate and rethink!

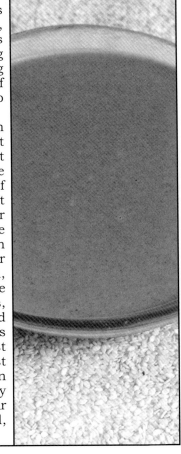

SUNFLOWER OIL	VITAMIN E 41.4 mg	CALORIES - total: 884 kcal. per 100 gram Saturated:9.7 g Poly:3.8 g Mono:83.6 g

Sunflower oil is composed of approximately 90 % unsaturated lipids and 10 % saturated lipids. The dominant unsaturated lipids are: linoleic acid 60 % and oleic acid 30 %. By using cold pressed sunflower oil with salads, you will obtain a very good supply of vitamin E, 41 mg and Omega 6, 63 g but only a trace of Omega 3, so add a teaspoon of linseed / flax oil to your sunflower oil bottle for greater benefits and balance. Sunflower oil is available at all supermarkets. It is produced via a chemical extraction process, such oil is best used for baking or frying but keep the 'cold pressed' oil specially for salad dressings. The vitamin E content of sunflower oil will help preserve the quality of the oil, as vitamin E retards oxidation and the formation of free radicals. Sunflower oil has hardly any taste and is suitable for cooking pancakes, scones and other delicate flavoured recipes. Let the sunshine in with sunflower oil.

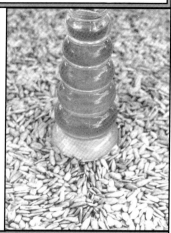

WALNUT OIL	VITAMIN E 0.4 mg	CALORIES - total: 884 kcal. per 100 gram Saturated: 9.1g Poly:63.3 g Mono:22.8 g

Walnut oil was once used exclusively for timber finishing but today the very good supply of Omega 3, 11. 5 g makes it a beneficial edible oil and ideal for those special salad dressings, keep the guests guessing, add a teaspoon of walnut oil to the waldorf salad and get the best of both worlds, or add a drop in the pancake mix, or the guacamole or dips. Walnut oil also provides an abundance of Omega 6 58 g and a fair supply of phytosterols 176 mg, for cholesterol reduction. Walnut oil is nearly 90% unsaturated with over 20% in the form of monounsaturated (oleic acid). Walnut oil is a well balanced oil for daily use. Serve up the waldorf, waiter!

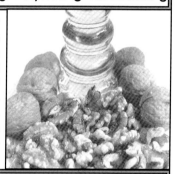

WHEATGERM OIL	VITAMIN E 149 mg	CALORIES - total: 884 kcal. per 100 gram Saturated:18.8 g Poly: 61.7 g Mono:15.1

Wheat Germ Oil is the most potent form of vitamin E 149 mg and it was the original source from which vitamin E was discovered. The whole wheat grain is an excellent food for your daily vitamin E requirements, however, very few people have tasted whole wheat and have a diet that is generally deficient in vitamin E foods. A small bottle, 200 ml of 'cold pressed' wheat germ oil should be an essential addition in the fridge, especially if you eat refined bread and refined foods, smoke and intend to protect yourself from polluted air. By taking one half teaspoon per day, twice a week, of cold pressed wheat germ oil you can be assured that your arteries and heart muscles will be given assistance for protection from pollution.

Wheat germ oil should also be part of every first aid kit and used primarily for skin irritations and prevention of wrinkly skin and for healing of scar tissue. For persons with heart problems, blood clots and other ailments, check with your medical practitioner before taking wheat germ oil. Wheat germ oil is a fair source of Omega 3, 5 g and over 60% of the oil is unsaturated with 15 % monounsaturated. Wheat germ oil provides an abundance of phytosterols 553 mg for protection from low density lipoproteins. Wheat germ oil is very rich in texture and is best used as a supplement, or as a first aid treatment for healing of damaged skin tissue. Wheat germ oil is ready, willing and waiting to heal.

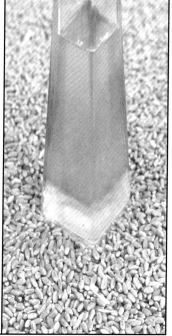

LIPIDS SUMMARY CHARTS

LIPIDS - 15 -20% DAILY DIET			TOTAL DAILY INTAKE OF LIPIDS - APPROX. FOOD QUANTITY / SERVE SIZE	MAIN FOOD GROUP PROPORTION		
Male 18 - 50 years 580 k.calories daily approx.		2,424 K.j per day approx.				
	K. CALORIES	Kilojoules		CARB.	PROTEIN	LIPID
Dairy foods	20%	116	485	200 ml. full cream milk, or, 150 g yoghurt, or, 30 g. cheddar cheese.	0	30	70
Nuts	30%	174	727	30 g almonds (25-30), or, 30 g brazil nuts (7-8) or, 30 g raw cashews (30).	0	40	60
Seeds	10%	58	242	20 g pepitas, or 20 g sesame seeds, or 20 g sunflower seeds.	0	60	40
Avocado	10%	58	242	half a small avocado.	30		70
Pure oil	10%	58	242	half a teaspoon of any cold pressed oil (canola or walnut oil are best).			100
Margarine	5%	29	122	one teaspoon of preferably canola based margarine.			100
Cooking oil	5%	29	122	one teaspoon of preferably peanut, olive or canola oil.			100
Other foods	10%	58	242	a small snack of 10 g. chocolate , or 15 g. potato chips.	30		70
TOTAL	100%	580 K.c.	2,424 K.j				

LIPIDS - 15 - 20% DAILY DIET			
Female 18 - 50 years 440 K.calories daily approx.		1,841 K.j per day approx.	
	K .CALORIES	kilojoules	
Dairy foods	20%	88	369
Nuts	30%	132	552
Seeds	10%	44	184
Avocado	10%	44	184
Pure oil	10%	44	184
Margarine	5%	22	92
Cooking oil	5%	22	92
Other foods	10%	44	184
TOTAL	100%	440 K.c.	1,841 K.j.

LIPIDS - 15 - 20 % DAILY DIET			
Teenagers 13 - 17 years 550 K. calories daily approx.		2,302 K.j. per day approx.	
	K .CALORIES	kilojoules	
Dairy Foods	20%	110	463
Nuts	30%	164	673
Seeds	10%	55	232
Avocado	10%	55	232
Pure oil	10%	55	232
Margarine	5%	28	119
Cooking oil	5%	28	119
Other foods	10%	55	232
	100%	110 K.c	2,302 K.j.

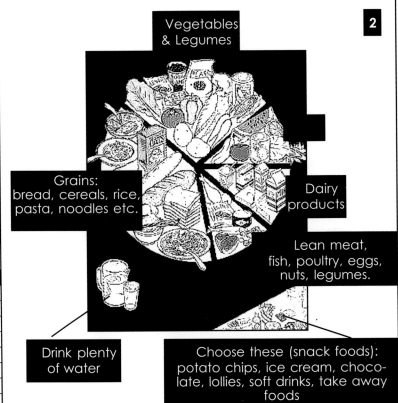

Vegetables & Legumes

2

Grains: bread, cereals, rice, pasta, noodles etc.

Dairy products

Lean meat, fish, poultry, eggs, nuts, legumes.

Drink plenty of water

Choose these (snack foods): potato chips, ice cream, chocolate, lollies, soft drinks, take away foods

Chart 1 provides a guide to the approx. amount of lipids (fats & oils), calories, kilojoules required per day, based on the USDA / R. D. I. dietary guide. It is not necessary to obtain all the foods listed in the chart, per day. This chart is designed to provide an indication of the total quantity of foods required per day to satisfy the 'nutritional appetite' for lipids. Some lipids are very beneficial and preferably, required daily. In chart two, produced by the Australian Commonwealth Department of Health and Family, it is clear that no specific mention of lipids is provided. This is mainly due to the inclusion of lipids with the group of dairy and snack foods plus the use of added cooking oils with meat, fish and poultry, plus other foods. When cooking, use cold pressed oils and moderate their use. Obtain a variety of the lipid groups every week. Obtain the pure oils with salads or bread and combine dairy with grains, legumes or vegetables.

MINERALS INTRODUCTION

Minerals perform a multitude of vital functions throughout the body.

There are 14 essential main minerals and 5 essential trace minerals, refer to page 6 for details.

Minerals are required for the construction of new cells. Every day the body builds new cells: blood, bone, connective, epithelium, muscular, nerve, skin and skeletal cells, refer to page 186. Minerals are the major building blocks for cells in addition to amino acids and fatty acids .

Throughout the following pages, over 200 specific functions of minerals is provided.

Minerals are the conveyer of vital electrical stimuli along nerves to activate the human body. Minerals are converted into organic salts via digestion. These organic salts are dissolved into body fluids such as water and blood.

Minerals have either positive or negative ions. Similar ions will repel and opposite charged ions will attract. For example, sodium and potassium are both positive ions, they repel each other.

The functions of all minerals is very complex. The interaction of positive and negative ions is essential for all body movements, such as relaxation and contraction of muscles, triggered by stimulus from the brain and nervous system. Minerals are vital for the acid - alkaline blood and body balance. Ideally, the diet should provide 75% alkaline forming foods and 25% acid forming foods.

The main alkaline forming foods are: fruits, vegetables, almonds, millet and brown rice. Most other foods are acid forming. Every food has both acid and alkaline minerals. A food is termed acid when the end product, after digestion, provides an acid ash or residue. The pituitary gland helps to control the acid - alkaline body balance. Let your dietary intake help the pituitary gland to provide an alkaline body balance, as it is vital for body healing.

Various common ailments can be attributed to a prolonged deficiency of a particular mineral, as described throughout the following pages.

Natural foods provide all the essential minerals and trace minerals. Processed foods are often depleted in their supply of minerals and especially the trace minerals.

Balance your life and body with the foods that give, not the foods that take away!

On pages 157 - 159, a list of minerals and their best food source is provided. Check through the list to see that you are obtaining at least a few of those foods from each mineral group regularly. Also refer to the individual foods throughout this book to obtain more details on the quantity of the minerals supplied and refer to the recommended dietary intake chart, as presented on page 96. The chart below provides a guide to the approx. percentage of minerals compared to body weight and also the various essential nutrients and their proportion with the human body composition. Minerals play a vital and constant role in the human system.

ELEMENTS & MINERALS BODY WEIGHT CHART			NUTRIENT COMPOSITION OF THE HUMAN BODY	
CARBON	18 %		CARBOHYDRATES	2 %
NITROGEN	3 %	96 %	PROTEIN	20 %
			LIPIDS	15 %
HYDROGEN	10 %		WATER	55 %
OXYGEN	65 %			
WATER H$_2$0	75%			
CALCIUM	2 %			
PHOSPHORUS	1 %			
POTASSIUM	0.4 %			
SULPHUR	0.25 %			
CHLORINE	0.25 %			
SODIUM	0.25 %			
FLUORIDE	0.20 %	4 %	MINERALS	7 %
MAGNESIUM	0.05 %			
IRON	0.008 %			
MANGANESE	0.003 %			
SILICON	0.002 %			
COPPER	0.002 %			
IODINE	0.00004 %			
			VITAMINS	1 %
ELEMENTS & MINERALS TOTAL BODY WEIGHT %	100 %		TOTAL NUTRIENT COMPOSITION	100 %

NOTE: All amounts in this book are measured in milligrams (mg) per 100 grams, unless stated otherwise.

CALCIUM - Ca - alkaline mineral

1 CIRCULATORY SYSTEM Calcium regulates the heart-beat and in combination with the mineral magnesium, it is vital for the nourishment of the cardiovascular system: heart, arteries, veins, capillaries. Tahini is one of the richest natural calcium foods plus it is full of vitamin E, also vital for the heart.

2 DIGESTIVE SYSTEM Calcium is essential for the involuntary muscular movements of the digestive system (peristaltic action). Natural bran is a good source of calcium, fibre and other minerals required to improve muscular tone in the intestines and thereby protects against constipation and for people with a constant meat diet, the need for proper elimination to avoid *bowel cancer* is vital, as meat contains no roughage or fibre content. Legumes, nuts, whole grains, seeds and vegetables are a very good source of roughage.

The parathyroid glands regulate the storage of calcium throughout the body in **3 GLANDULAR SYSTEM** combination with sunlight, vitamin D. Regular moderate sunlight is vital for healthy glands and for calcium metabolism.

5 MUSCULAR SYSTEM Muscles need calcium to contract and relax. Cramps are often due to a calcium deficiency as muscle fibres cannot contract or slide and mesh properly without a steady flow of calcium ions. Eating yoghurt the night before a big race can prevent cramps. During exercise muscles produce lactic acid and to avoid sore muscles, the lactic acid needs to be converted and eliminated. A bowl of yoghurt after the big race is first choice as it contains enzymes that convert lactic acid. For a good night's sleep, the calcium in acidophilus yoghurt is ideal.

6 NERVOUS SYSTEM Calcium combined with magnesium is required for the transmission of nerve impulses to muscles.

Almonds are an excellent magnesium and calcium food, plus they contain the balance of phosphorus, all vital for the heart muscles. A few almonds a day will help your muscles play.

8 SKELETAL SYSTEM Calcium is the most important bone mineral and with 200 bones in the adult skeleton, it is vital to ensure a regular supply of calcium with most emphasis for growing children and for women during pregnancy and lactation, plus the elderly. Various factors are important in regards to proper calcium absorption for a strong skeletal system. 1- bones become weak without exercise and weight bearing exercise or daily activities. For children they generally do enough jumping and other activities, however for the middle aged onwards, a regular daily walk or activity is essential to prevent the condition of osteoporosis or brittle bones. Excess rest in bed due to illness may also contribute. 2- From the age of 45 onwards, the parathyroid glands slow in activity and need a boost from fresh juices such as carrot, plus vitamin D to continue with proper control of calcium metabolism. 3- Excess protein and fat intake decrease the body's ability to use calcium, plus excess protein causes a loss of calcium via the urine. As meat is a very poor source of calcium, it is advised to restrict meat eating to avoid calcium deficiency problems. 4- Vitamin D - sunlight is vital for proper calcium absorption and strong bones. For the elderly, it is a good idea to make the effort to obtain at least 5 minutes moderate sunlight daily. For children and during lactation, extra moderate sunlight is vital for efficient use of calcium from the diet. 5- Bones need more than calcium, the minerals phosphorus and magnesium and vitamin A, C and D are essential. Natural foods are balanced. 6- The body can adjust calcium absorption depending on the supply; when excess calcium is taken the body may absorb only 20%, for people on a low calcium diet, they may absorb over 70% of the available calcium. Ideally the body needs a regular supply from the diet to maintain balance. 7- Over 95% of the body's calcium is contained in the bones, teeth and skeletal system. 8- The total calcium content of the body is entirely renewed over a six year period.

9- The daily intake of calcium during the last two months of pregnancy and during lactation must be increased from 1000 mg. per day to 1200 mg. per day, the same applies for adults from 50 onwards. A cup measure of acidophillus non fat yoghurt daily will supply approx. 450 mg. of calcium.

CALCIUM - *Ca - alkaline mineral*

12 GROWTH SYSTEM

Calcium is the dominant mineral for the growth system. Milk and dairy products are the most common source of calcium and they are very good sources of calcium however it is important that children obtain a good supply of fruits and vegetables to help cleanse the body of excess mucus produced from the digestion of dairy foods. In addition, excess drinking of chocolate milk inhibits the absorption of the mighty mineral calcium.

13 IMMUNE SYSTEM

Calcium is required to increase the body's general resistance to fight infections. Only when the calcium levels are low can a virus infection occur. The balance of calcium and phosphorus is affected by the continual intake of sugar.

14 JOINT SYSTEM

Calcium obtained from refined foods such as white bread, biscuits, some cereals and pasta, is converted from organic into inorganic by the heat and processing. Inorganic calcium can cause deposits within the joint system leading to improper repair of the joint tissues and eventually lead to conditions such as arthritis. Such foods as celery and lettuce contain natural sodium which helps keep calcium soluble within the bloodstream and thereby protects against excess inorganic calcium deposits around the joint system. The salad sandwich is balanced to protect your body. Foods such as grapefruit can help to disperse inorganic calcium from the joint system, as grapefruit contains salicylic acid. Refer to page (123)

20 REPAIR SYSTEM

Calcium foods are essential for the repair of bone fractures and in combination with a regular daily supply of vitamin D - sunlight, plus such foods as almonds, tahini and fresh vegetables for the nutrients phosphorus, magnesium, zinc, silicon, fluorine, copper and vitamin A and C, the repair of fractures and other bone and skeletal disorders can proceed effectively. Try a salad sandwich with natural cheddar cheese and a spread of tahini on the rye bread for a great bone repair lunch, whilst sitting outside enjoying your half hour in moderate sunlight, that's as good as it gets for natural bone repair on a regular daily basis.

CHLORINE - *Cl - acid mineral*

2 DIGESTIVE SYSTEM

Chlorine stimulates the production of hydrochloric acid in the stomach which is vital for the initial stage of protein digestion, converting protein into smaller units: proteoses and peptones. Chlorine also assists digestion of fats and it cleanses the body of excess fats. Tomatoes are an excellent source of organic chlorine but cooking them will destroy the chlorine content. Chlorine assists the function of the liver, protects against digestive problems and assists the distribution of hormones. It helps regulate the acid-alkaline balance of the blood. Common table salt contains sodium chloride, not organic chlorine. A deficiency of organic chlorine in the diet can lead to a sluggish liver and general body congestion and even heart disease. Most city water supplies contain added chlorine to kill water-borne bacteria, however, if taken regularly and sufficiently, it can destroy the valuable natural bacteria in the lower digestive system. A regular intake of acidophilus yoghurt will help prevent such disorders plus using boiled, filtered water or tank water will reduce the problem.

3 GLANDULAR SYSTEM

Chlorine is vital for the glandular system due to it's cleansing action on the bloodstream. The adrenal glands produce the hormone aldosterone, the salt retaining hormone. The liver controls the balance of aldosterone and when a poor supply of natural chlorine continues, it can affect the functions of the pancreas, spleen and gall bladder, as chlorine regulates their actions.

4 LYMPHATIC SYSTEM

Chlorine cleanses the lymph glands and blood, promoting the production of antibodies to fight infection, the development of cysts and fatty deposits within the bloodstream.

9 BLOOD SYSTEM

Chlorine purifies the blood and regulates blood pressure levels. The liver needs a regular flow of blood to maintain the functioning of the adrenal glands, the balance of salt levels and for correct fluid retention, otherwise conditions such as swelling, excess water retention, obesity and heart problems may develop. Mango, lettuce, spinach and avocado supply natural chlorine.

COPPER - *Cu. Alkaline min*

2 DIGESTIVE SYSTEM Copper is a vital trace mineral and an ingredient of many digestive enzymes, thereby promoting the functions of the digestive system. The copper content from natural foods after digestion is stored in the liver, kidneys, heart, brain, bones and muscles. Over half the copper is stored in the bones. Copper is required for the metabolism of fats.

9 BLOOD SYSTEM Copper is required with the mineral manganese for proper assimilation of iron. Due to the common use of copper pipes for water supplies in the home, excess copper intake can occur especially if supplements with copper are taken frequently plus the use of copper cooking pots and the excess intake of animal liver. Deficiencies of copper are not common but excess intake does occur. Excess copper can cause problems such as prolonged anaemia despite increases in the mineral iron, depression after childbirth, excess premenstrual stress especially if the pill is taken. Copper is required with iron in the development of blood haemoglobin. It is required for the conversion of ascorbic acid into the form of vitamin C and for protection from infection, especially the lungs as copper promotes tissue respiration and protects the lungs from infections. There is no RDA - recommended dietary allowance for copper but the average intake is approx. 2 mg. per day. A 100 gram serve of liver supplies approx. 9 mg. of copper, tahini supplies approx. 4 mg. per 100 gram. Copper is a very important blood mineral and vital for prevention of blood vessel ruptures and it may prevent the degeneration of heart muscles. The balance between the minerals zinc and copper is crucial, if excess of either occur, possibly due to supplements, the other mineral level will be lowered. Copper foods: tahini and most nuts.

19 BRAIN SYSTEM Copper can be the problem in some cases of schizophrenia, as the mineral zinc may be depleted in such patients, with excess copper balance. Excess copper, or insufficient zinc may be a cause in various mental problems. Natural foods supply balance. When an excess of vitamin C is taken regularly, copper metabolism may be reduced. Copper is also required for the central nervous system and glandular system.

FLUORIDE - *F- acid mineral*

8 SKELETAL SYSTEM Fluoride from natural foods is termed calcium fluoride, whereas fluoridated water contains sodium fluoride. It is deposited into some cities drinking water as an inorganic element. Research from 25 cities showed that fluoridated water increased the risk of various types of cancer by an average of approx. 40%. This research was conducted by Dr. J. Yiamoupannis, Science Director of the US National Health Federation. A caution by the U.S. Surgeon General warned hospitals not to use fluoridated water in kidney machines. The synthetic fluoride in drinking water can inhibit the functions of vitamin C and in regards to the skeletal system, vitamin C promotes hardening of the bones and tooth enamel. Excess fluoridated water intake can retard calcium absorption. Teflon based cookwear will increase synthetic fluoride intake, in contrast, aluminium cookwear will destroy the fluoride from city water but also from foods. Use filtered water, increase the intake of vitamin C and fluorine rich foods such as asparagus, apples, garlic, rice, cabbage and lettuce. Organic fluoride is essential strength and growth of bones. A prolonged fluoride deficiency can lead to curvature of the spine and decalcifying of bones.

9 BLOOD SYSTEM Fluoride from natural foods helps to increase the number of red blood cells. 90% of fluoride is contained in the bloodstream. Beetroot is tops on the list for blood building as it provides natural fluoride plus iron, manganese and copper, plus sodium, potassium, calcium, magnesium, chlorine and iodine, the full range of blood minerals. A fresh carrot and beetroot juice is one sure way to give your blood a boost.

15 OPTIC SYSTEM Fluoride promotes the optic system functions especially for the delicate iris of the eyes. Lettuce with asparagus, mayonnaise plus finely grated carrot will promote a sparkle to the iris of the eyes.

17 SKIN SYSTEM Fluoride foods promote a youthful skin and complexion. Rolled oats soaked in milk overnight, served with grated apple is the ideal regular breakfast for anyone, especially ageing super models, or mum's on a beauty diet.

IODINE - I Acid mineral

2 DIGESTIVE SYSTEM

Iodine is required for the rate of digestion and for the utilization of fats, as it is necessary for the oxidation of both fats and proteins, thereby promoting proper digestion. It also assists to regulate cholesterol levels and a prolonged deficiency may lead to obesity, however that is an unlikely reason for obesity, as iodine is only required in small amounts, but regularly. For people who live near the ocean and or eat fish regularly, a deficiency of iodine is less likely. Capsicum, eggs, pineapple and cheese all supply iodine. Kelp is the richest source of iodine with over 1% of it's weight in organic iodine. The average RDA is approx. 150 mcg (micrograms). Refer to RDA chart page 96.

3 GLANDULAR SYSTEM

Iodine is the major mineral for the thyroid gland and approx. 30% of all iodine is required by the thyroid glands for effective internal functions plus the control of general body metabolism, digestion and rate of hormone secretion. The thyroid gland produces the hormone thyroxine which is composed of 65% iodine and it's functions are for energy production, conversion of carotene into vitamin A, growth, healthy mental condition, skin, hair and nervous system. During pregnancy and lactation, iodine is vital for the development of the infants mental and physical development. The trace mineral selenium is also required for the production of the thyroxine hormone. A deficiency of iodine during pregnancy may increase the risk of miscarriage. The condition termed goitre which is an enlargement of the thyroid gland is caused mainly by a deficiency of iodine but may also be due to excess iodine. Kelp is the ideal natural food to create balance either way in the condition of goitre.

12 GROWTH SYSTEM

Iodine is a vital mineral for the growth system as thyroxine is required for body growth. A deficiency of iodine in infants can lead to a condition known as cretinism or commonly referred to as dwarfism, stunted growth and impaired mental development. Iodine is also required by the thyroid gland to keep the skin and hair in good condition, maintenance of the nervous system and for normal cellular growth. Kelp salt is the ideal way to share iodine in foods.

IRON - Fe- alkaline mineral

9 BLOOD SYSTEM

Iron is the main blood mineral, it is essential in the formation of rich red blood cells and 90% of the iron content in the body is stored in the bloodstream, the remainder is stored in the bone marrow until required in the formation of blood haemoglobin. Approx. 1 mg. of iron is disposed each day and for girls and women 15 mg. are required from the diet each day and during pregnancy 30 mg. per day. An additional 15 to 30 mg. are lost during the menstrual period and approx. 500 mg. are lost during childbirth. Men require 10 mg. and boys require 12 mg. per day. One of the ideal super iron-rich meals include ground pepitas, with finely chopped parsley, tomato and a dash of tahini salad dressing. For iron to be absorbed effectively, protein and vitamin C must be present and with the above salad, it has all the ingredients. Excess cooking depletes iron in foods. Pepitas supply 15 mg per 100 gram, parsley 9 mg. tahini 10 mg. Iron is vital for the supply of oxygen throughout the body via the haemoglobin from the lungs to the body tissues and myoglobin for the muscle cells. The mineral copper and the green matter in plants are also essential for iron activity. A deficiency of the mineral iron often shows as weariness, regular colds and inflammations and lack of energy. Some iron supplements are well balanced but nothing can beat the natural balance of natural foods. To obtain better value from the iron tablet, take it with a glass of fresh citrus juice, as the citric acid will promote the proper absorption of iron, via the linings of the lower intestines. Chelated iron tablets are three times more effective than non-chelated. For iron deficiencies such as anemia, it is vital to obtain more than tablets, as copper, vitamin E, B complex, manganese, calcium and protein are also required. Let Nature supply the full benefits. Excess iron from tablets, tonics, iron cookwear and animal organs can develop as excess iron is eliminated slowly from the body. Take it easy, naturally.

5 MUSCULAR SYSTEM

Iron is the delivery service for the supply of oxygen to the entire muscular system, as myoglobin. Iron can have 2 or 3 electrical charges which allows it to pick up an extra oxygen atom and then deposit the oxygen. Iron is the nucleus of every body cell and it is vital for cleansing the body cells of toxins.

MAGNESIUM - *Mg- alkaline*

1 CIRCULATORY SYSTEM Magnesium is vital for the transfer of nerve impulses to the heart muscles, keeping the heart rate steady and a deficiency may lead to high blood pressure, hardened arteries and chronic fatigue syndrome. As magnesium assists calcium balance and the action of vitamin D - sunlight, plus the metabolism of numerous minerals, it is essential to ensure a regular intake of magnesium foods, almonds. Such factors as excess alcohol, stress, nervousness and the fact that magnesium cannot be stored for long periods in the body all point to the need for magnesium foods in the daily diet.

2 DIGESTIVE SYSTEM Magnesium is involved in numerous digestive enzymes, it is required with calcium for the conversion of glucose into energy, the secretion and function of insulin. It is the natural anti-acid mineral and required for fat and protein metabolism.

5 MUSCULAR SYSTEM Magnesium protects against muscular cramps, as it promotes a steady flow of impulses from the nerves to the muscle tissues. If you exercise hard, let magnesium support your muscles.

6 NERVOUS SYSTEM Magnesium is the mighty nerve mineral, it promotes steady nerves by regulating the white nerve fibres which control the central nervous system. A magnesium deficiency can result in various nervous disorders, hyperactivity in children, irritability, heart attacks, neuralgia and depression. As processed foods are deficient in magnesium, it is vital to gain extra magnesium from natural foods such as wheat germ, almonds, tahini, avocado, bananas.

18 URINARY SYSTEM Magnesium keeps calcium and phosphorus soluble in the urinary tract thereby preventing kidney stone buildup.

19 BRAIN SYSTEM Magnesium is vital for nourishment of the white nerve fibres of the brain, it assists other nutrients to enter brain cells and it promotes memory and protect against mental illness.

MANGANESE - *Mn - alkaline*

2 DIGESTIVE SYSTEM Manganese assists in the digestion, absorption and utilization of the three main food groups: protein, carbohydrates and lipids. It is required for various digestive enzymes and reactions and it improves the absorption of the B complex vitamins and vitamin C. Processing of wheat and other grains can reduce the manganese content by 90% and animal product foods such as meat are a poor source of this mineral. Manganese is also required for the production of bile for fat digestion and insulin for carbohydrate/ glucose conversion into an energy source and to stabilize blood glucose levels. Wheat germ is a rich source of manganese.

3 GLANDULAR SYSTEM Manganese is a vital nutrient for the glands, the thyroid gland needs manganese and iodine to produce thyroxine, for body growth and metabolism plus the active control of 20 sets of body glands. Manganese is essential for regulating menstrual periods, during pregnancy and lactation for the production of milk from the mammary glands. Manganese is required in numerous hormones for both male and female reproductive glands. The majority of manganese is contained in the liver, pancreas and the adrenal glands.

6 NERVOUS SYSTEM Manganese foods improve the coordination of nerves and nerve impulse to the muscles. It promotes the effectiveness of the B complex vitamins and nourishes the nervous system.

8 SKELETAL SYSTEM Manganese is important for the growth of children as it is required for the stretching of bones to their normal shape and size as it is part of the connective tissues within bones. Most breakfast cereals and milk are a poor source of manganese, add a sprinkle of wheat germ to the 'boys' cereal and help them grow into proper shape.

9 BLOOD SYSTEM Manganese is a vital mineral in the formation of healthy red blood cells in combination with iron, copper and cobalt. A few pepitas ground and sprinkled on a salad provides the essential ingredients for the entire blood system. Manganese is also vital for the brain, memory and stability.

PHOSPHORUS- *P-acid mineral*

1 CIRCULATORY SYSTEM

Phosphorus is required for proper blood circulation and normal blood pressure, especially for people with very low blood pressure. Add sunflower seeds or wheat germ to your breakfast cereal. Phosphorus foods improve a poor complexion by stimulating blood circulation.

2 DIGESTIVE SYSTEM

Phosphorus is required for the utilization of fats, proteins and carbohydrates. The phosphorus in the outer portion of whole grains and legumes is termed phytic acid, it can reduce the absorption of calcium, zinc and iron but the enzyme phytase in the small intestine breaks down the phytic acid to allow it's absorption. The process of breadmaking, where yeast activates the gluten in the grain also reduces the phytic acid content. Refer to page 27 for more details.

6 NERVOUS SYSTEM

Phosphorus is essential for the maintenance and repair of the entire nervous system. Phosphorus foods strengthen the nervous system. If your nerves are at 'wits end', you may benefit greatly from a regular supply of rich phosphorus foods such as pepitas, tahini, peanuts or almonds.

8 SKELETAL SYSTEM

Approx. 90% of the body's phosphorus is contained in the bones, teeth and nails. It is totally renewed over a three year period. It is essential for healing of bone fractures and bone growth and may prevent poor teeth formation and limited growth in children. Cheese, tahini, nuts and wheat germ are a good source for children.

19 BRAIN SYSTEM

Phosphorus is required for a good memory, for creativity, proper concentration abilities, efficient mental activity and transfer of nerve impulses. Lecithin, refer page 137, a phosphorus compound obtained from corn or soy and as a supplement, is termed a natural relaxant and 28% of the brain matter is comprised of lecithin compounds. A lack of phosphorus leads to mental exhaustion. Excess sugar causes a phosphorus deficiency. Every cell and chemical reaction in the body needs phosphorus for transfer of hereditary characteristics and to reduce the onset of cancerous tissue formation.

POTASSIUM- *K- alkaline mineral*

1 CIRCULATORY SYSTEM

Potassium is vital for the circulatory system as it keeps the heart muscles in a healthy condition and helps to strengthen the muscles. In combination with iron, potassium promotes the use of oxygen in the body and to normalize heart muscle action, such as contractions and heartbeat rate. Potassium foods: dates, apricots, protect against hardening of the arteries and high blood pressure. During hot weather, potassium is lost in greater quantities compared to sodium/salt, via perspiration, a fresh peach and pineapple juice will restore the essential mineral potassium, soft drinks will actually cause a potassium imbalance due to their sugar and sodium/salt content, resulting in lethargy.

2 DIGESTIVE SYSTEM

Potassium is often destroyed by heat, cooking and processing plus alcohol, caffeine and salt also cause a loss of this alkaline mineral. Potassium is vital for the alkaline balance in the blood and as most diets are acid forming and include the above factors that reduce potassium reserves, the supply of such foods as dried apricots, peaches and raisins with breakfast or as a snack provides great benefits. Potassium is essential in the formation of glycogen - stored in the liver and converted to glucose when the body requires extra energy.

5 MUSCULAR SYSTEM

Potassium is the muscle mineral, it is required for stimulation of the nerves connected to muscles, repair of muscles and blood supply to muscles. It is vital for the heart muscles and for a steady heartbeat rate, as it regulates the muscle tone during activity and assists relaxation of muscles after exertion.

19 BRAIN SYSTEM

Potassium foods promote supply of oxygen to the brain, improving mental function. Potassium can prevent hypertension.

20 REPAIR SYSTEM

Potassium is a most effective healing mineral, especially for damaged heart muscles. Potassium regulates water balance and assists elimination of blood impurities via the kidneys. Cancer cells cannot live in a solution of potassium.

SILICON - Si - acid mineral

6 NERVOUS SYSTEM

Silicon provides an insulating surface around the individual nerve fibres, thereby protecting the nervous system. It is one of the most abundant minerals in the soil and plants struggle without traces of silicon. Leafy vegetables especially lettuce are an excellent source.

14 JOINT SYSTEM

Silicon is the forgotten mineral when considering the skeletal system and in particular, the joint system. It is vital for proper calcium metabolism, preventing the accumulation of inorganic calcium around the bone joints. Silicon forms into crystals which can break up the common uric acid crystals that result from excess protein, caffeine and tea intake, to mention a few. The uric acid crystals are then small enough to be eliminated, otherwise they tend to build around the bones and moving joints leading to the development of arthritis. The combination of the rich silicon content and fluoride in lettuce makes it one of the best foods to obtain regularly to offset the common arthritis. Of equal value is celery especially due to the rich natural sodium content and balanced potassium, plus the silicon content. For prevention and relief from further deterioration of arthritis, silicon rich foods are essential.

17 SKIN SYSTEM

Silicon is vital for efficient cell growth especially for hair growth and for the removal of dead skin cells. It promotes a healthy skin condition by opening pores and skin to allow toxins and grime to be discharged. It also promotes the formation of healthy red blood cells and blood circulation. For those men concerned with the possibility of baldness, due to hereditary reasons, extra silicon rich foods will help to cleanse the scalp and keep the skin cells open, to allow hair follicles to grow. Silicon is the major mineral in the building of hair, lettuce is really the best hair tonic as it is rich in silicon and chlorophyll, both vital ingredients for hair growth. For women, silicon foods will promote a clear skin condition and the hair quality that you dream about or see in magazines, as long as the diet is natural, you too can develop the look that shines with life. Silicon also protects against nervous exhaustion, mental fatigue, cancerous tissue formation and infections.

SODIUM - Na - alkaline mineral

1 CIRCULATORY SYSTEM

Sodium is required for normal blood pressure and consistency levels. It is vital for keeping other minerals soluble within the bloodstream and for prevention of hardened arteries. Natural sodium (sodium phosphate and sodium sulphate) as obtained from foods is balanced to provide a stable pressure within individual cells. Common table salt (sodium chloride) retains excess fluids at a rate of approx. 1 gram of salt to 70 grams of water, thereby increasing body weight. The sodium / potassium balance is the main factor in control of the body's fluid balance. Table salt is concentrated sodium without the essential balance of potassium to ensure correct cell pressure. As numerous processed foods contain added salt without a suitable balance of potassium, it is advised to restrict adding salt to meals, avoid salty processed foods and to increase the intake of potassium rich foods. The excess use of salt has lead to an increase in blood pressure and research has confirmed the direct link between salt and the risk of hypertension. Numerous foods in the average supermarket contain added salt such as cheese, chips, sauces, spreads, canned foods, bacon, butter, margarine and many more.

2 DIGESTIVE SYSTEM

Sodium is required for the production of saliva which is required for initial digestion of carbohydrate foods. Natural sodium provides an alkaline balance to the entire body, preventing disorders such as arthritis, ulcers and stomach acidity.

9 BLOOD SYSTEM

Natural sodium from foods such as celery, tomato, tahini, beetroot and carrots will promote normal blood pressure and protect against blood clots and thickening of the blood. Kelp salt is the richest source of natural sodium.

14 JOINT SYSTEM

Sodium preserves flexibility of joints and promotes movement of muscles. It keeps blood minerals soluble and protects against arthritis. Celery is the ultimate natural sodium food, apart from kelp and it is well balanced with potassium, to provide the perfect balance to the joint system. If you need to bend your body, natural sodium foods are ready to assist.

SULPHUR - *S- acid mineral*

2 DIGESTIVE SYSTEM

Sulphur promotes absorption of protein and conversion of amino acids. It stimulates the liver to produce bile for fat digestion and also for the pancreatic enzymes. It has a cleansing and antiseptic effect on the digestive system. It is an essential component in the production of insulin, required for conversion of the carbohydrates - glucose into energy. Sulphur is easily destroyed by cooking so it is advised to obtain fresh foods such as celery, garlic and coleslaw regularly, to help cleanse the digestive system.

3 GLANDULAR SYSTEM

Sulphur is vital for cleansing glands, production of enzymes, protecting against blood impurities and for the pancreas gland enzyme production.

4 LYMPHATIC SYSTEM

Sulphur cleanses the vital network of the lymphatic system. Such conditions as glandular fever and hepatitis are often caused by a buildup of toxins, from the diet and other factors, that clog the lymphatic system causing it to collapse. Garlic is one of the richest sulphur foods, it is natural medicine for ailments ending with 'itis'.

7 RESPIRATORY SYSTEM

Sulphur is a heat sensitive nutrient and in winter more than ever, people have cooked meals, the time when those nasty respiratory germs seem to attack. The common cold, bronchitis and tuberculosis have been successfully treated with raw garlic for years.

9 BLOOD SYSTEM

Sulphur is an excellent blood purifier, it provides oxygen to the blood and is required in the formation of blood plasma. It is contained in all body tissues and as part of blood haemoglobin, acting as an oxidising agent. Insulin is a sulphur compound and for diabetics, it is most valuable.

17 SKIN SYSTEM

Sulphur is a vital ingredient of the substance keratin, a protein substance within the outer skin layer. Sulphur foods promote a good complexion by cleansing the skin and scalp of acid toxins which are often the cause of acne and dandruff. For a complete skin rejuvenation, try a regular fresh carrot juice, or cucumber juice.

ZINC - *Zn*

2 DIGESTIVE SYSTEM

Zinc is often underestimated in it's nutritional benefits and requirements and as it is missing from common processed foods generally, it is likely that the addition of zinc rich foods will provide numerous benefits. Zinc is required as a vital component of numerous digestive enzymes, it is vital in the production of insulin and the proper action of insulin. Without zinc, insulin cannot be made or function. A deficiency of zinc can show as poor appetite and loss of taste and flavour in foods. Oysters are the richest source of zinc, over 60 mg. per 100 gram, so forget the supplement, try 2 or 3 oysters and get a massive dose of zinc. If you don't like oysters and most children don't, give them a sprinkle of wheat germ in the soup, cereal, burgers or a pancake regularly. Zinc is also required to break down alcohol and excess alcohol can lead to a zinc deficiency.

Zinc is essential for the prostrate gland, the manufacture of various male reproductive hormones and the development of the genital or-

3 GLANDULAR SYSTEM

gans in children. The story that oysters can promote libido is partially true as zinc is concentrated in the male sexual organs.

Zinc is vital for development of bones and teeth in children, for a prompt repair of fractures,

8 SKELETAL SYSTEM

general growth and the formation of cell proteins and bones which need a constant supply of zinc rich foods to grow, refer to page 159.

Zinc is essential for the development of the reproductive organs. Research showed that over half the boys in a US state were deficient

16 REPRODUCTIVE SYSTEM

in zinc. It is also required for the synthesis of DNA, the master cell code for life. Zinc supplements have been used to treat prostrate gland problems.

Zinc is vital for the production of keratin and finger nails are composed mainly of keratin.

17 SKIN SYSTEM

A deficiency can lead to poor nails, hair and skin condition. Zinc is important for the healing of burns, zinc cream is used to protect from sunburn.

COBALT

9 BLOOD SYSTEM

Cobalt is an essential trace mineral especially for the blood system as it is required for the development of red blood cells in combination with iron, manganese and copper. A lack of copper can occur in a diet without the addition of seafood or fish as most soils do not contain this trace element. A prolonged deficiency of copper can lead to impaired red blood cell production and anaemia.

Copper is part of the vitamin B12 structure and it also assists by breaking down cells that are not required for blood cell development. Cobalt also activates enzymes, body growth, nerves and is required for body healing.

CHROMIUM

2 DIGESTIVE SYSTEM

Chromium is often neglected as an essential mineral however it's known functions clearly indicate the importance of chromium in the diet. Chromium is essential for production of the enzyme GTF - 'glucose tolerance factor', vital for the manufacture and function of insulin, for the conversion of glucose into energy. A deficiency can easily occur with a diet high in sugar and refined foods as they are depleted in their supply of chromium and specifically because chromium is used up in the process of sugar-glucose conversion into energy, thereby draining the body of any reserves. A chromium imbalance can lead to high blood sugar levels and the condition of diabetes mellitus. Refined sugar supplies only .02 ppm (parts per million) of chromium and diets that constantly feed the body with sugar can progressively drain the chromium reserves. Such foods as egg yolks and cheese plus wholegrain breads supply good amounts of this mineral. A deficiency may also promote conditions such as heart attacks, high blood cholesterol, arteriosclerosis and high triglyceride levels. For a natural supplement, brewers yeast is very rich in chromium, black pepper and spices in general also add extra chromium to a meal. It is also required for fat metabolism and the synthesis of protein.

Diets that are full of refined foods and a constant intake of sugar from cups of tea and other sugar drinks can easily upset the balance of the blood - chromium levels.

MOLYBDENUM

2 DIGESTIVE SYSTEM

Molybdenum is required for the metabolism of fats, it is part of two enzymes: xanthine and aldehyde oxidase. The enzyme xanthine is required for the oxidation of fats. Molybdenum is used for proper elimination of waste and for the manufacture of genetic enzymes such as DNA. It may also be required for the utilization of iron. A deficiency of molybdenum is uncommon as it is available from both plants and animal products. The recommended daily intake averages 120 mcg. per day but currently no food evaluation charts are available. Legumes, green leafy vegetables, sprouts and seeds are a good source.

SELENIUM

10 CELLULAR SYSTEM

Selenium has numerous body functions and possibly the best known and vital one is the antioxidant quality in combination with vitamin E, promoting the body's use of oxygen and cell life. It delays the rate of oxidation of polyunsaturated fatty acids which helps preserve the condition of cells and skin tissues. It protects against the development of cancerous cells, promotes the production of thyroxine for regulating body metabolism and protects against premature ageing. Refined and cooked foods are depleted in their supply of selenium. Brazil nuts are the ultimate source of selenium with nearly 3,000 mcg per 100 grams. One brazil nut a day will easily supply all your selenium needs, fresh wheat germ with it's rich vitamin E supply will also provide ample amounts. Selenium has been successfully used in the treatment of kwashiorkor: a protein deficiency disease. It may also protect against heart disease, as it is required for production of the hormone prostaglandin for regulation of blood pressure.

VANADIUM

1 CIRCULATORY SYSTEM

Vanadium is an essential trace mineral, it promotes blood circulation and assists to inhibit the formation of cholesterol in the blood vessels, brain and central nervous system. Sea foods are the best source and trace amounts are available from vegetables depending on the soil condition.

MINERAL FOOD SOURCE CHARTS

CALCIUM - *alkaline mineral*

Nutrients for effective Absorption:
Iron, Magnesium, Phosphorus.
Vitamins: A,C,D,E,F Inositol & Protein

Nutrient Inhibiting Factors:
Lack of: *Sunlight, Exercise, Magnesium and Phosphorus.*
Refined foods, alcohol, chocolate, salt, oxalic acid, rhubarb, diuretics, antibiotics.
RDI: Refer page 96.

Parmesan cheese, Swiss cheese, Cheddar cheese, Tahini, Tofu, Carob powder, Almonds, Hazel nuts, Sardines, Brazil nuts, Yoghurt, Soft cheese, Parsley, Dried Figs, Sunflower seeds, Salmon, Corn tortillos, Spinach, Walnuts, Broccoli, Milk, Nuts, Wheat germ, Bran, Dried Apricots, Prunes, Peanuts, Chick peas.

PHOSPHORUS - *acid mineral*

Nutrients for effective Absorption:
Calcium, Manganese, Vitamins: A,D,F, & Protein

Nutrient Inhibiting Factors:
Excess: stress, sugar, magnesium, antacids, refined foods.
RDI: Refer page 96.

Rice bran, Pepitas, Wheat Bran, Almonds, Wheat germ, Tahini, Sunflower seeds. Brazil nuts, Parmesan, Soy bean, Peanuts, Pine nuts, Pistachio, Cashew nut, Walnuts, Cheddar, Vegetables, Legumes, Sardines, Salmon, Milk, Scallops, Whole grains, Nuts.

POTASSIUM - *alkaline mineral*

Nutrients for effective Absorption:
Sodium, Phosphorus, Sulphur, Chloride, vitamin B6.

Nutrient Inhibiting Factors:
Excess: salt, alcohol, coffee, stress, laxatives, diuretics, antibiotics.
RDI: Adults;
1,950 mg. - 5,460 mg.

Dried Apricots, Figs, Peaches, Raisins. Sultanas, Dates, Almonds, Legumes, Spinach, Garlic, Tuna, Walnuts, Avocado, Hazel nuts, Pine nuts, Sunflower seeds, Potatoes, Bananas, Parsnip, Peanuts, Parsley, Snapper, Nuts, Trout, Vegetables, Fruits, Mushrooms.

SULPHUR - *alkaline mineral*

Nutrients for effective Absorption:
Vitamin B group especially Thiamin & Biotin.

Nutrient Inhibiting Factors:
Cooking, high temperatures.

No RDI established.

Watercress, Scallops, Brazil nuts, Carrots, Crayfish, Prawns, Spinach, Peanuts, Sardines, Celery, Mussels, Berries, Crab, Cauliflower, Cabbage, Cucumber, Radish, Horseradish, Lettuce, Corn, Lemon, Lime, Peaches, Asparagus, Tomato, Avocado, Vegetables, Melons, Cheddar, Eggs, Almonds, Fruits.

CHLORIDE - *acid mineral*

Nutrients for effective Absorption:
Sodium & Potassium

Nutrient Inhibiting Factors:
Cooking, high temperatures.

No RDI established.
Adults safe level;
1,700 mg - 5,100 mg.

NATURAL CHLORINE; Tomato, Celery, Kelp, Lettuce, Asparagus , Cabbage, Parsnip, Radish, Turnip, Dates, Watercress, Avocado, Cucumber, Carrot, Berries, Beetroot, Leek, Pineapple, Bananas, Mango, Raisins.
ADDED CHLORIDE Olives, Cheese, Tuna, Peanut Butter, Bread.

SODIUM - *alkaline mineral*

Nutrients for effective Absorption:
Chloride, Potassium, Vitamin D.

Nutrient Inhibiting Factors:
excess salt, antibiotics, laxatives, diuretics.

RDI Adults:
920 mg. - 2,300 mg.

NATURAL SODIUM Celery, Spinach, Kale, Beetroot, Tahini, Carrots, Watercress, Parsley, Scallops, Cabbage, Coconut, Garlic, Lentils, Raisins, Turnip, Cashews, Eggs, Legumes, Broccoli, Brussels Sprouts, Fruits.
ADDED SODIUM Olives, Fetta Cheese, Butter, Cheese, Tuna.

MINERAL FOOD SOURCE CHARTS

MAGNESIUM - *alkaline mineral*

Nutrients for effective Absorption:
Calcium, Phosphorus, Vitamins: B6, C & D, & Protein

Nutrient Inhibiting Factors:
caffeine, alcohol, nicotine, diuretics, antibiotics.

RDI: Adults:
Men: 320 mg.
Women: 270 mg.
Pregnancy: 300 mg.
Lactation: 340 mg.

Wheat Bran, Almonds, Kelp, Wheat germ, Sunflower seeds, Pepitas, Cashew nuts, Tahini, Brazil nuts, Kelp, Carob powder, Hazel nuts, Pine nuts, Peanuts, Walnuts, Rolled Oats, Legumes, Spinach, Pecan nuts, Soy flour, Dates, Figs, Corn taco shells, Tofu, Sweet corn, Rye bread, Whole wheat, Brown rice, Parsley.

IRON - *alkaline mineral*

Nutrients for effective Absorption:
Vitamins; B12, C, E, Folate.

Nutrient Inhibiting Factors: excess caffeine & tannin. Antibiotics, antacids, aspirin, codeine.

RDI: Adult Men: 7mg.
Adult Women:
19 - 54: 12 mg -16mg.
Pregnancy: 22 - 36mg.

Mussels, Pepitas, Wheat Bran, Parsley, Rice bran, Miso, Wheat germ, Kelp, Tahini, Clams, Tofu, Liver, Carob, Raisins, Rolled Oats, Almonds, Broccoli, Spinach, Sunflower seeds, Beef, Cashews, Rye, Walnut, Chick peas, Lentils, Peanuts, Bread, Vegetables, Tuna, Dried fruits, Berries, Coconut, Peas, Apple, Tuna, Tofu, Salmon,

FLUORINE - *alkaline mineral*

Nutrients for effective Absorption: Calcium
Nutrient Inhibiting Factors:
Cooking in aluminium pots and saucepans.
No RDI.
Safe level approx.
3mg. - 4 mg.

Asparagus, Oats, Garlic, Apples, Rice, Cabbage, Beetroot, Watercress, Rice bran, Goats milk, Barley, Sweet corn, Millet, Wheat, Fish, Citrus, Cheddar cheese, Seafood, Tea, Spinach

MANGANESE - *alkaline mineral*

Nutrients for effective Absorption:
Calcium, Phosphorus, Copper, Zinc,
Vitamins: B1 & E.

Nutrient Inhibiting Factors:
RDI: Adults 2 - 5 mg.

Wheat germ, Bran, Brazil nuts, Chestnuts, Hazel nuts, Almonds, Oats, Walnuts, Garlic, Pepitas, Peanuts, Berries, Pineapple, Beetroot, Grapes, Legumes, Rye bread, Tomato, Tahini, Rice.

SILICON - *acid mineral*

No RDI established.

Lettuce, Parsnip, Asparagus, Spinach, Onions, Cucumber, Strawberry, Cabbage, Sunflower seeds, Fruits, Vegetables.

COPPER - *acid mineral*

Nutrients for effective Absorption:
Cobalt, Iron, Zinc
Nutrient Inhibiting Factors:
Excess zinc (oysters), vitamin C, manganese, molybdenum.
RDI Adults:
1.5 mg. - 3.0 mg.

Cashews, Tahini, Sunflower seeds, Brazil nuts, Hazel nuts, Pepitas, Almonds, Pine nuts, Walnuts, Oysters, Coconut, Peanuts, Oats, Wheat germ, Parsley, Dried fruits, Fruits, Vegetables. Soy bean, Macadamia nuts.

IODINE - *acid mineral*

Nutrients for effective Absorption:
Selenium
Nutrient Inhibiting Factors:
Cabbage, Turnips, Brussell Sprouts.

RDI Men: 150 mcg.
Women: 120 mcg.
Pregnancy: 150 mcg.
Lactation: 170 mcg.

Kelp, Watermelon, Cucumber, Spinach, Asparagus, Blueberry, Peanut, Bread, Clams, Butter, Capsicum, Strawberry, Seafood, Fish, Cheese, Dairy, Berries, Dried fruits, Peaches, Onions, Pineapple, Lettuce, Vegetables, Nuts, Seeds, Rice, Wheat.

MINERALS FOOD CHART

ZINC

Nutrients for effective Absorption:
Calcium, Phosphorus, & Copper.
Vitamins: A, D, B group.

Nutrient Inhibiting Factors:
Alcohol, Tea, Caffeine, HRT therapy,
Oral Contraceptives

RDI: Adults: 12 mg.
Pregnancy: 16 mg.
Lactation: 18 mg.

Oysters (65mg.)
Sunflower seeds (6.5 mg.)
Brazil nuts (4.1 mg.)
Almonds (3.8 mg.)
Scallops, Cashews,
Tahini, Parmesan,
Crab, Wheat germ,
Bran, Walnuts, Kelp,
Rye, Wheat, Olives,
Cheddar cheese,
Hazel nuts, Pepitas,
Garlic, Oats, Beef,
Miso, Sardines, Millet,
Egg yolk, Mackerel,
Maple syrup, Liver.

CHROMIUM

No RDI.

Safe Daily Intake:
50 mcg. - 200 mcg.

Egg yolks, Beef,
Cheddar cheese,
Wine, Rye bread.
Wholegrain bread,
Apples, Potatoes,
Oysters, Pasta, Butter,

SELENIUM

Essential associated Nutrients: Iodine, Vit. E
RDI. Adults:
Male: 85 mcg.
Women: 70 mcg.
Pregnancy: 80 mcg.
Lactation: 85 mcg

Brazil nuts (2,960 mcg.)
Wheat germ, Oysters,
Tuna, Fish, Seafood,
Sunflower seeds,
Wholemeal bread,
Eggs, Whole grains,

MOLYBDENUM

No RDI.

Safe Daily Intake:
75 mcg. - 250 mcg.

Kidney beans, Soy
beans, Peas, Beans,
Sprouted foods, Corn,
Apricots, Carrots,
Cauliflower, Cheese,
Coconut, Garlic.

VANADIUM

Fish, Seafood, Kelp,
Some vegetables

COBALT

Fish, Seafood.

ALCOHOL - C_2H_5OH

Alcohol is defined as a colourless, volatile, intoxicating and inflammable liquid.

After entering the digestive system, a portion of the ethyl alcohol is absorbed through the stomach lining, directly into the bloodstream. A special enzyme in the liver: alcohol dehydrogenase is designed to convert alcohol, however this is a slow process. Also, some people may lack the enzyme and be intolerant to alcohol. The liver converts ethyl alcohol into aldehyde, a colourless, volatile fluid of suffocating smell, obtained by the oxidation of ethyl alcohol. Another enzyme will convert aldehyde into a form of vinegar and once that is oxidised, the end product is carbon dioxide, a colourless heavy gas. The main body parts that are affected by alcohol are the brain and liver. Alcohol relaxes the brain but also destroys brain cells within the cerebellum, pineal gland and cerebral cortex. Alcohol also destroys liver cells when taken excessively over a prolonged period. A glass of red wine will relax the body and provide a good supply of antioxidants, refer to page 50. Alcohol and (smoking: page 160), deplete a variety of essential nutrients, as presented below.

ALCOHOL & SMOKING - PROBLEMS - CHART ONE		
NUTRIENT	**PROBLEMS**	**BENEFICIAL FOODS**
VITAMIN B1	Impaired learning cardiac damage mental problems	wheat germ peanuts brazil nuts yeast extracts
VITAMIN B2	mouth sores baldness nervous disorders ulcers, arthritis, poor skin condition weak eyesight	almonds cashews wheatgerm yeast extracts cheese bran
VITAMIN B3	poor skin condition headaches depression fatigue, indigestion nervous disorders	rice bran wheat germ peanuts yeast extracts nuts, fish sunflower seeds
VITAMIN B5	depression heart problems chronic fatigue poor liver function	sunflower seeds yeast extracts almonds peanuts
VITAMIN B6	headaches depression poor memory nervousness poor digestion	walnuts wheat bran yeast extracts oats rice bran
MAGNESIUM	arthritis nervousness blood clots mental illness	almonds wheat bran sunflower seeds wheat germ
ZINC	fatigue sterility prostrate problems	oysters sunflower seeds brazil nuts

Over one third of the world's population have a caffeine drink regularly. The average daily intake of caffeine is approx. 600 mg. This is approx. four cups of coffee, or 8 cups of tea, or two cans of fizzy cola drink. Most caffeine drinks go hand-in-hand with sugar.

The average can of fizzy drink contains about 5 teaspoons of sugar. The combination of both factors: caffeine and sugar is a recipe for health problems. The nervous system is dependant on a regular supply of B vitamins.

Caffeine restricts the absorption of B1 and induces the loss of B3. The B vitamin: inositol is inhibited by caffeine intake, refer to page 174. Sugar depletes the reserves of numerous B vitamins: B1, B2, B3, biotin and the minerals calcium, phosphorus and potassium. Caffeine increases: blood fatty acids, blood pressure and cholesterol. It causes an irregular heartbeat and may inhibit DNA repair and transfer, leading to infertility, particularly for women. It may increase the risk of osteoporosis in women as well as worsen the symptoms of PMS. It affects the brain development of the fetus and may cause breast cancer, insomnia, irritability and nervousness. On the other hand, research has shown positive factors in coffee, chocolate and tea, not sugar! This is mainly due to the antioxidants in coffee and chocolate. Also the compound that gives coffee it's aroma, termed trigonelline, promotes antibacterial activity.

Caffeine increases the levels of; cortisol: the anti stress hormone and endorphins: the natural painkiller, which may help to relieve headaches. Caffeine may reduce the risk of gallstones, dental cavities, Parkinson's disease, liver damage, asthma attacks and type 2 diabetes. Green tea is a rich source of the polyphenol; EGCG, or epigallocatechin gallate. It is a powerful antioxidant able to inhibit the growth of cancer cells, lower ldl cholesterol and protects against blood clots. Black tea and oolong tea contain far less EGCG, as it is depleted during processing.

Green tea may reduce the risk of heart disease in smokers. It may also protect against rheumatoid arthritis, infection, impaired immune function and cancer. Nearly 40% of the green tea leaf is polyphenols and the most important one is termed: flavan-3-ols, or catechin, or flavonols. Enjoy caffeine and tannin, drop the sugar and remember that pure water is the only vital drink.

Nicotine is a very addictive drug. After entering the lungs, the nicotine enters the bloodstream and stimulates the adrenal glands.

This causes an increased heartbeat, constriction of the arteries and an increased conversion of glycogen, from the liver, thereby providing an energetic burst. Nicotine also relaxes the muscles of the bronchi and lungs, causing 'lazy lungs'. The smoke and other chemicals in the cigarette damage lung tissues and arteries. Over a prolonged period, smokers may develop empysema, heart problems, circulatory problems, poor eyesight and nervous disorders. Depending on the duration of smoking, most smokers will develop health risk problems. Such conditions as recurrent colds, excess mucus, irritability, exhaustion and nervousness are common short term problems associated with smoking.

The average cigarette smoke contains at least 12 harmful compounds such as: carbon monoxide, cyanide and potassium nitrate. Nicotine can remain in the body and mind for many months, even years after a person has quit. There are many nicotine alternatives and they can be very helpful during the time of 'quitting'. A cleansing diet of fresh fruit and vegetable juices will promote the release of nicotine from the body and reduce the urge for nicotine. Refer to the chart below and to the chart on page 159 for a list of nutrients that smoking depletes.

Smoking is the habit you wish you never took up, it takes over your life and quitting is so tough, it's not worth all that smoke and puff!

SMOKING - HEALTH PROBLEMS - CHART TWO		
NUTRIENT	PROBLEMS	FOODS
VITAMIN C	poor eyesight infections increased cholesterol skin problems poor blood condition wrinkly skin cancer weak arteries colds and flus	red capsicum guava green capsicum blackcurrants chillies, berries parsley, lemon oranges, papaya kiwi fruit, pineapple broccoli
NUTRIENTS & FOODS TO HELP PROTECT AGAINST SMOKING		
SULPHUR	cleanses the respiratory system	garlic, carrrot juice
Beta Carotene	protect respiratory system from infections.	carrot juice sweet potato
Beta Cryptoxanthin	decreased risk of lung cancer	pumpkin
VITAMIN E	antioxidant protects cells	wheat germ oil sunflower seeds
VITAMIN C	antioxidant protect the arteries	capsicum, guava.

Vitamins were discovered to be an essential food item over a century ago, some vitamins have only recently been discovered. The name vitamins is derived from the Latin for live - 'vita', plus 'amine', from the word for a nitrogen containing compound. The word vitamins was introduced by a Polish chemist, Casimir Funk who recognized the existence of 'food substances' during the mid 1930's. The original discovery of individual vitamins was usually due to their availability from natural foods. Vitamins are the most intricate food substances, they are in minute portions and provide enormous benefits for protection and for activating numerous body functions. Food processing, heat and cooking deplete many vitamins and the effects of stress, illness and various risk factors greatly increases the need for numerous vitamins to be obtained regularly from a variety of natural foods. Vitamins are added to common processed foods to offset the development of well recognized ailments and vitamin supplements are purchased in an effort to balance the inadequate dietary intake. One estimate showed that 80% of people are not absorbing vitamin tablets effectively, as the small intestine may create a barrier against such chemically isolated substances. Only naturally produced vitamin supplements provide some benefits and only natural foods can provide the complete answer to vitamin requirements.

Throughout this chapter on vitamins there are over 200 recognized benefits associated with the world of vitamins and over 200 common ailments are directly related to a prolonged vitamin deficiency. There is no life without vitamins and only natural foods provide the 'essential food substances' with their unique ability to protect from illness.

With 17 vitamins known to be essential for life, it is a 'big ask' to expect good health from a diet of processed foods, cooked foods, canned foods and no natural foods, it really is pushing the limits of human nature and the results are evident with the increasing number of illnesses, hospital beds and regular sick days.

Let your diet be full of life and healing benefits from the variety of 100 natural foods. Vitamins are alive, active and ready to transform your life and health into a positive state, just add exercise and fresh water.

VITAMIN A

13 IMMUNE SYSTEM Vitamin A is most important in fighting infections as it provides strength to cell walls (mucous membranes) which protect the inner part of cells from attack by germs, pollution, viruses and bacteria.

Vitamin A improves the functions of the white blood cells. Vitamin A increases immunity to disease and decreases the symptoms of colds and the flu, as it retards the spread of infection.

Carotenoids from plant sources provide powerful antioxidant action to protect cells from the effects of free radicals from cooked oils and processed foods.

Beta carotene is the most potent antioxidant carotenoid. Smoking depletes the store of carotenoids in the body.

Carotenoids improve cellular connections and may therefore prevent the development of cancerous cells. The antioxidant action of carotenoids may also prevent cancer formation. A prolonged deficiency of carotenoids increases the risk of diseases.

17 SKIN SYSTEM Vitamin A is vital for the growth of healthy skin and hair and especially for the repair of damaged skin tissues and reduction of scar tissues. Vitamin A is required for the removal of dead skin cells.

Teenage acne is usually due to changing hormonal balance, especially the pituitary gland, plus such factors as emotional stress and a poor diet, rich in cooked fats, or chocolate and processed foods, all contribute to the temporary problem.

Vitamin A can assist to balance hormonal function, cleanse skin tissues and rebuild damaged tissues. A regular carrot juice will be hard to beat for skin benefits, especially as it is the sweetest source of organic sulphur, the ultimate skin cleansing mineral. Cooked foods lack the mineral sulphur as it is a heat sensitive nutrient. Carrots are the ultimate vitamin A - beta carotene food. Beta carotene obtained from fresh juices has no known bad side effects.

NOTE: All amounts in this book are measured in milligrams (mg) per 100 grams, unless stated otherwise.

161

VITAMIN A (R.E.) - *Retinol / Carotene - fat soluble*

16 REPRODUCTIVE SYSTEM

Vitamin A is required for the synthesis of R.N.A., a nucleic acid that assists the transmission of hormones and chemical messages for the reproduction of hereditary characteristics. A deficiency of vitamin A can lead to impaired reproduction. It is essential during pregnancy and additional amounts of 400 - 500 R.E. are vital during lactation. Intake of vitamin A: (carotenoids) is safe from natural foods but caution from supplements, especially during pregnancy as birth defects have been reported due to excess vitamin A supplement intake. Carrot juice is safe, it also promotes the flow of mother's milk. Carotenoids are vital for the reproductive system in women.

12 GROWTH SYSTEM

Vitamin A is essential for all cellular and bone growth and for effective use and the metabolism of the minerals: calcium and phosphorus. Apricots, mango, peaches, pumpkin and cantaloup are all very good sources of carotenoids to help children's bone growth.

15 OPTIC SYSTEM

Vitamin A is essential in the formation of visual purple which illuminates objects in dim lighting. The retina stores vitamin A within four optic pigments, the one used in dim lighting is termed rhodopsin, the other three optic pigments are collectively termed iodopsins and required for normal daylight vision.
Vitamin A is also required for peripheral or side vision and correct colour vision. A deficiency of vitamin A can lead to poor vision, cornea disorders and a prolonged deficiency may cause blindness.

2 DIGESTIVE SYSTEM

Vitamin A is required for the secretion of gastric juices which are required for protein digestion. Low protein diets may restrict the effective use of vitamin A. For people having difficulty in digesting fats, a deficiency of this vitamin may persist. Alcohol consumption causes a loss of vitamin A via the liver.
Sweet potato and pumpkin are an excellent source of vitamin A - carotene.

7 RESPIRATORY SYSTEM

Vitamin A protects the delicate internal linings of the throat, mouth, trachea, nose and lungs from infection, pollution, dust and smoke. Vitamin A increases resistance to disease of the mucous membranes against germs, viruses and infections. There are three forms of conversion from food based vitamin A - retinyl palmitate, into useable vitamin A which is a fat soluble compound, the most effective form for the respiratory system is: retinoic acid which is essential for the health of tissues within the lungs and trachea, termed mucosal tissues, they protect against invading airborne germs, viruses and bacteria. The other forms of retinyl palmitate are: retinol and retinal.

5 MUSCULAR SYSTEM

Vitamin A is required for the growth of muscular tissues and for the repair of damaged tissues. Retinoic acid from food based vitamin A is required for the synthesis of glycoproteins to assist the joining of cells within tissues.

Vitamin A is a fat-soluble vitamin that can be stored in the liver for a few days or weeks, depending on conditions of stress and illness.

There are two main forms of vitamin A:
PREFORMED VIT. A - retinol (animal source)
PROFORMED VIT. A - carotenoids (plants)
In 1974, the USDA introduced a way to calculate both forms of vitamin A, termed;

RETINOL ACTIVITY EQUIVALENTS:
1 R.E. = 1 mcg - retinol
1 R.E. = 6 mcg. - beta carotene
1 R.E. = 3.333 (I.U.) International Units

There are a few forms of carotenoids from plants that the body can convert into vitamin A, the most easily converted is beta carotene.

About one third of the carotene content in food is converted into useable vitamin A. When starch foods are cooked, the carotene content is easier to absorb.

Diabetics may be unable to convert carotene from plant foods into useable vitamin A. Cod liver oil, fish oils, liver, butter, cheese all provide vitamin A.

VITAMIN C - ascorbic acid - water soluble

17 SKIN SYSTEM

Vitamin A is required daily for numerous functions such as the development of collagen, the substance that holds skin cells together. Such conditions as dry skin, wrinkles, easy bruising and splitting hair may all be due to a prolonged vitamin C deficiency, or intermittent supplies that cause the body to go without for a few days. Vitamin C is vital for prevention and relief from skin infections that are often caused by burns and wounds and sports injuries.

13 IMMUNE SYSTEM

Vitamin C is the most active water soluble antioxidant and in order to maintain a strong immune system, daily intake of vitamin C rich foods is essential, especially for people who smoke, or suffer from stress related conditions. Vitamin C is the most well known and self administered vitamin, especially to offset colds and winter viruses. Human cells when subjected to a solution of vitamin C were able to produce increased amounts of interferon, a substance that the body produces to protect cells from viruses. Normal to high levels of vitamin C supplements 100 - 1,000 mg per day in the form of ascorbic acid assist the activity of the white blood cells to protect against harmful bacteria, however, excessive amounts of vitamin C, (over 3,000 mg.) can retard the activity of the white blood cells and deactivate the functions of vitamin B12. Also, calcium absorption can be hindered by excess intake. Vitamin C increases the number and activity of white blood cells with normal intake from natural foods and ideally it needs bioflavonoids, such as the white pith in citrus or capsicum, to be fully active and effective. Vitamin C protects cells from oxygen-based damage with ailments such as cancer and cardiovascular disease. When children are due to have vaccinations, ensure their vitamin C levels are adequate. High doses of vitamin C have proved effective against toxins in pesticides and nitrates which are associated with cancer formation. Vitamin C promotes the absorption of iron and for body cleansing and elimination of toxins, both vitamin C and iron rich foods are essential.

3 GLANDULAR SYSTEM

Vitamin C is essential for the health of the adrenal glands and during conditions of stress, vitamin C is released from the adrenal glands. The liver requires vitamin C for elimination of toxins. Numerous enzyme reactions require vitamin C for the functioning of the pituitary, adrenals and ovaries. Vitamin C protects against glandular infections such as tonsillitis, glandular fever and mumps.

15 OPTIC SYSTEM

Vitamin C is required daily for the health of the optic system. The lens of the eyes needs vitamin C and a prolonged deficiency may cause poor vision. A healthy lens is always supplied with vitamin C.

2 DIGESTIVE SYSTEM

Vitamin C is required to convert cholesterol into bile acids. It is also vital for effective absorption of the mineral iron from dietary intake and the subsequent storage in the bone marrow. Vitamin C protects against excess acidity and it promotes the storage of folate for blood development and prevention of anaemia. Ideally, vitamin C foods are best obtained at most meals of the day, especially breakfast. Fat molecules that are transported around the body require vitamin C for protection from oxidation.

OTHER SYSTEMS

Vitamin C is required for the health of the nervous system. Vitamin C is termed the 'youth vitamin' as it preserves skin tissue but also because the older we are, the more vitamin C is required. Vitamin C can last in the body for 10-20 hours under normal conditions but such factors as stress, smoking, injury, virus, disease, colds and infections can reduce vitamin c levels.

Vitamin C in combination with bioflavonoids, are vital for strength of arteries and capillaries. Vitamin C is important in the proper formation of children's teeth and for their growth and bone formation. Such medications and drugs as aspirin, cortisone, antibiotics, nicotine, and oral contraceptives diminish the body's store of precious vitamin C.

VITAMIN E - *d alpha tocopherol - fat soluble*

Vitamin E is the common name for a group of fat soluble substances known as tocopherols and tocotrienols. Their chemical structure is similar with tocotrienols being more unsaturated. There are four main types of each: alpha, beta, delta and gamma. The most potent form of vitamin E is natural *d* alpha & *d* gamma tocopherol and tocotrienol. Numerous types of vitamin E supplements are available, however, to be sure that it is natural vitamin E, the label must read: *d* alpha tocopherol or tocotrienol. Synthetic vitamin E is referred to as *dl* alpha tocopherol, it is esterified to stabilize storage and may be less than 50% effective. A combination of both tocopherol and tocotrienols ensures the complete benefits.

1 CIRCULATORY SYSTEM — Vitamin E assists blood circulation by enlarging blood vessels and arteries which provide both oxygen and nourishment to all body cells. Persons with high blood pressure or rheumatic heart disease are best to consult their medical practitioner before taking vitamin E supplements. Vitamin E (tocotrienols in particular) lower blood cholesterol. Vitamin E protects against narrowing of carotid arteries and may reverse the condition.

10 CELLULAR SYSTEM — Every cell in the body lives by burning up oxygen to produce energy and warmth. Vitamin E regulates this action and prevents cells from burning out too quickly. The normal life of a healthy red blood cell is 120 days, a deficiency of vitamin E can reduce cell life to 70 days. Vitamin E improves the number, activity and potency of the male sperm cells. Vitamin E preserves the walls of the red blood cells and prevents their destruction from oxidative stress. In addition, vitamin C, selenium, vitamin B3 and the amino acid glutathione must be available to offset oxidative stress.

Vitamin E is also essential for the transfer of cellular information within cells and to other cells and as vitamin E is fat soluble, it links to fat membranes within and outside cells to protect against oxidation thereby promoting life and gaining the title of the anti-ageing vitamin.

5 MUSCULAR SYSTEM — Vitamin E increases the power and activity of muscles and improves their endurance by increasing the supply of oxygen and the lifespan of muscular cells. Vitamin E strengthens the heart muscles. Sunflower seeds are the ultimate E food.

7 RESPIRATORY SYSTEM — Vitamin E protects the lungs from pollution, smoke, ozone and other environmental chemicals due to the powerful anti-peroxidase action of both tocopherols and tocotrienols, in combination with vitamin C, selenium and B3.

2 DIGESTIVE SYSTEM — Vitamin E helps regulate the body's use of fats and protein from the daily diet. The common daily use of mass produced margarine and polyunsaturated fats greatly increases the need for vitamin E. Low vitamin E levels may lead to diseases of the pancreas, gallbladder, liver, bladder, nervous disorders and celiac disease.

16 REPRODUCTIVE SYSTEM — Vitamin E promotes the activity of the ovaries and assists normal menstruation; reduced bleeding, dryness and irritation of the genital passages. Vitamin E promotes blood supply to the unborn baby and may offset the possibility of miscarriage. Vitamin E improves the potency of the male sperm cell and it is vital for normal fertility in both male and female. The synthetic female hormone: oestrogen is a vitamin E antagonist and an increased dietary intake of vitamin E is vital for maintenance of vitamin E functions. The name tocopherol is derived from the Greek words: *tocos*-childbirth and *pherin* - to bring forth.

3 GLANDULAR SYSTEM — Vitamin E promotes the function of the pituitary and adrenal glands in the production of hormones and protects hormones from oxidation. Natural vitamin E foods such as almonds and cosmetic creams containing (*d* alpha tocopherol - tocotrienols)

17 SKIN SYSTEM — protect the skin from ultraviolet radiation from sunlight. Natural vitamin E foods and creams are also very beneficial for the healing of burns and damaged skin tissues.

VITAMIN D - *lumisterol calciferol*

8 SKELETAL SYSTEM Vitamin D is produced by the action of sunlight on skin cells which converts cholesterol into a form known as cholecalciferol, or pro vitamin D. It is transferred to the liver and converted into the form of calciterol, or active vitamin D. The parathyroid glands use calciterol to control calcium metabolism, activated by the hormone PTH (parathyroid hormone) to ensure a constant supply and level of calcium in the blood. Vitamin D also assists in the absorption of phosphorus, a diet low in iron may reduce vitamin D absorption.

During winter especially, adequate sunlight is required, preferably at least 15 minutes per day. In summer, especially in the tropical areas, it is best to avoid sunlight during the hours of 11am till 3 pm, due to the intense ultraviolet radiation. Vitamin D can be stored in the body for many days but during times of constant indoor work, cloud or rain, or snow, it is best to obtain vitamin D from cod liver oil, fish or eggs. For adults over 50, an increase intake of vitamin D from moderate sunlight and foods is required to protect against increased dental diseases and also to protect against the development of osteoporosis.

2 DIGESTIVE SYSTEM Vitamin D is essential for good digestion and the metabolism of numerous minerals and vitamins. The thyroid gland requires vitamin D for the control of digestion.

12 GROWTH SYSTEM Vitamin D is essential for children's growth and children require nearly twice as much vitamin D as adults, but beware of midday sun and wear a hat during summer and at lunch or play.

3 GLANDULAR SYSTEM Numerous glands such as the thyroid, parathyroid, pituitary, pineal and adrenal glands require vitamin D for their activity and production of hormones.

6 NERVOUS SYSTEM The nervous system requires nutrients that are activated by the action of vitamin D, such as the minerals phosphorus, calcium and magnesium.

VITAMIN K - *menadione*

9 BLOOD SYSTEM Vitamin K is the key factor for the process of blood coagulation and the clotting time of blood. A substance known as prothrombin in the blood is formed by the action of vitamin K. At the site of abrasion or bleeding, the converted form of thrombin acts on the fibrinogen of plasma and converts it into a substance termed fibrin, which traps the red cells into a mesh, forming clots. Vitamin K has proved effective in reducing blood loss during menstruation. Vitamin K is referred to as the anti-haemorrhagic vitamin or simply the band-aid vitamin. Vitamin K is required for blood circulation and it assists the functions of the liver and heart. Vitamin K in combination with vitamin C has been effective in the prevention of excessive blood loss after operations.

2 DIGESTIVE SYSTEM Vitamin K is required for the conversion of carbohydrates into the form of glycogen which is stored in the liver and converted into glucose when activity levels increase or dietary intake is insufficient. Vitamin K is absorbed from the upper section of the small intestines and in combination with bile it is transferred to the liver until required for blood clotting.

OTHER FACTORS Vitamin K is best obtained from fresh green leafy vegetables, especially lettuce. Such factors as freezing and prolonged cooking deplete the supply of vitamin K, for this reason, spinach when cooked or frozen is not the best source of vitamin K, but fresh spinach is the ultimate source. Vitamin K is a fat soluble vitamin and the older we are, the more vitamin K is required. Vitamin K protects the liver from lead pollution.

DEPLETING FACTORS Regular use of aspirin, antibiotics, mineral oils and exposure to x rays can destroy the vitamin K intestinal bacteria within the human body. Natural acidophilus yoghurt is ideal to obtain as it helps restore natural bacteria to the intestines and promotes the production and synthesis of internal vitamin K. Babies are given vitamin K at birth to promote healthy development of blood cells.

VITAMIN F - Omega 3 - alpha linolenic acid
Omega 6 - linoleic acid   (essential fatty acids)

Vitamin F is the collective term for the essential fatty acids: alpha linolenic acid or Omega 3 and linoleic acid or Omega 6. Both Omega 3 and Omega 6 cannot be produced by the body and must be supplied with the diet. They are essential to life and must be balanced to ensure good health. Excess intake of Omega 6 is fairly common mainly due to margarine and vegetable oils, but the intake of Omega 3 is often inadequate. An excess of Omega 6 interferes with the unique functions of Omega 3. The ideal dietary intake of the essential fatty acids is 1 part Omega 3 with 2 parts Omega 6. Generally speaking, the average diet may obtain a 1 part Omega 3 to 25 parts Omega 6. This huge imbalance is due to a few factors: the big increase in margarine consumption and the wide availability and excess intake of Omega 6 foods, plus the limited natural sources of Omega 3. Such foods as pepitas (pumpkin seed kernels), walnuts, flax seeds and canola oil are an excellent source of Omega 3, fish, seafood, egg yolk, pecan and hazel nuts are a good source. Apart from those foods, there are only a few that provide Omega 3. The ideal diet must contain a good proportion of rich Omega 3 foods.

Refer to page 134 for the Omega 3 & Omega 6 food source chart.

17 SKIN SYSTEM The skin system is dependant on a regular supply of Omega 3 to protect against dry or itchy skin, as Omega 3 helps to maintain resilience and lubrication to skin cells. Omega 3 foods promote healthy hair and hair growth and supple, youthful skin.

10 CELLULAR SYSTEM The cellular system requires Omega 3 in particular to retain water and vital nutrients. As cells are primarily composed of fats. The supply of fats from the diet greatly dictates the condition of individual cells. Excess saturated fats cause cells to become hard and to lack fluidity and storage of nutrients. Omega 3 protects against tumours and breast cancer by retarding the action of enzymes that damage cells. Omega 3 is vital for the cells of the nervous system, development of sex hormones and for healthy intestinal bacteria.

13 IMMUNE SYSTEM Omega 3 is the key nutrient to offset inflammatory conditions such as back pain, asthma, bowel inflammation, rheumatoid arthritis, auto-immune diseases, joint stiffness, swelling, chronic fatigue and atherosclerosis. An excess of Omega 6 dietary intake in comparison to Omega 3 intake can lead to prolonged inflammatory conditions, as Omega 6 fats promote inflammatory reactions in molecules, in contrast, Omega 3 help produce hormones termed prostaglandins. Omega 3 is converted by the body into eichosapentaenoic acid (EPA) and docosahexaenoic acid (DHA), both these prostoglandins reduce inflammation. Both EPA & DHA are obtained directly from salmon, herring, tuna and halibut. Catch the O3 benefits with fish.

19 BRAIN SYSTEM Omega 3 is vital for brain development, especially DHA Omega 3, no wonder fish is termed a 'brain food'. The brain is composed of 60% fat. The brain requires large amounts of DHA Omega 3, especially in the first two years of life. Research shows that infants from mother's having a high Omega 3 blood level, had advanced levels of learning and attention spans. Mother's milk does transfer DHA to the baby, when the mother's dietary intake includes Omega 3 foods such as walnuts, salmon and pepitas. Post natal depression may be linked to a deficiency of Omega 3 (DHA), as the baby will obtain as much as necessary from the mother, possibly leading to a chronic DHA deficiency. In addition, mental health conditions such as depression, mood swings, bipolar disorder, schizophrenia and dementia can be traced to a deficiency of Omega 3. Brain cell receptors require Omega 3 to help direct a smooth and efficient neuron signal connection within a very complex brain system and integrated nervous system. Omega 3 promotes concentration. Omega 3 promotes low cholesterol levels, regular heartbeat, reduced blood pressure and protection from coronary disease. Omega 3 also helps thin the blood, preventing blood clots and strokes.

1 CIRCULATORY SYSTEM

Meat supplies no Omega 3, except for venison and buffalo meat.

Vitamin P is often referred to as flavonoids or bioflavonoids. Nearly all bright coloured red, orange, blue and yellow fruits and vegetables contain flavonoids. There are a few groups of flavonoids: anthocyanins, anthocyanidins, dihydroflavonols, flavonols, flavanones and isoflavones. Within these groups there are numerous other forms of flavonoids, for example within the group of flavonols the common forms are hesperidin, rutin and quercetin. Within the group of flavanones the common forms are apigenin found in chamomile and luteolin. Some foods are a unique source of a particular flavonoid. Most flavonoids provide an antioxidant activity and help prevent cellular damage.

The immune system functions are greatly enhanced by flavonoids, mainly **13 IMMUNE SYSTEM** due to the fact that they increase the antioxidant activity of vitamin C. Within citrus fruits and capsicum, the white pith is full of flavonoids. Bottled orange juice may contain vitamin C, usually added, but the supply of flavonoids is often lacking. Numerous functions of vitamin C are dependant on the presence of flavonoids. During conditions of stress and inflammation, due to injury, flavonoids regulate the activity of the immune system to protect against over-activity of cells, which can lead to excess inflammation. In conditions such as with joint inflammation, back injuries, spinal inflammation, various allergies, viruses and tumours, flavonoids reduce the pain and symptoms due to a decrease in reactive cell activity. Isoflavones found in legumes block the enzymes that can produce excess of the natural female hormone: oestrogen, thereby reducing the risk of developing breast and ovarian cancer. The flavonoid quercetin, in apples, may help alleviate allergies by retarding histamine production. Flavonoids protect against high blood pressure, as they block the action of the enzyme: angiosten. In addition, **1 CIRCULATORY SYSTEM** flavonoids such as rutin, found in buckwheat are most beneficial for strengthening blood capillaries and may protect against varicose veins and the entire vascular system by helping to develop strong cells.

15 OPTIC SYSTEM Flavonoids may provide protection from cataracts, especially with diabetics, as excess blood sugar levels produce alcohol sugars that can cause clouding of the eyes or cataracts. Flavonoids assist by blocking the digestive enzyme aldose-reductase from converting galactose into the harmful form of galacticol.

17 SKIN SYSTEM The flavonol: anthocyanidin helps to strengthen and connect strands of collagen skin protein. Flavonoids can also protect against skin infections, bacteria and fungus such as tinea which can also be alleviated by drops of tea tree oil.

3 GLANDULAR SYSTEM Isoflavones such as genistein found in soy products and some legumes can block enzymes that cause tumour growths in uterine, breast and prostate cancer, reducing the risk of ovarian and breast cancer.

9 BLOOD SYSTEM Flavonoids can protect against recurrent nose bleeding, easy bruising and platelet aggregation. Flavonoids may also be required to prevent the development of leukaemia and haemophilia. Flavonoids regulate the permeability of blood capillaries.

Flavonoids regulate the activity of cells such as B cells, T cells, NK cells and **10 CELLULAR SYSTEM** most cells especially for the proper functioning of the immune system. Flavonoids provide antiviral activity and may help in cases of the HIV and herpes virus, by retarding the activity of cells and other bacteria that attempt to develop. Flavonoids also provide antibiotic action and protect against harmful bacteria. Refer to page 175 for food sources. Flavonoids protect LDL cholesterol from possible oxidation by the action of free radicals.

OTHER FUNCTIONS Flavonoids may help relieve the condition of rheumatism due to their anti-inflammatory action. Flavonoids protect against the common cold in addition to the action of vitamin C and the mineral iron. Flavonoids are destroyed by processing.

NON ESSENTIAL VITAMINS & CO - FACTORS

VITAMIN T

Vitamin T is often referred to as the 'sesame seed vitamin' and it is often neglected in nutrition books because it is not a true vitamin. It is described as a food factor and apart from sesame seeds, tahini, and egg yolks are the only known source. Vitamin T assists in the formation of blood platelets and normal blood coagulation.

Vitamin T may be a factor in protection against anaemia and haemophilia. Vitamin T helps promote memory abilities and may improve a failing memory. Tahini is the richest source of vitamin T.

VITAMIN U

Vitamin U is also termed a non-essential vitamin and was first discovered in cabbage. Vitamin U has provided relief for peptic and stomach ulcers. Cabbage also contains sulphorane which destroys the helicobacter pylori bacterium that is a cause of peptic and duodenal ulcers. Regular use of coleslaw can provide protection from bacteria causing ulcers.

VITAMIN B13 - orotic acid

Vitamin B13, supplied in root vegetables, is required for the effective use of folic acid and vitamin B12. Vitamin B13 has been used effectively in cases of multiple sclerosis and chronic hepatitis, as it is vital for cell regeneration and transfer of nutrients into cells. It is also required for brain functioning, the nervous system and production of genetic material.

VITAMIN B17 - laetrile

Vitamin B17 was discovered in 1958, restricted due to the cyanide compound. It has been used in the treatment of cancer. Apricot kernels supply B17.

COENZYME Q - ubiquinone

Coenzyme Q was discovered in 1957 and has proved to be a vital nutrient but it is not considered essential, as the body can manufacture this compound antioxidant under normal conditions.

Coenzyme Q is required for protection of the heart muscles from oxidation, especially in conditions such as angina, high blood pressure and arrhthmia. Coenzyme Q is vital for the conversion of fats into useable energy and within the circulatory system, fats that 'hang around' may cause problems such as blood clots, coronary arterial disease and heart failure.

The cellular system uses coenzyme Q for activating energy production from fats and other substances within cells. Coenzyme Q protects cells from oxidation during this process of energy production and it has proven to reduce cell damage by nearly 90%, when provided in supplemental form. Coenzyme Q assists the antioxidant funcions of vitamin E by recharging the activity of vitamin E, even after it has exerted it's activity on cells as a protector against free radicals. Coenzyme Q is required by cells for growth and maintenance and for protection of the DNA structure within cells. A deficiency of coenzyme Q may lead to cancer of the lungs, breasts, colon, kidneys, prostate and pancreas.

Coenzyme Q stimulates the immune system and also increases resistance to disease. In clinical trials with a high dosage of coenzyme Q, over a 3 year period, reduced symptoms of breast cancer and use of painkillers were reported. The ability to absorb coenzyme Q declines with age. The best food source of coenzyme Q are soy oil, sardines, mackerel, fish, peanuts, beef, organ meats, nuts, spinach and broccoli.
A healthy body can make all the coenzyme Q required. Supplements may assist in cases of a deficiency due to age or depleted abilities to produce coenzyme Q, or diet.

VITAMIN B1 - *thiamine*

6 NERVOUS SYSTEM

Vitamin B1 is a water soluble vitamin and required daily for the health of the nervous system. The body can only store limited amounts and during conditions of stress, physical exercise and depression, increased intake of B1 is essential. The nervous system requires B1 for the development of the myelin sheaths which are a fat layer covering nerve endings. A deficiency of B1 can result in damage to the nerve endings. In addition, B1 is essential for the production of neurotransmitters termed acetylcholine, to activate muscle action and a deficiency may lead to sciatica, muscle cramps, poor coordination, tiredness, lack of concentration and learning abilities.

The heart muscles require B1 for proper muscle tone and prevention of congestive heart failure. Intake of alcohol depletes the reserves of this vitamin and excess intake of alcohol can increase the need for B1 from 10 - 100 times the normal daily requirement.

The process of digestion is dependant on a regular supply of B1, as the enzyme pyruvate dehydrogenase is formed with B1 and required for the conversion of glucose into energy. For protein digestion, vitamin B1 is required for the production of hydrochloric acid. The substance allinin in garlic and onions increases the absorption of thiamine. A deficiency of B1 can lead to loss of appetite, anorexia plus accumulations of fat in the arteries, constipation and stomach ulcers.

Vitamin B1 is vital for children's growth as it helps increase their appetite and absorption of nutrients from foods. It is essential to increase the intake of vitamin B1 during pregnancy and lactation and it is vital for adult fertility. Thiamine increases oxygen absorption within blood which promotes mental functions and physical activity. Yeast extracts, sunflower seeds and rice bran are an excellent source. Intake of caffeine, antibiotics and the pill deplete B1, as they act as diuretics and remove water soluble vitamins.

VITAMIN B2- *riboflavin*

15 OPTIC SYSTEM

Vitamin B2 is vital for the optic system as it promotes cell respiration and the body's use of oxygen and the recycling of enzymes that protect the body from oxidation. The substance glutathione is required for prevention of oxygen damage to cells and vitamin B2 assists by promoting the reuse of this antioxidant protein molecule. A deficiency of B2 may result in cataracts, sensitivity to light, blurred vision, itching eyes, burning sensation in eyes and dimness of vision.

17 SKIN SYSTEM

Vitamin B2 is required for healthy skin condition as it protects against oxidation of skin cells and promotes cell respiration, cellular growth and a youthful complexion. A deficiency of B2 may result in conditions such as cracked skin near the corners of the mouth, dermatitis, acne, oily skin, peeling skin and sore lips, tongue and mouth. A deficiency may also contribute to baldness and weight loss. Alcohol, stress and excess physical exertion can lead to a deficiency plus antibiotics, the pill and various drugs cause a loss of vitamin B2. Vitamin B2 is required for the secretion of

2 DIGESTIVE SYSTEM

protein digestive enzymes and the absorption of numerous nutrients. B2 is absorbed via the small intestine and transported in the blood to body tissues. Vitamin B2 promotes the supply and conversion of other B vitamins such as B3, B6 and folate plus vitamin K into an active form. Vitamin B2 is essential for the production of energy from carbohydrates, proteins and lipids. It attaches to protein enzymes and promotes oxygen and energy production especially in the heart and skeletal muscles. Riboflavin or vitamin B2 is stable to heat and cooking, acids and air but it is destroyed by light and alkalis plus processing destroys over 70% of the original B2 content. Most processed grains such as bread, pasta and flour have added B2. Such foods as almonds, malt and yeast extracts are a very good source of vitamin B2.

B2 protects against baldness, anaemia, migraine and lack of energy. It is vital during pregnancy and lactation and for children's growth and development.

VITAMIN B3 - *niacin*

17 SKIN SYSTEM

Vitamin B3 is important for healthy skin condition but excess intake of B3 supplements can cause a redskin rash. A deficiency can also lead to dermatitis, cataracts and skin allergies.

3 GLANDULAR SYSTEM

The hormone insulin is dependant on a regular supply of vitamin B3 for blood sugar regulation and proper insulin activity. B3 is an essential ingredient in the production of both male and female sex hormones for reproduction. Vitamin B3 promotes a peaceful nights sleep and it is a vital component in the genetic process as it is required for the production of DNA: deoxyribose nucleic acid. Yeast extracts are a good source.

2 DIGESTIVE SYSTEM

Vitamin B3 is essential for the conversion of fats and the regulation of fat levels of the blood, as it controls the release of fats for energy production and the production of cell membranes. It is also required for the production of cholesterol within the liver and helps to lower blood cholesterol levels when obtained in high doses. Vitamin B3 is required for the efficient use of protein and a deficiency may lead to indigestion, constipation, diarrhoea and varied digestive disturbances. Vitamin B3 is a most stable B vitamin, it is not destroyed by cooking, heat, acids, alkali, air or light. An excess intake may occur from taking B3 supplements and eating too many peanuts, as 100 grams of peanuts supplies over 20 mg and the daily RDA for men is 19 mg. The upper tolerable level from supplements is 35 mg and 200 grams of peanuts supplies 40 mg. Conditions of stress, trauma, fever, intake of the contraceptive pill and excess alcohol consumption can lead to a vitamin B3 deficiency. Vitamin B3 assists the functions of the digestive enzymes and it is vital for conversion of all food groups into useable energy and for the storage of starch glucose in the liver as glycogen. A deficiency of B3 can show as muscular weakness, poor appetite and various digestive disorders. Vitamin B3 is vital for the brain and normal mental functions and a prolonged deficiency may lead to Alzhiemer's disease and other age related mental conditions. B3 is also obtainable via conversion of tryptophan.

VITAMIN B5 - *pantothenic acid*

2 DIGESTIVE SYSTEM

Vitamin B5 is essential for the transport of fatty acids within body cells. Vitamin B5 transfers fats from the watery cytoplasm within cells to the place where body fat is produced, the mitochondria. The transport of these fats is supported by a protein which requires the availability of vitamin B5 to function. Vitamin B5 is also required for the release of energy from stored fats and for the synthesis of cholesterol. Other fat molecules that are responsible for the transfer of chemical messages into cells require vitamin B5 for their synthesis. The word 'panto' means everywhere and without doubt vitamin B5 is in every cell, it is essential for white blood cell production and for the utilization of carbohydrates and proteins as well as the functions of vitamin B2. A deficiency of vitamin B5 may lead to abdominal pains, kidney damage and ulcers. Sunflower seeds are an excellent source.

3 GLANDULAR SYSTEM

Vitamin B5 is essential for the health of the adrenal glands and it is required for the production of the hormone: adrenaline for protection from stress. Vitamin B5 is destroyed by cooking, processing and up to a 70% loss in frozen foods. Vitamin B5 may protect against chronic fatigue syndrome and arthritis.

6 NERVOUS SYSTEM

Vitamin B5 is essential for the growth and development of the nervous system. A deficiency of vitamin B5 often shows as fatigue and weakness as nerve disorders produce weak muscle action and pins and needles in the hands and feet. Vitamin B5 has beneficial effects in conditions such as insomnia, psychosomatic disorders, cramps, depression, apathy, unstable heart action and chronic fatigue syndrome.

10 CELLULAR SYSTEM

Vitamin B5 is required for the production of antibodies to fight infection, it protects cells against radiation and is essential for the development of healthy fats in cells. Vitamin B5 assists cells to make chemical changes such as with hormone production and to protect cells from chemical breakdown. Vitamin B5 promotes healthy skin, hair and also assists the functions of the liver.

VITAMIN B6 - *pyridoxine*

6 NERVOUS SYSTEM

Vitamin B6 is also referred to as the 'vitality' vitamin, it performs a wide variety of functions and participates in the activity of over 100 enzyme reactions and it is vital for the nervous system. Vitamin B6 is vital for the development of amines which transfer nerve responses throughout the nervous system. A deficiency of B6 can lead to headaches, poor memory, decline of intelligence, irritability, convulsions, nervousness, depression, confusion, over-sensitivity and it has also been used effectively in the treatment of Parkinson's disease. Vitamin B6 is a vital component in the production of the nerve transmitters: epinephrine, seratonin, norepinephrine and melatonin. Excess vitamin B6 supplementation can be detrimental to the nervous system. Walnuts and wheat germ are an excellent source of vitamin B6.

2 DIGESTIVE SYSTEM

The digestive system requires vitamin B6 for the conversion of energy from amino acids and for the production of gastric juices for protein digestion. In addition, vitamin B6 is required in the construction of amino acids, it is a water soluble vitamin and vital for the conversion of tryptophan into niacin and the absorption of vitamin B12 plus the metabolism of carbohydrates, especially the conversion of glycogen: stored glucose in muscle cells and the liver, into useable energy. Vi-

17 SKIN SYSTEM

tamin B6 is referred to as the anti-dermatitis factor and a prolonged deficiency of B6 may also contribute to eczema and acne. Garlic is full of B6 plus sulphur compounds to cleanse the skin, yeast extracts are also a good source of B6.

3 GLANDULAR SYSTEM

The master gland of the body, the pituitary gland requires B6 to promote normal metabolism. The contraceptive pill, oestrogen and some medications can deplete the reserves of vitamin B6, plus processing and cooking can cause up to a 95% loss in the B6 value. The development of white blood cells, haemoglobin and adrenaline all require vitamin B6, it is vital during pregnancy to offset nausea, helps rid the blood of harmful toxins and is required for DNA manufacture.

VITAMIN B12- *cobalamin*

9 BLOOD SYSTEM

Vitamin B12 is a water soluble vitamin and stored in the liver, kidneys and various body tissues, it is vital for the proper formation of red blood cells as it assists the development of DNA which provides the genetic information for the reproduction of healthy red blood cells. The mineral cobalt has a central role in the development of vitamin B12, hence the name cobalamin. Foods rich in folate and iron, such as parsley, protect against red cell retardation and anaemia.

2 DIGESTIVE SYSTEM

Within the stomach a special mucoprotein termed 'the intrinsic factor' is essential for vitamin B12 to be absorbed later in the small intestine. Some auto-immune ailments prevent the mucoprotein from functioning and a deficiency of stomach acids: hydrochloric acid may also reduce the transfer and release of B12 from foods, both conditions may lead to pernicious anaemia. Excess use of antacids and stomach ulcer medications are a cause of the above conditions. Vitamin B12 is also required for the metabolism of carbohydrates and fats plus the utilization of amino acids throughout the body.

6 NERVOUS SYSTEM

Vitamin B12 is an important component with the formation of the protective layer of nerve cells: myelin sheaths. Vegan mother's need to be aware that numerous infant and children's nerve and muscular problems can develop from a deficiency of vitamin B12 foods.

OTHER FACTORS

Plants, animals and humans cannot produce vitamin B12, it is made by bacteria, algae, moulds, yeasts and fungi. For strict vegans, foods such as fermented tofu, tempeh, miso, shoyu and tamari, plus mushrooms, kelp, comfrey, dulse, kombu, nori, brewers yeast, torulla yeast and some organic vegetables may provide a trace of vitamin B12. For vegetarians, such foods as yoghurt and cheese will provide a good supply of vitamin B12. Seafood such as clams, oysters and fish are an excellent source of B12. Vitamin B12 is heat sensitive and up to 80% can be lost in cooking. Vitamin B12 can be recycled in the body for several years.

VITAMIN B15 - *pangamic acid*

1 CIRCULATORY SYSTEM Vitamin B15 has not been classified as an essential vitamin however there are functions that it participates with such as the improved utilization of oxygen, and blood circulation. Vitamin B15 also helps protect against carbon monoxide pollution and this function is reliant on vitamins A and E. B15 has provided improvement in conditions of angina, hypertension, arteriosclerosis and heart conditions due to the cholesterol lowering and extended cell life and oxygen benefits. Vitamin B15 has proved effective in the treatment of hypoxia: shortage of oxygen.

13 IMMUNE SYSTEM Vitamin B15 functions as a detoxifying agent against cancer causing chemicals and especially against environmental pollutants. Vitamin B15 has been used as a preventative treatment for cancer and the original source was from apricot kernels, discovered in 1951 by Drs Ernst Krebs. Other sources are pepitas, brewers yeast, sesame seeds, tahini, oats and whole brown rice. Vitamin B15 extends cell life and works as an antioxidant. One study showed that B15 greatly enhanced the body's ability to inhibit the growth of HIV type one. Another study showed a four fold increase in antibody response to supplementation of vitamin B15. Vitamin B15 may also provide benefits in cases of hepatitis, cirrhosis of the liver and emphysema.

6 NERVOUS SYSTEM Vitamin B15 helps to stabilize emotional and mental problems and as a supplement it proved beneficial in cases of autism. One study showed a considerable improvement in the speech of mentally impaired children plus better concentration and interest in toys and games. Vitamin B15 is water soluble and it is not classed as essential to life, but it has many important functions. Vitamin B15 has been used in the treatment of Alzheimer's disease, diabetes, liver disease, alcoholism, trauma, stress, senility and athletic injuries. Excessive perspiration causes a loss of B15 and for cuts and bruises from exercise accidents, it helps in their healing. Vitamin B15 assists in protein synthesis, is beneficial for prevention of premature ageing and helps to neutralize alcohol cravings.

BIOTIN - *co-enzymeR (vitamin H)*

10 CELLULAR SYSTEM Biotin is essential for the production of healthy cells and tissues, in particular the skin cells. Biotin activates the enzyme: acetyl Co-A carboxylase which is required for the construction of fats within the cell membranes. Biotin also assists in the maintenance and repair of bones and during pregnancy and lactation, additional intake of biotin foods is vital to protect against cot death and various birth defects. One study showed that nearly 50% of pregnant women were deficient in this vitamin. Such factors as the consumption of raw egg white, which contains avidin a glycoprotein, inhibits the absorption of biotin, plus a deficiency of vitamin B5 can also lead to a biotin deficiency.

17 SKIN SYSTEM Biotin is vital for the production of healthy skin cells and a prolonged biotin deficiency may lead to seborrheic dermatitis in adults and cradle cap in infants. Baldness may also be due to a prolonged biotin deficiency. Legumes have biotin. Biotin is essential for the conversion of fatty foods into individual cells, as it activates the enzyme that is vital for cell construction.

2 DIGESTIVE SYSTEM Biotin also promotes the conversion of sugar: blood glucose into the form of useable energy. Biotin protects against digestive disorders such as irritable bowel syndrome, ulcerative colitis and diarrhoea. Biotin can be synthesized by intestinal bacteria when favourable conditions exist. Antibiotics and mineral oils may upset the intestinal bacteria. Most processed cereals have no biotin, oats are full of biotin. Such nutrients as folic acid, vitamin B5 and B12 plus protein and carbohydrates need biotin for their full effectiveness and utilization. A biotin deficiency may contribute to an overweight condition, as it is essential for the conversion of fats.

6 NERVOUS SYSTEM Biotin is vital for the nervous system and may protect against the development of poor muscle and nerve coordination, seizures, muscle cramps and poor muscle tone. Biotin is also required for the distribution of carbon dioxide from the lungs, in combination with the amino acid lysine. Biotin is stable to oxygen, cooking and light.

CHOLINE

2 DIGESTIVE SYSTEM Choline is a water soluble vitamin with the ability to convert fats into smaller water soluble substances, similar to the role of bile. This function promotes the distribution of fat soluble nutrients into the bloodstream and into developing cells which are primarily made of fats. The name 'chole' is taken from the Greek word meaning bile. Choline needs the other B complex vitamins to be effective, especially folate, vitamin B3 and the 'hard to get' amino acid methionine.

6 NERVOUS SYSTEM Choline is essential for the nervous system, it is the main component of acetycholine, a neuromuscular transmitter and vital for prevention and treatment with such conditions as Parkinson's disease, attention deficit disorder, Alzheimer's disease, autism, poor memory, hyperactivity and various nervous conditions. Most processed foods are deficient in choline. The substance termed lecithin, obtained from corn or soy beans, available as a supplement is vital for replenishment of choline reserves, as the body can only produce lecithin when it has sufficient choline.

19 BRAIN SYSTEM The brain needs lecithin to function properly, over 28% of brain matter is composed of lecithin and research has shown that mentally impaired persons brain-lecithin content is often as low as 19%. Stress and nervousness rapidly use up the lecithin reserves, it is nature's tranquilizer, it promotes a good nights sleep and protects against fatigue and insomnia.

1 CIRCULATORY SYSTEM Lecithin is also referred to as phosphatidylcholine. Choline is vital for reduction of blood homocysteine levels which are a major cause of coronary heart disease. Choline is essential for the conversion of homocysteine into a harmless form. Choline assists the liver to convert fats and promote their even distribution and to control harmful triglycerides. A deficiency can lead to cardiovascular disease, renal failure, hardened arteries, high blood pressure, weak blood capillaries, high cholesterol, infertility, liver disorders and obesity. Choline is made with intestinal bacteria.

FOLATE- *folic acid, vitamin Bc*

9 BLOOD SYSTEM Folate is essential for the development of red blood cells in combination with cobalt, iron, manganese, vitamin B12 and C. Increased folate intake is vital during pregnancy, it is required for reproduction and in the formation of genetic cells such as DNA & RNA which cannot divide properly without folate. It is vital for prevention of blood disorders such as cardiovascular disease, macrocytic anaemia and poor circulation. Folate is vital for prevention of high blood levels of homocysteine which are produced during cell production. A folate deficiency may also contribute to childhood leukaemia. Fresh spinach is full of folate.

19 BRAIN SYSTEM Folate reduces the blood levels of harmful homocysteine and protects against such conditions as dementia and Alzheimer's disease. One report showed a fourfold increase in these ailments when folate levels were low and homocysteine levels were high. Folic acid is destroyed by high temperatures, cooking and lengthy storage, plus antibiotics, alcohol, the pill and excess acids also reduce folate levels. Increased folate intake is required during periods of infection, mental fatigue, depression, insomnia and irritability. Folate is vital for the correct transfer of nerve messages, termed neurotransmitter and for the process of cellular growth and reproduction.

10 CELLULAR SYSTEM Folate is vital for the production of new cells and numerous conditions related to a deficiency include the skin, such as vitiligo, gingivitis and cleft palate. Various forms of cancer are related to a folate deficiency such as lung, cervix, intestinal and oesophagus cancer. Foods such as sunflower seeds, asparagus and wheat germ are a very good source of folate, a name derived from the Latin word for foliage or leaf. All leafy green vegetables supply fair amounts of folate.

12 GROWTH SYSTEM Folate is vital for children's growth and infants require more folate than adults. Protein is required for proper folate absorption. Most breakfast cereals have added folate plus yeast extract spreads are a concentrated source.

INOSITOL - myoInositol

1 CIRCULATORY SYSTEM Inositol is a water soluble B complex vitamin and required for the health of arteries, as it increases their elasticity thereby protecting against hardened arteries. Such foods as mandarins and oranges supply Inositol and the other vital nutrient for the arteries, vitamin P. Inositol is also important for the metabolism of fats and cholesterol and may help reduce blood cholesterol levels. Similar to choline, Inositol assist the movement of fats from the liver and muscles and it is a component of the cell membrane and required for the transfer of hormones and nerve impulses within cells.

6 NERVOUS SYSTEM Inositol is often considered as a non essential vitamin because it can be made by the body from intestinal bacteria and glucose. For people who regularly consume caffeine drinks including tea, chocolate, cola drinks and coffee, it really is an essential vitamin as caffeine destroys Inositol. A deficiency of inositol can lead to a deteriorating nervous system including conditions of anxiety, insomnia and nervousness. Inositol is required within fat cells to assist in nerve transmission and the proper formation of cell membranes.

10 CELLULAR SYSTEM Inositol is an essential component in the proper formation and construction of new cells. Within the brain, intestines, eyes and bone marrow, Inositol is vital for the health of individual cell membranes, it regulates the contents of cells and promotes their function. Inositol is also necessary for hair growth and a prolonged deficiency may be a key factor contributing to baldness. Diabetics have an increased excretion of inositol and it may protect against the development of peripheral neuropathy.

16 REPRODUCTIVE SYSTEM Inositol is essential for reproduction and a prolonged deficiency, possibly caused by excess caffeine intake or antibiotics may cause infertility in either male or female. Inositol is also required for the proper control of oestrogen levels and it may provide protection against the development of breast lumps. Inositol is required for proper uterine contractions and hormone-cell transfer.

P.A.B.A. para-aminobenzoic acid

17 SKIN SYSTEM P.A.B.A. is a component of folic acid, it is a vitamin within a vitamin and can be made by intestinal bacteria in the intestines and is therefore not considered as an essential vitamin, however, such factors as the intake of antibiotics and sulpha drugs can destroy the natural bacteria that are required to produce P.A.B.A. and other B complex vitamins. Various skin and hair conditions may be due to a prolonged deficiency of P.A.B.A., as it protects natural hair and skin colour, prevents premature greying of the hair, ageing and wrinkling of the skin. A general B complex deficiency also contributes to these factors. In the skin pigmentation disorder known as vitiligo, P.A.B.A. has been used successfully in treatment under supervision, however other factors such as lack of vitamin C, B5 and a deficient supply of hydrochloric acid within the stomach, may all contribute to the condition. P.A.B.A. is world famous now for it's role as a sun block. It protects against sunburn and as a cream, may be used to treat conditions of sunburn. P.A.B.A. protects the skin from ultraviolet radiation and promotes the repair of skin blotches caused by excess sunlight or ultraviolet lamps. Excess use of sunscreens may reduce the production of vitamin D within the skin surface. Ideally, moderate sunlight is obtained regularly but in summer, caution to exposure between the hours of 11am to 3 pm.

P.A.B.A. can be stored in tissues and when the body has no further stores, due to the excess use of antibiotics or sulpha drugs, conditions such as fatigue, irritability, nervousness and depression may develop.

6 NERVOUS SYSTEM

P.A.B.A. is required for the metabolism of individual amino acids and it helps promote the use of protein. It has been used under supervision to assist infertile women to become pregnant, after a 3 to seven month intake.

OTHER FACTORS

Excess intake of P.A.B.A. may cause liver damage. P.A.B.A. promotes the effects of cortisone and may prevent the development of abnormal fibrous tissues and connective tissue disorders and eczema.

VITAMIN A - *retinol - carotene*

Nutrients for effective Absorption:

Calcium. Phosphorus and Zinc Vitamins C. E. F. B group.

Nutrient Inhibiting Factors:

strenuous exercise. stress and alcohol, antibiotics, low fat intake.

Dandelion greens, carrot juice, carrots, apricots (dr.), Kale, Collard, Sweet potato, Parsley, Spinach, Turnip greens, Chives, Watercress, Mango, Peach (dr.), Cantaloupe, Endive, Apricot, Broccoli, Lettuce, Papaya, Prune, Pumpkin,

VITAMIN C - *ascorbic acid*

Nutrients for effective Absorption:

Calcium and Magnesium. Vitamins: P and A

Nutrient Inhibiting Factors:

Heat. Oxidation. Smoking, Pollution. Aspirin and Alcohol

Acerola Cherry, Guava, Red Capsicum, Chillies, Blackcurrants, Kale Leaves, Parsley, Collard Leaves, Kale, Oranges, Turnip Greens, Dock, Green Capsicum, Broccoli, Lemon, Brussell Sprouts, Mustard Greens, Watercress, Strawberry, Spinach.

VITAMIN D - *lumisterol calciferol*

Nutrients for effective Absorption:

Calcium and Phosphorus Vitamins: A, C, F, B group.

Sunshine
Outdoor living
Cod liver oil, salmon, halibut, sardines, eggs, butter, margarine.

VITAMIN K - *menadione*

Nutrients for effective Absorption:
Vitamin C
Nutrient Inhibiting Factors:
freezing, heat, x-rays, warfarin, radiation, pollution,

Spinach, Lettuce, Peas, Parsley, Watercress, Celery, Broccoli, Oats, Wheat germ, Berries, Asparagus, Cabbage, Vegetables, Legumes, Sprouts, Cucumber.

VITAMIN E - *d alpha tocopherol*

Nutrients for effective Absorption:

Manganese and Sulphur Vitamins: C & B group

Nutrient Inhibiting Factors:

Processing, freezing, cooking, laxatives.

Wheat germ oil, Sunflower seeds, Almond Oil, Almonds, Hazel nuts, Wheatgerm Sunflower oil, Safflower oil, Soy oil, Wheat sprouts, Nuts, Corn oil, Walnuts, Canola oil, Olive oil, Sesame oil, Tahini,

VITAMIN F - *essential fatty acids*

Omega 3	Omega 6
Walnuts, Pepitas, Canola oil, Linseed, Flaxseed, Sunflower oil, Pecan nuts, Soy oil, Sunflower seeds, Salmon, Sardines, Tuna, Herring, Mackerel, Trevally, Trout, Mullet, Prawns, Anchovies, Egg yolk, Fish, Seafood.	Canola oil, Walnuts, Pecan nuts, Hazel Nuts, Almonds, Olive oil, Tahini, Sunflower oil, Peanuts, Soy Oil, Sunflower seeds, Pepitas, Brazil nuts, Macadamia nuts, Cashews, Soy beans, Poultry, Meat, Margarine, Dairy foods.

VITAMIN P - *flavonoids*

Nutrients for effective Absorption:
Vitamin C.
Nutrient Inhibiting Factors:
Processing, heat, cooking, oxygen, light.

Citrus pith and peel, Capsicum pith, Buckwheat, Berries, Blackcurrants, Cherries, Blueberries, Apricots, Grapes, Mulberries.

VITAMIN T

Tahini, Sesame seeds, Egg yolks.

COENZYME Q

Soy oil, Fish, Peanuts, Beef, Organ meats, Spinach, Broccoli.

VITAMIN U

Cabbage, Coleslaw, Sauerkraut.

P.A.B.A.

Citrus fruits, Oats, Wheat germ.

VITAMIN FOOD SOURCE CHARTS

VITAMIN B1 - *thiamine*

Nutrients for effective Absorption: Vitamin C and B complex, Sulphur.
Nutrient Inhibiting Factors: Alcohol, tobacco, stress, refined foods and drinks, processing, cooking, antibiotics, tannin, caffeine, antacids.

Rice bran, Oat bran, Yeast Extracts Wheat Germ, Tahini, Peanuts, Brazil nuts, Sunflower seeds, Cashews, Pistachio, Rye, Legumes, Malt, Pine nuts, Macadamia, Walnuts, Chestnuts, Wholemeal bread, Breakfast cereals.

VITAMIN B2 - *riboflavin*

Nutrients for effective Absorption: Vitamin C and B group.
Nutrient Inhibiting Factors: Alcohol, light, tobacco, drugs, stress, processing, the pill, antidepressants.

Almonds, Wheatgerm, Yeast extracts, Millet, Bran, Parsley, Cashews, Liver, Soy flour, Cheese, Avocado, Legumes and sprouts, Peach, Apricots, Nuts, Dates, Eggs, Oats,

VITAMIN B3 - *niacin*

Nutrients for effective Absorption: Vitamin C and B group
Nutrient Inhibiting Factors: Alcohol, stress, tobacco, processing.

Rice bran, Peanuts, Wheat bran, Wild rice, Yeast extracts, Nuts, Sunflower seeds, Fish, Legumes, Pepitas, Tahini, Tuna, Salmon, Mushrooms, Dates, Wheatgerm, Millet.

VITAMIN B5 - *pantothenic acid*

Nutrients for effective Absorption: B complex.
Nutrient Inhibiting Factors: Processing, cooking, caffeine, drugs, alcohol.

Sunflower seeds, Yeast extracts, Almonds, Wheat bran, Peanuts, Wheat germ, Liver, Mushrooms, Eggs, Nuts, Cashews, Pepitas.

VITAMIN B15

Apricot kernels, Oats, Pepitas, Dried yeast, Rice bran, Tahini, Rye, Wheat germ, Grains.

INOSITOL

Oranges, Grapefruit, Lecithin, Peanuts, Whole grains, Pecan, Melons, Onions, Peas.

VITAMIN B6 - *pyridoxine*

Nutrients for effective Absorption: B complex, especially B1, B2 & B5.
Nutrient Inhibiting Factors: Alcohol, smoking, light, oxidation, processing.

Walnuts, Wheat bran, Yeast extracts, Oats, Rice bran, Dried yeast, Wheat germ, Pepitas, Sunflower seeds, Soy, Salmon, Tuna, Liver, Mackerel, Soy, Pecan, Bananas, Peas, Dates, Hazel nuts, Peanuts.

VITAMIN B12 - *cobalamin*

Nutrients for effective Absorption: Cobalt, Folate, Iron.
Nutrient Inhibiting Factors: Antacids, air, alcohol, laxatives, light, oral contraceptives,.

Seafood, Clams, Fish, Liver, Egg yolk, Kidney, Yoghurt, Cheese, Milk, Meat, Tuna, Skim milk, Oysters, Salmon. Refer to page 171 for more information.

BIOTIN - co-enzyme R - *vitamin H.*

Nutrients for effective Absorption: B complex.
Nutrient Inhibiting Factors: Food processing, Avidin - egg white.

Walnuts, Almonds, Peanuts, Dried yeast, Sunflower seeds, Oats, Pecan nuts, Tahini, Liver, Oysters, Sardines, Mushrooms, Soy, Wheat, Yoghurt.

CHOLINE - *thiamine*

Nutrients for effective Absorption: B complex, Inositol
Nutrient Inhibiting Factors: Alcohol, processing.

Lecithin, Corn, Soy, Barley, Cabbage, Cauliflower, Eggs, Dried yeast, Tahini, Spinach, Wheat germ, Legumes, Potatoes.

FOLATE - *folic acid- vitamin Bc*

Nutrients for effective Absorption: Vitamin C, B complex: B12 & B6.
Nutrient Inhibiting Factors: Heat, light, air, Antibiotics, alcohol, Oral contraceptives.

Dried yeast - extracts, Sunflower seeds, Mint, Corn, Wheat germ, Asparagus, Parsley, Spinach, Almonds, Cashews, Hazel nuts, Green vegetables, Legumes, Oat bran.

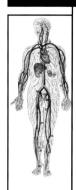

This chapter on the human Body Systems includes;

MAIN BODY SYSTEMS

1 - Circulatory
2 - Digestive
3 - Glandular
4 - Lymphatic
5 - Muscular
6 - Nervous
7 - Respiratory
8 - Skeletal

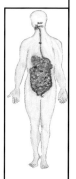

SUB SYSTEMS

9 - Blood
10 - Cellular
11 - Elimination
12 - Growth
13 - Immune
14 - Joint
15 - Optic
16 - Reproductive
17 - Skin
18 - Urinary
19 - Repair

Within each section, a basic guide to the main function of the system is provided plus the vital nutrients required and their natural food source.

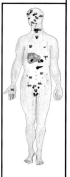

It will be clear from this information that numerous minerals and vitamins are required by each body system.

The human body is a very complex structure and only the basic body functions are provided in this chapter.

By appreciating these functions we can be encouraged to help the body obtain the nutrients and foods that support the numerous needs of individual body systems and sub systems.

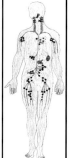

This information is provided as a guide only, it is not to be used for personal diagnosis of any condition. Seek the advice of a qualified medical practitioner or naturopath.

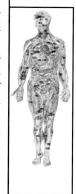

On pages 195 - 198, a list of ailments is provided on the left hand column.

Under the heading of body systems on each page, a coded number will represent the specific system or systems that are affected by each particular illness.

Refer back to the body system's in this section to gain information on the nutrients required and the best food source of those nutrients.

Various factors can lead to the onset of illness, sometimes taking many years to be noticed. On page 194 there is a list of nearly 50 individual risk factors. It is likely that without risk factors, there would be a significant decrease in numerous common ailments.

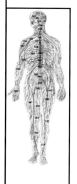

On pages 195 - 198 a list of the risk factors that are common with specific ailments are provided to provide a better understanding of a specific ailment. Some risk factors are hard to overcome as they are part of the daily lifestyle, or they may be passed on via hereditary traits.

Other risk factors are caused by habit forming drugs or substances. Ideally, for any ailment, it is best to eliminate or at least reduce all the risk factors and to increase the intake of foods that may benefit the individual body systems. The human body works hard to keep in a healthy state but when the risk factors continue, eventually illness may develop.

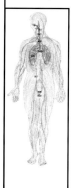

Fortunately there are natural foods that can provide an abundance of specific nutrients, antioxidants and other substances to help overcome some illness.

With this information we can help to avoid illness and to improve our diet. Exercise is also an important factor in the whole equation of health.

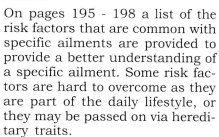

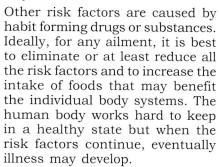

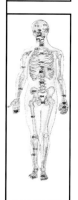

1 - superficial temporal
2 - occipital
3 - maxillary
4 - vertebral
5 - facial
6 - lingual
7 - common carotid
8 - subclavian
9 - arch of aorta
10 - superior vena cava
11 - heart
12 - superior mesenteric
13 - inferior vena cava
14 - liver
15 - renal
16 - kidneys
17 - spleen
18 - radial
19 - ulnar
20 - common iliac
21 - hypogastric
22 - external iliac
23 - femoral
24 - saphenous
25 - popliteal
26 - post. tibial
27 - anterior tibial
28 - saphenous
29 - dorsalis pedis
30 - dorsalis venous
31 - arcuate

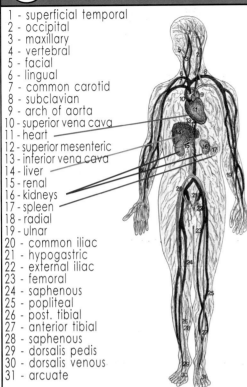

main body function

| HEART |
| LIVER |
| KIDNEYS |
| SPLEEN |
| ARTERIES |
| VEINS |

The heart pumps blood at 72 beats per minute - adult, 90 beats minute - children - 110 beats / min. infants.

The heart pumps approx. 7,500 litres per 24 hours.

The heart pumps blood throughout the entire body and it takes only 10 seconds for a complete cycle.

The liver removes toxins from the bloodstream at a rate of at least one and a half litres every minute.

The kidneys are a pair of filters with remarkable ability to regulate the amount of blood salt and acid levels. The kidneys filter blood at the rate of 1.3 litres per minute with millions of tiny tubes termed nephrons. The spleen destroys old red blood cells and blood platelets and provide lymphocytes for new blood.

The blood leaves the heart via the pulmonary artery and enters the lungs where oxygen is added. The combined network of arteries and veins within the circulatory system measure approx. 96,000 kilometres. Veins carry oxygenated blood throughout the body.

vital nutrients

Calcium regulates and assists the smooth functioning of the heartbeat. Magnesium and calcium nourish the circulatory system.

Phosphorus is essential for proper blood circulation, regulation of blood pressure levels and heart muscle contractions.

Potassium is essential for the heart muscles, proper blood circulation, heart muscle contractions and a regular heartbeat.

Iron is required to carry oxygen.

Magnesium assists nerve impulses for the heart.

Silicon assists blood circulation

Iodine protects against heart palpitations.

Sodium maintains blood pressure.

Vanadium regulates blood circulation.

Vitamin E promotes the ability of red blood cells to carry oxygen, it assists the heart muscles to use oxygen more efficiently and protects against blood clots.

Vitamin C and P promote strong blood capillaries.

Vitamin B15 protects against hardened arteries.

beneficial natural foods

tahini, cheese, *almonds*, hazel nuts, *sunflower seeds*, dried apricots, walnuts, spinach.	
pepitas, sunflower seeds, *tahini*, brazil nuts, cashew nuts, walnuts, *almonds, lecithin.*	
dried apricots, dried fruits, fresh wheat germ, legumes, *almonds*, sunflower seeds.	
pepitas, *tahini*, parsley.	
brazil, *tahini, almonds*, cashew.	
lettuce, spinach, strawberry.	
kelp, watermelon, capsicum.	
celery, olives, spinach, cheese.	
fresh fish, tuna, kelp, seafood	
sunflower seeds, tahini, almonds, hazel nuts, fresh wheat germ, peanut, apples, *lettuce, walnuts*, brazil nuts.	
guava, capsicum, citrus fruits.	
pepitas, *tahini*, oats, wheatgerm.	

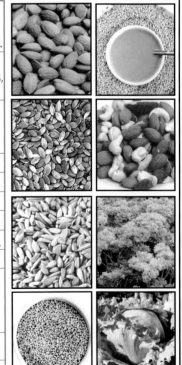

32 - parotid gland
33 - submandibular
34 - sublingual gland
35 - mouth / tounge
36 - oesophagus
37 - stomach
38 - pylorus
39 - duodenum
40 - gall bladder
41 - pancreas
42 - liver
43 - jejunum
44 - ileum
45 - small intestine
46 - colon
47 - caecum
48 - appendix
49- sigmoid
50 - anus

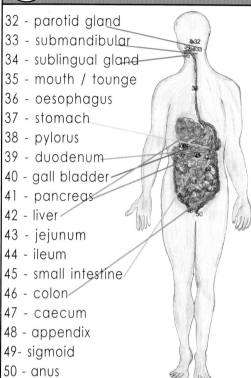

main body function

SALIVARY GLANDS The three pairs of salivary glands produce the enzyme ptyalin, required for the initial conversion of cooked starch, into the form of maltose.

STOMACH The stomach produces an enzyme: pepsin from a combination of the enzyme pepsinogen and hydrochloric acid, for the initial conversion of protein foods.

PANCREAS The pancreas produces an enzyme: trypsin, for the conversion of protein (proteoses and peptones) into peptides assisted by the gall bladder which produces bile. This takes place within the duodenum and also the conversion of fats and oils (lipids) are converted by the enzyme lipase (pancreas) plus bile into fatty acids and glycerol.

GALL BLADDER

DUODENUM

SMALL INTESTINE In the small intestine, the enzyme amylase converts uncooked starch into maltose, plus, the maltase converts maltose into glucose. Also within the small intestine, the jejunum, converts peptides into amino acids, they pass into bloodstream and go to the liver. The colon collects all the unused food materials and disposes of the waste via the rectum.

LIVER

COLON

vital nutrients

Calcium is essential for the involuntary muscular movements of the digestive system, termed peristaltic action.
Phosphorus is required for the movement of fatty acids and phospholipids and distribution of fats.
Sodium: stimulates the production of carbohydrate digestive enzymes such as saliva.
Sulphur: keeps the digestive system clean, for pancreatic enzymes, insulin and protein digestion.
Chlorine is essential for the production of the protein enzyme pepsin, in the stomach.
Magnesium: ingredient of enzymes for protein and carbohydrate digestion and glucose conversion.
Manganese: production of bile, insulin and essential for metabolism.
Copper: protein metabolism, enzyme component.
Iodine: thyroid gland, digestion, body metabolism.
Zinc: component of insulin and many enzymes.
Chromium: glucose conversion, insulin activity.
Vitamin D: essential for digestion and metabolism.
Vitamins: B complex, vitamins A and K.

beneficial natural foods

tahini, acidophillus yoghurt, almonds, hazel nuts, sunflower seeds, dried apricots, walnuts,

pepitas, sunflower seeds, *tahini*, brazil nuts, cashew nuts, *garlic*.

celery, olives, spinach, cheese, eggs, beetroot, carrots. *pears*.

brazil nuts, scallops, crustacea, *garlic*, onions, spinach.

tomato, *celery*, lettuce, cabbage, *papaya*, radish.

brazil nuts, *tahini*, pepitas, almonds, cashews, *bananas*.

fresh wheat germ, hazel nuts, nuts, oats, *garlic*, seeds, *apples*.

tahini, sunflower seeds, cashew.

fish, seafood, kelp, spinach.

wheat germ, sunflower seeds.

eggs, whole grains, cheese.

regular moderate sunlight.

refer nutrient charts.

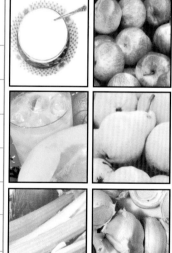
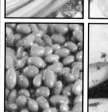

51 - pineal
52 - pituitary
53 - lacrimal
54 - ceremonius
55 - ebner
56 - thyroid
57 - parathyroid
58 - thymus
59 - mammary
60 - adrenal
61 - fundus
62 - mucous
63 - ovaries
64 - prostrate
65 - testes
66 - sweat
67 - sebacious
68 - epithelium
69 - digestive

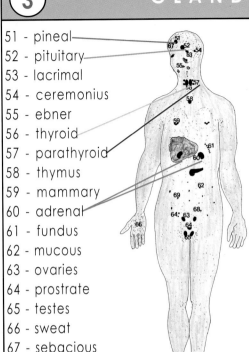

main body function

| PINEAL GLAND |
| PITUITARY GLAND |
| THYROID GLAND |
| PARA-THYROID GLANDS |
| ADRENAL GLANDS |

51- pineal: coordinates sensory consciousness
52- the pituitary gland controls: metabolism, lactation, sex hormones, para and thyroid and the pancreas.
53- produces moisture for the eyes and tears.
54- produces wax to protect the ears.
55- produces water solution for the tongue.
56- thyroid: produces the hormone thyroxine which control growth, mental development, nervous activity and general metabolism.
57- parathyroid control calcium metabolism.
58- early children's development/ reproductive organs
59- produces colostrum during lactation.
60- adrenal glands secretes adrenaline for digestion, stress control, glucose production and heart rate.
61- produces hydrochloric acid/stomach.
62- assists excretion of toxins from digestion.
63- oestrogen hormone for fertilization/menstruation.
64- prostatic fluid for production of semen.
65- produces the male hormone testosterone.
66- produces the fluids: appocrine and eccrine for sweating.
67- produce sebum for healthy skin and hair.
68- produces enzymes to assist digestion.
69- absorbs nutrients, water and enzymes.

vital nutrients

Calcium blood levels and storage of calcium are regulated by the parathyroid glands, dependant on supply of vitamin D.

Sulphur is vital for the function of the pancreas gland, for insulin production and the fat digestive enzymes: lipase and trypsin.

Chlorine is required by the reproductive organs plus it is an essential mineral for cleansing.

Manganese is required by the mammary glands for lactation, by the thyroid gland with iodine for production of the hormone thyroxine. It is required for manufacture of insulin with the mineral zinc.

Iodine is essential for the thyroid gland to produce the hormone thyroxine required for metabolism, growth, nerves, skin, hair and energy levels.

Bromine levels are controlled by the pituitary gland. This trace mineral is required for stable emotions especially during menopause and the 'mid life crisis'.

Vitamin C protects against glandular infections.

Vitamin D activates the glandular system.

Vitamin E and B complex are vital for all the body's glands.

beneficial natural foods

tahini, cheese, almonds, hazel nuts, sunflower seeds, dried apricots, walnuts, spinach.

carrot juice, carrots, spinach, garlic, onions, cucumber, lettuce, celery, tomato, figs.

tomato, celery, lettuce, cabbage, mango, carrots, peach.

hazel nuts, pecan nuts, walnuts, pine nuts, pepitas, *beetroot, pineapple,* grapes, parsley, *lettuce, tahini, garlic,* legumes.

fish, seafood, kelp, spinach, ionized salt, *watermelon, cucumber,* spinach, berries.

watermelon, rockmelon, honeydew melon, *cucumber,* celery, asparagus, *tomato, lettuce,* carrots, garlic, peach.

berries, *tomato, peach, orange.*

regular moderate sunlight.

tahini, almonds,

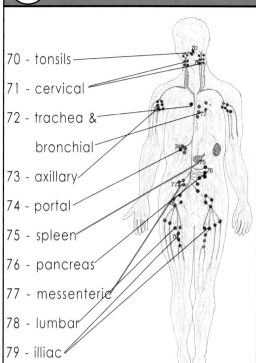

70 - tonsils

71 - cervical

72 - trachea & bronchial

73 - axillary

74 - portal

75 - spleen

76 - pancreas

77 - messenteric

78 - lumbar

79 - illiac

main body function

SPLEEN

The Lymphatic system is best described as the body's processing, protection and filtration system, as the lymphatic glands process fats, expel worn out blood corpuscles and protect against bacterial invasion. The spleen is the largest organ of the body's lymphatic system, it is termed not 'essential' to life, however it functions to eliminate old red blood corpuscles and blood platelets. It stores iron from the worn out cells and produces bilirubin required as part of bile, to breakdown fats. The spleen also participates in producing antibodies and to fight infections, it also produces some of the blood lymphocytes.

MESSENTERIC

The lymphatic glands of the small intestine are termed mesenteric glands, they are vital for absorption of fats from the diet which are then conveyed by the lymphatic system (the secondary circulatory system) via the thyroic duct to the liver which removes the hydrogen from fats and then returns the 'unsaturated fats' to the fat stores of the body. When the lymph glands become clogged, illness results.

vital nutrients

Chlorine is involved in regulating the blood acid - alkaline levels, it also stimulates the functions of the liver and is vital for cleansing the blood and reduction of fatty deposits.

Iron is required to eliminate toxic waste from the bloodstream, thereby protecting the lymphatic system from impurities and inflammation.

Sulphur provides a cleansing and antiseptic effect on the digestive system and the lymphatic glands of the small intestines (mesenteric glands)

Phosphorus is found in every cell and is required for the transfer of nutrients through cell walls. Lecithin is a phosphorus compound and used for the conversion and movement of fats throughout the lymphatic system.

Vitamin E reduces oxidation of fats thereby it protects the lymphatic system from toxins.

Vitamin F, in particular linoleic acid is required for cholesterol control and protection from high blood pressure.

Biotin and B complex required for fat metabolism.

Choline is vital for the control of cholesterol and fats.

beneficial natural foods

tomato, celery, lettuce, cabbage, watercress, cucumber, *carrots*, berries, beetroot, mango, *pineapple*, lime, guava, dates.

pepitas, wheatgerm, kelp, parsley, tahini, *wheatgrass*, *sunflower seeds, almonds*.

carrots, figs, dates, garlic, onions, cabbage, *pineapple*, celery, *tomato, wheatgrass*.

bran, pepitas, wheat germ, *sunflower seeds*, brazil nuts, tahini, almonds, peanut, *walnut*, lecithin granules, oats, hazel nuts, sprouts, parsley, *garlic*.

wheat germ oil, tahini, *almonds*, hazel nuts, wheat germ, *seeds*.

sunflower seeds, almonds, avocado, strawberry, nuts, tahini, peanut, fish, *walnuts*.

walnuts, *almonds*, seeds, rice.

lecithin, green vegetables, seeds, tahini, corn, soya grits.

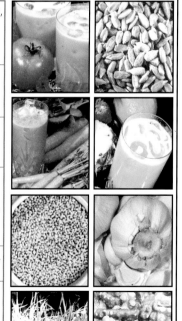

80 - frontalis
81 - temporal
82 - occipitalis
83 - facial
84 - orbicularis oculi
85 - buccinator
86 - masseter
87 - digastic
88 - levator
89 - scalene
90 - omo-hyoid
91 - sterno-mastoid
92 - trapezius
93 - deltoid
94 - pectoral major
95 - biceps
96 - brachialis
97 - pronator
98 - brachioradilis
99 - flexor carpri radialis
100 - flexor carpri ulnaris
101 - sublimis
102 - thenar
103 - hyponar
104 - acromion process
105 - pectoralis minor
106 - serratus anterior
107 - lattissimus dorsi
108 - serratus anterior
109 - linear alba
110 - external oblique
111 - gluteus medius
112 - gluteus maximus
113 - rectus femoris
114 - vastus externus
115 - vastus internus
116 - tibialis anterior
117 - soleaus
118 - peroneus longus
119 - transversus
120 - internal intercostal

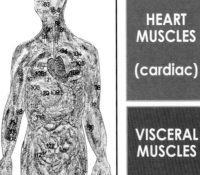

HEART MUSCLES (cardiac)

VISCERAL MUSCLES (stomach)

SKELETAL MUSCLES (legs, arm spine)

main body function

The muscular system covers most parts of the body and approx. 40% of body mass is muscle. Muscles are made from millions of fibres and covered by tissues termed fascia. Muscles are connected to the skeletal system by tendons. Nearly all muscles have an opposite: to lift and to lower. There are about 650 muscles in the adult human body.

The three main types of muscles are: heart muscles - cardiac muscles visceral muscles - stomach and bloodstream, skeletal muscles - legs, arm and spine.

A muscle is described as an organ which produces motion by the action of the nervous system and contraction of muscle fibres.

The two main types of muscle fibres are striated and smooth fibres.

Large voluntary muscles are composed of approx. 80% water and 20% protein. Muscles require heat to perform and approx. 75% of energy used by muscles is for heat production, 25% for muscle action.

vital nutrients

Potassium is the 'muscle mineral', it is required for stimulating nerves connected to the muscles. It is vital for repair and the conditioning of muscles.

Calcium for regulating the heartbeat, muscular growth and contraction.

Iron is the foundation mineral of myoglobin, it supplies oxygen to the muscle cells and activates muscular contractions.

Magnesium provides the connection between muscles and nerve stimuli. It helps protect against cramps and assists muscular contractions.

Manganese is required for muscular strength and muscular coordination as it stimulates proper transfer of nerve impulses to the muscular tissues.

Copper is required for elastin, muscle stretching.

Selenium preserves muscular elasticity.

Sodium is required for muscular enlargement.

Vitamin E is the muscle vitamin, it promotes oxygen supply and endurance to muscles and it promotes blood circulation.

Vitamin A and B complex are all vital for the muscular system.

beneficial natural foods

rice bran, wheat bran, pepitas, *wheat germ, sunflower seeds, almonds, hazel nuts, tahini, brazil nuts, cashews, banana.*

tahini, acidophilus yoghurt, almonds, nuts, sunflower seeds.

pepitas, *almonds, parsley, tahini, sunflower seeds, kelp, rice bran, wheat germ, tofu.*

brazil nuts, *tahini, pepitas, almonds, sunflower seeds, wheat germ, bananas,*

fresh wheat germ, hazel nuts, oats, garlic, peanuts, tahini, sunflower seeds, coconut.

tahini, cashews, sunflower seeds.

brazil nuts, *wheat germ, tuna*

celery, olives, spinach, cheese.

wheatgerm oil, *tahini, almonds, sunflower seeds, hazel nuts, wheat germ,* peanuts, pecans.

refer to nutrient charts.

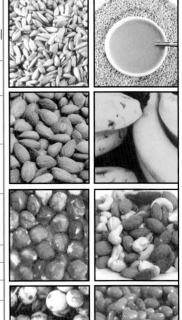

128 - frontal
129 - parietal
130 - occipital
131 - temporal
132 - cerebellum
133 - temporal lobe
134 - mid brain
135 - medulla
136 - cervical
137 - pheneric
138 - radial
139 - ulnar
140 - thoracic
141 - lumbar
142 - sacral
143 - femoral
144 - coccygeal
145 - filum
146 - sciatic
147 - gluteal
148 - sciatic
149 - femoral
150 - obturator
151 - saphenous
152 - lateral
153 - anterior tibial
154 - sural
155 - brachial
156 - circumflex
157 - radial
158 - ulnar
159 - median
160 - ulnar

CENTRAL NERVOUS SYSTEM

PERIPHERAL NERVOUS SYSTEM

SYMPATHETIC NERVOUS SYSTEM

SPINAL COLLUMN

BRAIN

main body function

There are three main parts to the nervous system: the central nervous system: (spinal cord and brain), the peripheral nervous system: (organs and muscles) and the sympathetic nervous system: (brain and nerves). The nervous system works constantly to coordinate every movement: conscious and subconscious. During sleep the nervous system relaxes thereby allowing nerve endings to repair, to receive nutrition and to be ready for when we wake to provide the many actions and reactions from physical, subconscious and emotional involvement including the functions of the brain: memory, thought, speech, vision and sight interpretation and sense awareness such as : pain, excitement and pleasure. There are 31 pairs of spinal nerves each connecting to various different parts of the body. Nerve cells are called neurons and they transmit messages. The brain is the master controller of nearly all nervous system interactions and the speed of message transfer varies from over 200 kilometres per hour to less than 4 kilometres per hour.

vital nutrients

Magnesium is the 'nerve mineral', it regulates the white nerve fibres and the central nervous system. It protects against nervous exhaustion.

Phosphorus is vital for conditioning the responses of the nervous system and protects against nervous stress. The grey matter of the brain is composed of phosphorus compounds termed lecithin and phospholipids.

Manganese nourishes the nerves, maintains nerve impulses and coordinates nerve transmission.

Silicon insulates nerve fibres, protects from stress.

Potassium assists to coordinate nerves and muscles and impulses and stimulation to the brain.

Vitamin C protects against nervous stress.

Vitamin D maintains a healthy nervous system

Vitamin B1 promotes memory and concentration.

Vitamin B2 protects against nervous stress.

Vitamin B3 nourishes the nervous system.

Vitamin B5 promotes strong nerves.

Vitamin B6, B12 and *Choline* protect the nerves.

beneficial natural foods

sunflower seeds, brazil nuts, *tahini, almonds, pepitas,* cashew, pine nuts, carob, *peanuts,* hazel nuts, oats.

pepitas, sunflower seeds, tahini, brazil nuts, cashews, *almonds, sunflower seeds, walnuts,* cheese, wheat germ, bran, soy milk, *peanuts,* soy grits, yeast.

wheat germ / bran, *walnuts,* pine nuts, pecan nuts, *pepitas.*

lettuce, oats, strawberry.

raisins, wheat germ, sultanas, *almonds, walnuts,* dates, garlic.

capsicum, citrus, berries, fruit.

moderate regular sunlight.

yeast extracts. *seeds, tahini.*

yeast extracts, *almonds,* seeds.

yeast extracts, *nuts,* seeds.

yeast extracts, *almonds,* nuts,

yeast extracts, *walnuts,* tuna, cheese, *seeds,* avocado, fish.

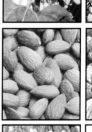

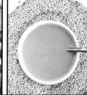

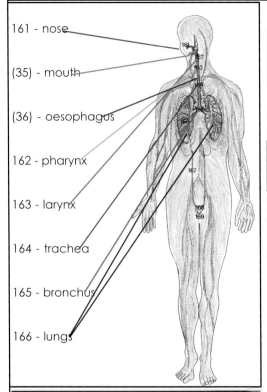

161 - nose

(35) - mouth

(36) - oesophagus

162 - pharynx

163 - larynx

164 - trachea

165 - bronchus

166 - lungs

NOSE

MOUTH

OESOPHAGUS

PHARYNX (tonsils)

LARYNX

TRACHEA BRONCHI

LUNGS

main body function

The nose contains minute hairs and membranes that are full of blood and allow the inhaled air to warm to body temperature before reaching the lungs.

The mouth is primarily for ingesting food and drinks and for speech, however air can be inhaled but it is less protected from dust, compared to the nose. The oesophagus is a muscular tube, approx. 25 cm. long, lined with mucous membranes extending from the pharynx to the stomach, it is for food intake.

The pharynx is divided into three parts: naso, oral and larylgeal pharynx. The naso pharynx is positioned at the back of the nasal cavity, their function is to protect against bacteria. The larynx is for speech and as an air passage. The trachea is the windpipe, approx 12 cm. length, it separates into two tubes passing into the bronchi which are similar to the structure of the trachea. The lungs absorb oxygen and exhale the carbon dioxide.

vital nutrients

Sulphur is required for cleansing the respiratory system and for tissue respiration in the process of new cell development. Garlic oil contains approx. 80% sulphur content.

Iron is essential for the transfer of oxygen throughout the body, in the form of myoglobin for the transfer of oxygen to muscles.

Potassium combined with the mineral phosphorus are required for the supply of oxygen to the brain which sends impulses to the diaphragm and the muscles surrounding the rib cage, to breathe, inhale and exhale. During 24 hours the lungs inhale/exhale approx. 14,000 litres of air.

Vitamin A is essential for protection of the internal linings of the mouth, throat, nose and lungs from infection, dust and smoke. Mucous is produced to eliminate toxins from the respiratory system.

Vitamin C is essential for tissue respiration and to defend the respiratory system from bacteria.

Vitamin E is required for repair of damaged lung tissues and promotes oxygen within body cells.

B complex vitamins. Refer pages 168 - 173.

beneficial natural foods

garlic, onions, horseradish, radish, *carrot juice*, carrots, raw cabbage, coleslaw, scallops, brazil nuts, crustacea, peanuts, figs, dates, spinach, tomato.

pepitas, almonds, parsley, *tahini*, *sunflower seeds*, kelp, wheat germ, tofu, rice bran.

rice bran, wheat bran, *pepitas*, wheat germ, *sunflower seeds*, *almonds*, hazel nuts, *tahini*, brazil nuts, cashews, peanuts, walnuts, parmesan cheese, raisins, *parsley*, pinenuts, garlic.

carrot juice, carrots, parsley, guava, *mango*, pumpkin, *papaya*, sweet potato, cheese, butter, apricots, cantaloupe.

guava, capsicum, *parsley*, *mango*, currants, *papaya*, citrus.

wheat germ oil, *tahini*, almonds, *sunflower seeds*, wheat germ.

B complex tablet daily.

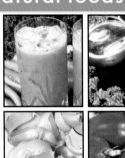
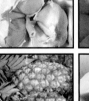

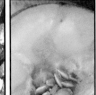

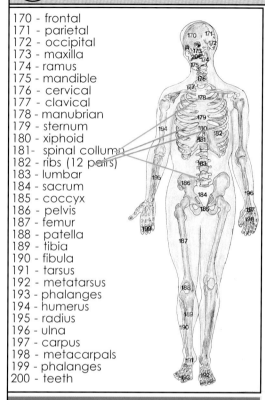

170 - frontal
171 - parietal
172 - occipital
173 - maxilla
174 - ramus
175 - mandible
176 - cervical
177 - clavical
178 - manubrian
179 - sternum
180 - xiphoid
181- spinal collumn
182 - ribs (12 pairs)
183 - lumbar
184 - sacrum
185 - coccyx
186 - pelvis
187 - femur
188 - patella
189 - tibia
190 - fibula
191 - tarsus
192 - metatarsus
193 - phalanges
194 - humerus
195 - radius
196 - ulna
197 - carpus
198 - metacarpals
199 - phalanges
200 - teeth

SPINAL COLUMN

BONES

RIBS

TEETH

main body function

The human skeleton is the frame to the body with a total of approx. 200 bones for adults and 350 bones with infants. The name skeleton comes from the Greek work for 'dried up', however bones contain approx. 30% water. The skull has over 20 different bones.

The inner part of bones is made from a protein: collagen, the outer layer is made mainly from the minerals calcium, phosphorus, silicon, fluorine and magnesium. The spinal column is the central part of the skeletal system, supporting the head and consisting of 33 bones with two main groups: flexible (7 cervical are at the top, 12 dorsal, 5 lumbar) fixed (5 sacral, 4 coccyx).

The ribs are arranged in twelve pairs and the 'true' ribs are the top seven pairs. The ribs protect the vital organs within such as the heart, liver and lungs.

By the age of two the first set of 20 'milk teeth' are formed and progressively from the age of 6 to 25 the permanent 32 teeth are formed. Teeth are made from calcium, phosphorus, magnesium and zinc.

vital nutrients

Calcium is the main bone mineral and the total calcium content of the body is renewed over a 6 year period. About 90% of the calcium within the body is in the skeletal system.

Phosphorus is essential for repair of bone fractures. To function efficiently calcium (2.5) must be balanced with phosphorus (1) and 80% of the body's phosphorus is within the skeletal system.

Magnesium is essential for proper absorption of both calcium and phosphorus and approx. 70% of magnesium is stored within the skeletal system.

Silicon is essential for calcium metabolism, it also provides strength to the bones and protects the bones from uric acid crystals, as it assists their elimination from around bone joints.

Vitamin C is essential in the formation of collagen, the protein substance within every bone. Vitamin C is required daily to assist in the growth and maintenance of bones.

Vitamin D - sunlight is vital for strong bones and bone growth in children. It is essential to ensure an adequate amount of sunlight especially in winter.

beneficial natural foods

tahini, acidophillus yoghurt, almonds, hazel nuts, walnuts, sunflower seeds, dried apricots, *cheese,* milk, chick peas.

pepitas, sunflower seeds, tahini, cheese, cashews, *almonds, walnuts,* wheat bran, oats, rice bran, peanut, wheat germ.

almonds, wheat germ, rice bran, cashews, brazil nuts, *tahini, walnuts, sunflower seeds.*

lettuce, oats, barley, asparagus, rice bran, spinach, parsnips, onions, dates, *strawberries, sunflower seeds,* cucumber.

guava, blackcurrants, *capsicum,* citrus fruits, rockmelon, broccoli, parsley, papaya, *berries,* kiwi fruit, mango, spinach, tomato.

regular direct sunlight in winter, moderate direct sunlight in autumn and spring. In summer, caution with midday direct sun.

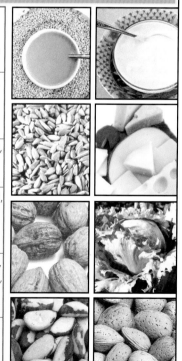

main body function

The blood system is the carrier of all nutrients in the form of : oxygen, glucose, amino acids, minerals, water, vitamins and enzymes. Blood is our lifeline and over a period of 2 months the entire body's blood cells are renewed.

The main functions of blood are:
1- removes waste via the liver and kidneys.
2- transfer chemical messages as hormones.
3- supply antibodies to areas of infection.
4- conveys oxygen to all body tissues and organs.
5- defend the body via the action of white cells. 6- carry all nutrients for body nourishment. 7- maintains physical and mental abilities.

Blood is composed of: 55% Plasma, 45% Cells. Plasma contains 90% water, 10% solids in the form of minerals and protein. Cells contain 95% red cells, 3% platelets and 2% white cells. Blood contains 16 mineral elements and the average person holds 6 litres of precious blood.

beneficial nutrients

Potassium - eliminates blood impurities, reduces high blood pressure, improves blood circulation.
Sodium - keeps minerals soluble within the bloodstream and controls blood pressure.
Sulphur - provides oxygen to the blood, required for development of blood haemoglobin.
Chlorine - purifies the blood and regulates blood pressure.
Fluorine - increases the number of blood cells.
Iron - vital for blood haemoglobin production.
Manganese - formation of red blood cells with iron and copper.
Cobalt - maintains red blood cells.
Other essential nutrients for the blood system: chromium, vanadium, Vitamin C, Vitamin F, Vitamin K, Vitamin P, B complex Vitamins.

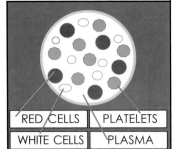

RED CELLS | PLATELETS
WHITE CELLS | PLASMA

natural foods

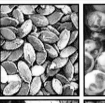
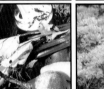

10 CELLULAR SYSTEM

main body function

The diagram on the left shows the six main types of cells. A cell is defined as a small mass of protoplasm containing a nucleus with the following abilities:
1 -assimilation of nourishment
2 - growth and repair
3 - reproduction
4 - excretion of waste
5 - power of movement

Protoplasm consists of the following substances: 1- organic compounds as protein, 2 - fatty substances, 3 - carbohydrates, 4 - inorganic salts and 5 - water.

Within the structure of every living cell there is a code stored in the D.N.A. (deoxyribonucleic acid) molecule with the unique ability to issue instructions for the reproduction of identical new cells via the R.N.A. (ribonucleic acid) at the outer boundary of cells. There is a constant flow of nutrients within each cell and that occurs millions of times a day within the body. All cells require a combination of glucose, minerals, vitamins, oxygen and water.

beneficial nutrients

Sodium - regulating fluids from either side of cell walls.
Sulphur - cell respiration, new cells.
Chlorine - cell membranes.
Fluorine - increases red blood cells.
Iron - nucleus of every cell and transports oxygen to muscle cells.
Magnesium - activates protein and carbohydrates within cells.
Silicon - vital for cell growth with the hair, skin and eyes, promotes red blood cell and bone development.
Cobalt - maintains body cells.
Chromium - movement of glucose-blood sugar into cells.
Vitamin A - skin, digestive, respiratory , bone and urinary cells, also transfer of genetic material.
Vitamin C - vital for skin cells.
Vitamin E - promotes cell life and cell respiration.
Vitamins: F, K & B complex.

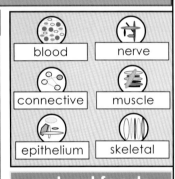

blood | nerve
connective | muscle
epithelium | skeletal

natural foods

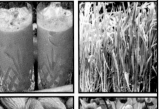

11

ELIMINATION SYSTEM

main body function

There are two main parts to the elimination system: digestive system and excretory fluids elimination.

After the process of digestion within the stomach and small intestine, the remaining food 'chyme' passes into the large intestine, it is approx. 1.5 meters long and has five main parts: the caecum, the transverse colon, descending colon, pelvic colon and the rectum. Digestive elimination requires a fair portion of roughage to function efficiently. Such foods as fruits, vegetables, legumes and whole grains are ideal foods to assist the elimination system.

The excretory fluids system includes the kidneys, skin, liver and lungs. The kidneys remove excess urea (protein) via the urine. The skin removes excess moisture. The liver removes nitrogen, old red blood cells and toxic substances. The lungs expel carbon dioxide and water. Mucus is produced within the body to expel toxins from the respiratory system and from the digestive system. Fasting is beneficial.

beneficial nutrients

Sodium eliminates carbonic acid from the lungs and waste inorganic elements from the body.

Chlorine removes toxins from the liver, blood and respiratory system.

Sulphur eliminates toxins from digestion and the skin and blood.

Iron in combination with copper eliminate waste from the blood.

Silicon cleanses the skin, removes uric acid from the blood.

Potassium assists the colon and the kidneys and skin to remove waste.

Magnesium removes kidney stones.

Manganese removes excess sugar from the blood, via the urine.

Phosphorus assists the kidneys and the elimination of excess acids.

Choline eliminates excess fats.

natural foods

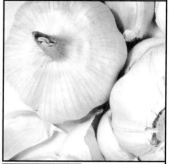
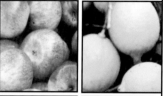

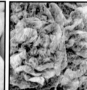

12

GROWTH SYSTEM

main body function

The growth system has numerous main stages;

1. A single cell to 3 months when all cells are formed.
2. In the first year the baby will triple in weight and double in height and brain size. 3. from 2 years - 10 years, the child grows in height, on average 7.5 cm. per year. 4. from 11 years to 20 years the rapid growth stage occurs with approx. 8 cm height increase in boys in the first few years, with girls height increase of approx. 6 cm. per year during adolescence.

The pituitary gland is the most important controller of growth, it produces a hormone - somatotrophin for body growth and other hormones to stimulate the growth of the thyroid gland - thyrotrophic hormone, thereby increasing the body's metabolism rate. The adrenal glands and the sex glands are stimulated by various hormones produced by the pituitary gland. The thymus gland functions from birth till approx. the age of seven, for development of the reproductive and immune system.

beneficial nutrients

Calcium is the main growth mineral however it requires numerous other minerals and vitamins to function efficiently. Calcium is required for growth of bones, skin, teeth, blood and hormone development.

Phosphorus is required in a 2.5 parts calcium to 1 part phosphorus ratio for growth of bones and nerves.

Potassium for muscle growth.

Iodine is essential for the thyroid gland which controls both body and mental growth.

Fluorine assists strong bone growth.

Magnesium assists development of strong bones, teeth and nerves.

Iron for blood haemoglobin growth.

Other essential factors are the daily supply of protein, Vitamin A and sunlight.

natural foods

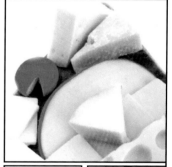
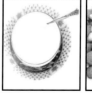

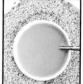

main body function

The immune system is constantly on the alert for any invading germs, bacteria, viruses and infections. The first line of defence are the white cells of the blood, also known as phagocytes which multiply rapidly to destroy the infection, bacteria or virus. The second line of defence comes from the lymphatic system which produces lymphocyte cells and they have a powerful disease fighting ability, they produce antibodies which attempt to prevent bacteria and viruses from reproducing. The phagocytes ingest the captured bacteria and dispose of them. The spleen plays a major role, it produces antibodies, lymphocytes and destroys worn out blood cells. The most common ways for bacteria and viruses to enter the body are through the diet, water and the inhaled air. The lymphatic system consists of a wide ranging network of lymp-nodes in the neck, groin, armpits, digestive system and also within the spleen. The lymph-nodes are like filters, collecting infections which the white cells and antibodies destroy.

beneficial nutrients

Iron strengthens the immune system by replacing worn out blood cells in combination with copper and the mineral manganese.
Potassium assists the kidneys to remove fluid waste and infections.
Calcium increases the body's ability to fight infections.
Chlorine removes toxic waste.
Vitamin A promotes the immune system's ability to fight infections and increases resistance to toxins.
Sulphur prevents infections.
Vitamin C protects against toxins and infections by increasing the supply of white blood cells.
Vitamin P activates vitamin C.
Vitamin D activates all nutrients.
B complex Vitamins (B5 & B6) assist in the production of antibodies.

natural foods

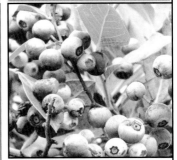
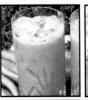

main body function

The joint system performs an incredible variety of movements. The three main types of joints are: 1. fixed joints: skull bones. 2. slightly moveable: pelvis, collar bone. 3. freely moveable: hands, feet, knees, spine, hip, neck, shoulders, wrist, elbows, jaw and ankles.
The most common problem with the joint system is the condition of arthritis, there are two main types of arthritis: osteoarthritis and rheumatoid arthritis. Osteoarthritis causes a loss of cartilage linings around the moving joints, often caused by years of wear and tear, incomplete nutrition, insufficient rest and work under stessful conditions and excess body acidity. Rheumatoid arthritis causes the joints to become inflamed and painful, the exact cause is uncertain but conditions of prolonged emotional stress, anger and resentment may trigger the condition. Excess intake of refined foods may cause inorganic calcium to buildup around joints and replace tissues which results in the deterioration of joint flexibility.

beneficial nutrients

Sodium (celery), not table salt, keeps calcium soluble in the blood, preventing a buildup of calcium. It also reduces acidity in the blood.
Potassium helps to balance the acid-alkaline levels of the blood.
Chlorine maintains healthy joints as it purifies the blood of toxic waste.
Sulphur eliminates body toxins.
Vitamin C is essential for production of collagen and synovial fluid plus it protects against inflammation.
Vitamin E repairs damaged tissues, improves circulation, cell nourishment and body flexibility.
Vitamin F repairs damaged tissues.
Vitamin S repairs damaged tissues and promotes cellular growth.
Salicylic acid in grapefruit reduces the buildup of inorganic calcium.

natural foods

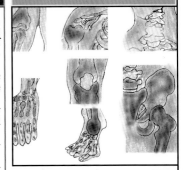
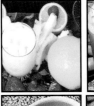

main body function

The Optic system provides the view to the world and the incredible range of colours, shapes and objects.

Light enters the eyes through the cornea - lens which focuses and passes light through the pupil which regulates the amount of light within the iris, the coloured part of eyes.

Muscles within the eye (ciliary muscles) cause the lens to bulge or flatten and transfer light to the retina. Within the retina, millions of light receptors termed cones (colour) and rods (black and white) build an image which is then transferred to the brain for final evaluation, via the optic nerve. The eyes are protected by the eyelid: blinking which keeps the eye moist and clean, eyebrows keep sweat from the eyes and eyelashes keep dust away from the eyes. The optic system can become strained by poor lighting or excess use with computers, television screens and excess ultraviolet sunlight. Protection of the eyes is vital to maintain good vision for many years.

beneficial nutrients

Vitamin A is essential for peripheral (side vision), colour vision and night vision. Protects against eye infections and a prolonged deficiency can lead to blindness.
Fluorine assists the function of the iris and promotes sparkle to eyes.
Silicon repairs damaged tissues.
Zinc is stored within the eyes and a deficiency can lead to poor sight.
Calcium assists to prevent cataracts.
Vitamin C is essential for the lens of the eyes and nourishment of eyes.
Vitamin P assists vitamin C functions.
Vitamin B2 promotes clear vision.
Vitamin B5 nourishes the eyes.
Vitamin B6 protects against eye strain and cataracts.
Choline prevents glaucoma.

natural foods

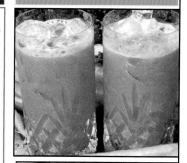
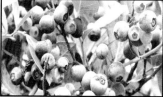

main body function

The reproductive system develops during puberty for boys (12-15) for girls (12-14). From birth till the age of seven, the thymus gland initiates the development of the reproductive organs. At puberty, the pituitary gland produces a hormone (GTH) which stimulates the production of the male (testosterone) hormone and the female (oestrogen) hormone.

The female is born with all the eggs (ova) that are required during the reproductive years. It takes about 46 days for the male sperm to mature and millions are produced everyday.

The combination of the male sperm and female egg create a transformation of life from 23 chromosomes into 46 chromosomes producing a fertilized egg.

Once pregnancy has occurred, it takes approx. 36 weeks for the baby to be born.

The reproductive life for the male can last for 70 to 80 years but for the female, the onset of menopause during the late 40's will be the end to the reproductive cycle.

beneficial nutrients

Chlorine assists in the distribution of the reproductive hormones.
Iron is essential during pregnancy and menstruation.
Manganese is vital for the glands of the reproductive system and for production of milk, sex hormone production and menstrual cycles.
Zinc is essential for the reproductive organs and protects against sterility and prostrate problems.
Chromium assists cell growth.
Selenium enhances vitamin E.
Vitamin E is the life vitamin, it is essential for cell division at conception and protects against sterility, miscarriage and premature birth.
Vitamin A is required for the transfer of heriditary characteristics.

B complex vitamins are vital, refer (169-174).

natural foods

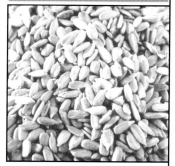
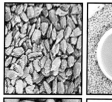

main body function

The skin supports a number of important functions by providing a protective layer to the body which keeps out bacteria, water and sunlight. The skin has sensitivity to heat, cold, pain and pressure thereby providing a warning signal and temperature gauge. The outer layer of skin (epidermis) contains no blood vessels and is in fact dead skin. The next layer under (dermis) is living skin and consists of fibrous and connective tissues, sweat glands, nerve fibres, oil glands (sebaceous) and blood vessels. The sebaceous glands produce sebum which keeps the skin supple and the hair oiled. The body has approx. 3 million sweat glands which balance body temperature via sweating (pores open) cools the body, and, when cold, the sweat glands contract due to the blood vessels and muscles contracting. Vitamin D is the only nutrient that is available without food intake, as the skin surface, via a substance termed (ergosterol) can absorb vitamin D and transform it into a useable form within the body.

beneficial nutrients

Phosphorus is part of every skin cell and it is vital for skin repair.
Sulphur cleanses the skin.
Chlorine rejuvenates the skin.
Fluorine preserves a healthy skin and hair condition.
Silicon eliminates toxins from the dermis layer, repairs damaged skin and removes dead skin.
Copper for skin and hair pigment.
Iron promotes a healthy skin complexion.
Selenium preserves skin elasticity and assists the action of vitamin E.
Vitamin E assists growth and repair of skin.
Vitamin C, P and F help develop collagen.
Vitamin E promotes healthy skin life, essential for healing of skin tissues.
B complex: B2, B3, B5 and P.A.B.A.

natural foods

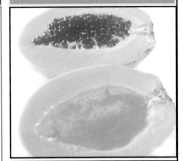

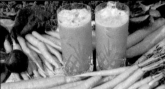

main body function

The urinary system filters and eliminates waste liquids and the kidney's, a pair of highly efficient filters cleanse approx. 1 litre of blood per minute (adults). Blood enters the kidneys via the renal artery which transfers blood via millions of capillaries (glomerulus) under high pressure, into a capsule (Bowman's). Red and white cells, fat and protein molecules and platelets are too large to pass into the 'Bowman's capsule', they bypass and re-enter the bloodstream via the renal vein.
Plasma containing water, amino acids, glucose, salts and urea can pass into the capsule and then through the long system of tubes (tubule), the next filtration stage of the kidneys. Nearly 99% of the water and all the nutrients are re-absorbed into the bloodstream. The remaining substances are mainly water (96%), solids (2%)- chlorides, phosphates, sulphates and oxalates, and urea (2%) - end product of protein digestion. All these substances plus toxins and some drugs are passed from the kidneys via the urine.

beneficial nutrients

Potassium cleanses the kidneys, regulates the body's water balance.

Magnesium maintains minerals in a soluble state, preventing stones.

Sodium also regulates the body's water balance with potassium.

Manganese: formation of urea.

Vitamin A protects against inflammation of the prostrate gland and kidney stones.

B complex, B6 protects against kidney stone formation.

Choline: for healthy kidneys.

Vitamin C protects against inflammation of the urinary system caused by phosphatic crystals as it can dissolve the crystals.

Vitamin E stimulates the elimination of urine and may benefits reduction of oedema.

natural foods

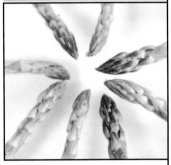

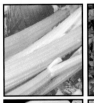

main body function

The brain is the control centre for actions, reactions and sensations. The brain has two main parts: the higher centre which controls memory, will, thoughts and consciousness. The cortex or cerebral hemisphere is the main part of the brain (80%), it consists of grey matter, or 10 million nerve cells, the centre of thoughts, intelligence, memory, speech, hearing, vision and the direction of physical actions.

The lower centre (cerebellum) controls unconscious actions such as balance, posture and movement. The brain stem controls respiration, heart rate, blood vessel size, swallowing, production of saliva and digestive enzymes. Also within the brain are three glands: pituitary - produces growth hormones, sex hormones, milk hormones and as the 'master gland' it controls other glands: thyroid, adrenal, pancreas and sex glands. The pineal gland is the spiritual centre of the brain. The thalamus gland is responsible for feelings of pain. The hypothalamus gland regulates body temperature, blood, water and salt balance.

beneficial nutrients

Phosphorus transfers nerve impulses and is essential for brain function.

Magnesium is required for memory, nourishment and regulating the white nerve fibres of the brain and spinal cord and for steady nerves.

Manganese nourishes the nerves and brain and promotes memory.

Iodine is essential for speech and mental functioning and during pregnancy it promotes mental and physical development of the child.

Bromine protects against mental depression and emotional stress.

Vitamin T promotes a good memory and concentration.

Vitamins B1, B3, B5, B6, B12, B15 and folic acid promote memory, concentration, mental stability, sleep and emotional stability.

natural foods

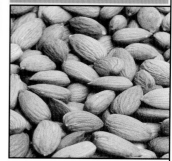
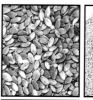

main body function

The repair system is constantly working to rebuild damaged liver cells, cuts, abrasions and the various internal organs. The body is usually able to repair when adequate time is allowed plus suitable treatment depending on the severity of the condition, plus, the supply of essential healing nutrients.

Generally speaking, all the body systems are in a constant state of repair and for some conditions that have developed over many years of hard living and lack of suitable nutrition, the benefit from increased nutrition, rest and proper treatment will provide relief and sometimes completely cure the condition.

For children, healing occurs at a faster rate compared to adults, provided they are given a proper diet. The human body has a genuine interest and ability to repair, even if nobody else cares, your body will relish proper daily repair nutrition. Refer to the ailment charts for help on healing of specific body parts.

Let nature be your true healer.

beneficial nutrients

Calcium assists bone repair in combination with vitamins D, A and C, plus the minerals phosphorus, magnesium, fluorine and zinc.
Iron repairs the blood.
Fluorine strengthens bone repairs.
Zinc is vital for repair of burns or wounds as it combines with white cells to remove injured tissues.
Copper is essential for repair of bones, skin, muscles and nerves.
Vitamin A is essential for repair of damaged skin, tissues and bones.
Vitamin C is vital for repair of wounds, varicose veins, bruises, fractures, acne and all tissues.
Vitamin D is essential for general body repair and bone fractures.
Vitamin E is vital for skin, tissue and general repairs.

natural foods

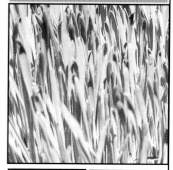

This section on ailments and healing and nutritional needs is designed to provide a wide range of common ailments and the most suitable natural foods, supplements and other factors to assist with either the prevention or healing of specific ailments.

The information is provided as a guide only, it should not be interpreted as a cure for any ailment or condition. Obtain advice and guidance from a qualified medical practitioner, naturopath or therapist for a diagnosis and suitable treatment.

On pages 193 - 194, a list of 312 factors are provided as the *key index* to reference the charts on pages 195 - 198.

The charts provide a list of 92 ailments with the main body systems that are affected, for example; page 195 abscess: number 17 - skin system, number 13 - immune system. Refer to the pages from the skin system (190) and immune system (188) for details on the essential nutrients for maintenance of the body system and other factors such as the foods that supply the required nutrients for the individual body system and the main function of the body system.

Every ailment affects at least one human body system and usually at least 2 - 3 Body systems are in need of repair, correct food intake, specific nutrients and other factors, as presented in the column on the right hand side of each of the following pages with the heading nutritional needs.
Most ailments can benefit from natural foods, supplements and nutrients.
Let nature protect and heal your body.

The main reason for nearly all ailments is due to the health risk factors and within the key index on page 194, a total of 49 risk factors are listed with their name and a colour code for reference with the charts on pages 195 - 198. For example; abscess: *risk factors*: infection, bacteria and hygiene- poor. For effective healing, the risk factors must be eliminated from the diet and lifestyle, or controlled by suitable treatment as listed on the nutritional needs column or from proper medical advice.
The sample code below is a guide to the way the charts on pages 195 - 198 are presented. This chart sample below is on page 195.

ABSCESS	
17	SKIN SYSTEM
13	IMMUNE SYSTEM
I	INFECTION
B	BACTERIA - POOR
H	HYGIENE
41	VITAMIN A
42	VITAMIN C
148	WHEAT GRASS JUICE
227	TEA TREE OIL

AILMENT	BODY SYSTEM'S		RISK FACTORS			NUTRITIONAL NEEDS			
ABSCESS	17	13	I	B	H	41	42	148	227

KEY TO AILMENTS & HEALING CHARTS

BODY SYSTEMS	BS	VITAMINS	VIT	FRUITS	FRU	LEGUMES	LEG
1 - CIRCULATORY	1	41 - A	41	81 - PAPAYA	81	120 - CAROB	120
2 - DIGESTIVE	2	42 - C	42	82 - ORANGES	82	121 - CHICK PEA	121
3 - GLANDULAR	3	43 - D	43	83 - PEACHES	83	122 - GREEN BEAN	122
4 - LYMPHATIC	4	44 - E	44	84 - PEARS	84	123 - KIDNEY BEAN	123
5 - MUSCULAR	5	45 - F	45	85 - PINEAPPLE	85	124 - LENTILS	124
6 - NERVOUS	6	46 - K	46	86 - PLUMS	86	125 - LIMA BEAN	125
7 - RESPIRATORY	7	47 - P	47	87 - TOMATO	87	126 - MUNG BEAN	126
8 - SKELETAL	8	48 - T	48	88 - WATERMELON	88	127 - PEANUTS	127
9 - BLOOD	9	49 - U	49	VEGETABLES	VEG	128 - PEAS	128
10 - CELLULAR	10	B1	50	89 - ARTICHOKE	89	129 - SOY BEAN	129
11 - ELIMINATION	11	B B2	51	90 - ASPARAGUS	90	NUTS	NUT
12 - GROWTH	12	B3	52	91 - BEETROOT	91	130- ALMONDS	130
13 - IMMUNE	13	C B5	53	92 - BROCCOLI	92	131 - BRAZIL NUT	131
14 - JOINT	14	O B6	54	93 - BR. SPROUTS	93	132 - CASHEW NUT	132
15 - OPTIC	15	M B12	55	94 - CABBAGE	94	133 - HAZEL NUT	133
16 - REPRODUCTIVE	16	P B15	56	95 - CARROTS	95	134 - PECAN NUT	134
17 - SKIN	17	L BIOTIN	57	96 - CAPSICUM	96	135 - PISTACHIO	135
18 - URINARY	18	E CHOLINE	58	97 - CAULIFLOWER	97	136 - WALNUT	136
19 - BRAIN	19	X FOLIC ACID	59	98 - CELERY	98	SEEDS	SEED
20 - REPAIR	20	INOSITOL	60	99 - CUCUMBER	99	137 - PEPITAS	137
MINERALS	MN	P.A.B.A.	61	100 - GARLIC	100	138 - SESAME	138
21 - CALCIUM	21	FRUITS	FRU	101 - LEEK	101	139 - SUNFLOWER	139
22 - PHOSPHORUS	22	62 - APPLES	62	102 - ONIONS	102	SPROUTS	SPR
23 - POTASSIUM	23	63 - APRICOTS	63	103 - LETTUCE	103	140 - ALFALFA	140
24 - IRON	24	64 - AVOCADO	64	104 - PARSLEY	104	141 - BEAN SPROUTS	141
25 - CHLORINE	25	65 - BANANA	65	105 - PARSNIPS	105	142 - BUCKWHEAT	142
26 - SODIUM	26	66 - BERRIES	66	106 - POTATOES	106	143 - LENTIL	143
27 - SILICON	27	67 - CHERRIES	67	107 - PUMPKIN	107	144 - MUNG	144
28 - SULPHUR	28	68 - CURRANTS	68	108 - RADISH	108	145 - SESAME	145
29 - MAGNESIUM	29	69 - DATES	69	109 - WATERCRESS	109	146 - SUNFLOWER	146
30 - MANGANESE	30	70 - FIGS	70	110 - SILVERBEET	110	GRASS JUICE	GJ
31 - COPPER	31	71 - GRAPEFRUIT	71	111 - SPINACH	111	147 - BARLEY	147
32 - IODINE	32	72 - GRAPES	72	112 - ZUCCHINI	112	148 - WHEAT	148
33 - ZINC	33	73 - GUAVA	73	GRAINS	GR	DAIRY	DR
34 - COBALT	34	74 - KIWIFRUIT	74	113 - BARLEY	113	149 - BUTTER	149
35 - FLUORINE	35	75 - LEMONS	75	114 - CORN	114	150 - CHEESE HARD	150
36 - SELENIUM	36	76 - LIMES	76	115 - MILLET	115	151 - CHEESE SOFT	151
37 - MOLYBDENUM	37	77 - MANGO	77	116 - OATS	116	152 - CREAM	152
38 - VANADIUM	38	78 - MELONS	78	117 - RICE	117	153 - MILK COWS	153
39 - BROMINE	39	79 - NECTARINE	79	118 - RYE	118	154 - MILK GOATS	154
40 - CHROMIUM	40	80 - OLIVES	80	119 - WHEAT	119	155 - YOGHURT	155

KEY TO AILMENTS & HEALING CHARTS

POULTRY	POU	SUPPLEMENTS		HEALTH BENEFITS		HEALTH RISK FACTORS	
156 - CHICKEN	156	193 - APPLE CIDER VINEGAR	193	234 - BALANCED DIET	234	274 - RADIATION	RA
157 - DUCK	157	194 - ACIDOPHILLUS	194	235 - EXERCISE	235	275 - REFINED FOODS	R
158 - EGGS	158	195 - ASCORBIC ACID	195	236 - FASTING	236	276 - SALT - EXCESS	Q
159 - EGG YOLK	159	196 - B COMPLEX	196	237 - RELAXATION	237	277 - SMOKING	T
160 - TURKEY	160	197 - BREWERS YEAST	197	238 - SLEEP	238	278 - STINGS / BITES	BS
MEAT	MT	198 - COCONUT MEAL	198	239 - SUNSHINE	239	279 - STRESS - PHYSICAL	SB
161 - BACON	161	199 - CORN FLOUR	199	240 - SWIMMING	240	280 - STRESS - NERVOUS	S
162 - BEEF	162	200 - DANDELION COFFEE	200	241 - WATER	241	281 - SUGAR - EXCESS	X
163 - HAM	163	201 - DRIED FRUITS	201	242 - YOGA	242	282 - SUNLIGHT - LACK	S
164 - LAMB	164	202 - ECHINACEA	202	HEALTH RISK FACTORS		283 - TOXINS - AIR	TX
165 - PORK	165	203 - EUCALYPTUS OIL	203	243 - ALCOHOL	A	284 - TOXINS - FOOD	TF
166 - RABBIT	166	204 - HONEY	204	244 - ANTIOBIOTICS	AB	285 - TOXINS - OILS	TO
167 - VEAL	167	205 - LECITHIN	205	245 - ALERGY	AG	286 - UNKNOWN	N
FISH	FISH	206 - LICORICE	206	246 - BACTERIA	B	287 - VIRUS	VR
168 - BASS	168	207 - MAPLE SYRUP	207	247 - CAFFEINE - EXCESS	C	288 - VITAMINS - LACK	V
169 - COD	169	208 - MISO	208	248 - CHEMICALS	CH	289 - VITAMIN B - LACK	L
170 - FLOUNDER	170	209 - MOLASSES	209	249 - CONTAGIOUS	CG	290 - X RAYS	XR
171 - HADDOCK	171	210 - MUESLI	210	250 - DIET - DEFICIENT	D	291 - YEAST INTOLERANCE	YS
172 - HERRING	172	211 - MUSHROOMS	211	251 - DISEASE	DS		HRB
173 - MACKEREL	173	212 - MUSTARD	212	252 - DRUGS	DR	292 - ALOE VERA	292
174 - PERCH	174	213 - NORI	213	253 - EXERCISE - LACK	E	293 - ANISEED	293
175 - PIKE	175	214 - OATMEAL	214	254 - FATS - EXCESS	F	294 - BASIL	294
176 - SALMON	176	215 - PASTA	215	255 - FEVER	FE	295 - CALENDULA	295
177 - SARDINES	177	216 - PECTIN	216	256 - FOOD ADDITIVES	Z	296 - CAMOMILE	296
178 - SNAPPER	178	217 - PITA BREAD	217	257 - FOOD POISOINING	FP	297 - COMFREY	297
179 - SHARK	179	218 - PROPOLIS	218	258 - FUNGUS	FG	298 - DANDELION	298
180 - TROUT	180	219 - PUMPERNICKEL	219	259 - GLUTEN	G	299 - GINGER	299
181 - TUNA	181	220 - RICE BRAN	220	260 - HERIDITARY	HR	300 - GINSENG	300
SEAFOOD	SFO	221 - RICE FLOUR	221	261 - HYGEINE - POOR	H	301 - LAVENDER	301
182 - CAVIAR	182	222 - ROYAL JELLY	222	262 - INFECTION	I	302 - MINT	302
183 - CLAMS	183	223 - SOY FLOUR	223	263 - INFLAMMATION	IF	303 - PENNYROYAL	303
184 - CRAB	184	224 - SOY MILK	224	264 - INJURY	IJ	304 - ROSEHIP	304
185 - LOBSTER	185	225 - SOY SAUCE	225	265 - JUICE - LACK	J	305 - ST.JOHN'S WORT	305
186 - OYSTERS	186	226 - TAHINI	226	266 - MEAT - EXCESS	M	NATURAL OILS	NOL
187 - PRAWNS	187	227 - TEA TREE OIL	227	267 - MILK - EXCESS	K	306 - CORN OIL	306
188 - SCALLOPS	188	228 - TEMPEH	228	268 - MINERALS - LACK	U	307 - OLIVE OIL	307
189 - SHRIMP	189	229 - TOFU	229	269 - OBESITY	O	308 - SAFFLOWER OIL	308
		230 - VINEGAR	230	270 - OLD AGE	OA	309 - SESAME OIL	309
190 - AGAR	190	231 - WHEAT BRAN	231	271 - OVEREATING	OE	310 - SUNFLOWER OIL	310
191 - KELP	191	232 - WHEAT GERM	232	272 - PRESERVATIVES	PR	311 - SOY OIL	311
192 - SPIRULINA	192	233 - YEAST	233	273 - PROTEIN - LACK	P	312 - WHEAT GERM OIL	312

AILMENT	BODY SYSTEM'S	RISK FACTORS	NUTRITIONAL NEEDS
ABSCESS	17 13	I B H	41 42 148 227
ACNE	17 3 4	H D R X F	33 196 41 VEG JUICE FRU JUICE 100
ADENOIDS	3 4 7 13	D I L E R	95 JUICE 239 100 HYDROGEN PEROXIDE GARGLE
ANEMIA	9 2	D U R P L	137 24 42 139 91 196
ANGINA PECTORIS	1 9 7	S T F Q A	44 205 312 85 142 103
ARTERIOSCLEROSIS	1 9 2 11	E S T O F	205 41 42 44 36
ARTHRITIS	14 8	S R Q G D	44 FISH 71 240 98 234
ASTHMA	7 6 13	Y K L R S	95 100 85 136 203 130
BAD BREATH	2 7 11	E D G I T	236 194 235 234 241
BALDNESS	17 10 20 1	D L S R HR	103 235 148 196 116
BRONCHITIS	7 13	Y I T D K	100 148 85 239 95 41
BRUISING	1 20 10	O D L V E	142 312 96 91 42
CANCER	13 10 9 20	D V U J L	148 100 147 95 42 VEG
CELIAC DESEASE	2 11	G R D	LEG FRU NUT VEG 194
CHICKEN POX	13 17 20	V H J	238 196 42 95 237 81
CIRCULATION	1 5 9	E D F J W	235 312 205 240 226
CHOLESTEROL	9 1 2 4	F M K S R	205 LEG VEG NUT
COLITIS	11 2 20	S IF F AG D	MN VIT 81 194 62
COMMON COLD	7 13 11 4	K V IF J TX S	95 239 96 202 42 146 304
CONSTIPATION	11 2 6	D S R L E	84 216 FRU 241 LEG
CROUP	7 13 11	I V K R D	INHALE STEAM 85 JUICE 237 63 203
CYSTIC FIBROSIS	3 2 7	N P E	196 312 148 239
CYSTITIS	7 11 13	B I D W	88 JUICE 66 JUICE 241 99 JUICE

AILMENT	BODY SYSTEM'S	RISK FACTORS	NUTRITIONAL NEEDS
DANDRUFF	17 3 10 11	V D B H L	196 95 JUICE 139 100 227
DERMATITIS	17 10 6 20	IF S CH AG	241 96 196 237 42
DIABETES	2 3	X OE D HR R S K	196 42 312 40 116 33
DIARRHEA	11 2 3	B S H D Z	120 65 155 106 62 237 201
DIVERTICULITIS	2 20 11 6	IF B D R H	220 62 201 214 241
ECZEMA	17 6 20 13	S CH AG HR B D	FISH 226 VEG 196 FRU 95 JUICE
EDEMA - OEDEMA	18 2 1 11	Q L E D O	98 JUICE 234 65 312 130 235
EMPHYSEMA	7 11 10	T E Y I	95 JUICE 148 235 312 85 JUICE
EPILEPSY	6 19	IJ TF AG K HR U	237 NUT 234 VEG FRU JUICES
FEVER	13 4 1	I V B TX	75 JUICE FRU JUICES 195 238 202 239
GALLSTONES	2 11 4	F X AG D O	205 307 75 JUICE VEG
GASTRITIS	2 11 10	A C D Z B	81 94 65 148 95 JUICE
GASTROENTERITIS	2 13	B TX VR AG A	236 302 TEA 100 238
GLAUCOMA	15 3	HR IJ DS IF	95 JUICE 195 FRU 66 FISH 196
GOITER	3 2 11 4	U TX I D	191 KELP TABLETS 139 131
GOUT	14 9 2 11	M A D O C	241 122 FRU JUICES 98 88
HAY FEVER	15 6 11 13	AG Y CH HR TX	95 JUICE 75 JUICE 100 HORSE-RADISH
HEADACHE	19 6 9 13 11	S SB I AG E TO	FRU JUICES 130 237 62 235 137
HEART ATTTACK	1 6 2	D F E O S	205 85 JUICE 100 42 136 312
HEMMORRHOIDS	11 2 5	SB D E R C	292 81 235 142 237
INDIGESTION	2 6	OE S F D A	237 62 241 206
INFECTION	13 4 10 20	IJ DS B H	95 JUICE 148 227 42 204 295 EYE 218
INSOMNIA	6 19	S E C D X	296 196 103 239 155 235

AILMENT	BODY SYSTEM'S					RISK FACTORS						NUTRITIONAL NEEDS					
JAUNDICE - HEPATITIS A	9	11	17	2		V D F A R			H			91 JUICE	95 JUICE	238	87 JUICE	205	VEG
KIDNEY STONES	18	2	9	3		M A W R D						241	VEG. JUICES	FRUIT JUICES	237		
LEUKEMIA	9	13	10			RACH X R D VR						148	91 JUICE	95 JUICE	VEG	FRU	
MEASLES	13	7	4	17		IF VR FE TX CG						237	FRUIT JUICES	VEG. JUICES			
MENINGITIS	19	9	13			VR FE B IF						MEDICAL TREATMENT		95 JUICE			
MONONUCLEOSIS - GLANDULAR FEVER	4	3	13	9		D IF H VR						238	95 JUICE	VEG. JUICES	42	196	
MULTIPLE SCLEROSIS	6	19				VR DS R S D						196	130	136	312	FISH	137
NEPHRITIS	18	1	20			IF S E D R						VEG	FRU	241	LEG		
NEURITIS	6	13	5			M IF L IJ FP						75 JUICE	196	VEG	NUTS		
OBESITY	2	11	3	4	1	E OE F M K						235	FRUIT JUICES	241	VEG. JUICES	236	
OSTEOARTHRITIS	14	10	8			SB U OA E R						71 JUICE	98 JUICE	312	239	65	
OSTEOPOROSIS	8	16	20	10		U OA E A T						239	NUTS	235	224	297	242
PARKINSONS D.	6	19	5			SB S L DS TX						54	196	148	136	50 45 239 44	
PNEUMONIA	7	13	10			IF B VR V T						95 JUICE	VEG. JUICES	239	148	FRU	
POLIO	6	5	13			VR H IF						VEG. JUICES	148	95 JUICE	196	239	
PROSTATIS	18	16	13	3		S H IF OA C						137	91 JUICE	44	NUT	87	
PSORIASIS	17	10				HR D U TX						239	139	FISH	95 JUICE	312	
R.S.I. REPETATIVE STRAIN INJURY	5	6	14	1	19	SB S D						237	312	240	NUT	226	239
RHEUMATISM	5	14	13			IF D U OA S						98 JUICE	239	226	136	130	
RHEUMATOID ARTHRITIS	14	13	5			S IF OA D V						100	138	299	139	235	312
SCALDS- BURNS	17	10	13	20		FIRE HEAT						BATHE IN COLD WATER SEEK MEDICAL HELP					
SCIATICA	14	5	8	6		SB IJ IF						237	226	240	196	65 242	FRUIT JUICES
SHINGLES	6	13	17	10		VR D S OA						196	239	42	295	81	148

197

AILMENT	BODY SYSTEM'S	RISK FACTORS	NUTRITIONAL NEEDS
SINUSITIS	7 13 4 11	K D B R V	100 111 95 JUICE / VEG. JUICES 239 85 JUICE
SLIPPED DISC BACKACHE	14 8 5 6	IJ E O	237 312 240 226 239 65 235
STOMACH ULCER	2 6 10	D S T A K Q C	81 94 241 194 237 95 JUICE 206 100
STRESS	6 19 3	E L C T X	237 238 196 235 239 130 240 62 137 88 103 296
STROKE	1 19 7 5 9	S D Q E T	205 237 196 312 FRUIT JUICES 65 FISH
SUNBURN/STROKE	17 10 20	SUN EXPOSURE W	241 81 GEL 292 44 301 295 CALAMINE LOTION
SWOLLEN GLANDS GLANDULAR FEVER	3 4 9 13	VR V D J	95 JUICE 237 100 42 VEG. JUICES 85
SEXUALLY TRANSMITTED DISEASE (STD)	16 17 3 13 9	I H C G V R	148 100 42 147 202 218 96
THROMBOSIS	1 9 5	E O D T X	142 85 JUICE 42 98 JUICE 235 71 312
THRUSH	2 13 16 17	AB DR X FG YS	194 155 100 295 227
TINEA	17 13 10	FG H C G B	239 227 301 196 234
TONSILLITIS	4 7 13	VR B IF J D	85 JUICE 42 95 JUICE 204 HYDROGEN PEROXIDE GARGLE
TUBERCULOUS	7 13 4	I VR K D B T	95 JUICE 148 100 FRUIT JUICES 75 JUICE 85 JUICE
ULCERS	17 20 13	HF AG H S D	81 312 155 292
(URTICARIA) HIVES-NETTLE RASH	17 13 10	DR Z S AG BS	42 102 295 296 96 100
VAGINITIS	16 13 20 17	IF B YS CH D	194 155 193 100 227
VARICOSE VEINS	1 5 9 7	E O HR V	142 98 JUICE 42 237 96 71
VENEREAL DISEASE	16 18 20 13	DS CG I H	148 202 96 42
VIRUSES	7 13 9 4	CG F K D J	85 JUICE 100 104 42 148 VEG. JUICES
WARTS	13 9 17	VR S X CG	227 75 OIL
WHOOPING COUGH	7 13 4	B I K D	85 JUICE 96 95 JUICE 241 63 204 239
WORMS	2 11	IF H M CG	100 137 95 JUICE
WOUNDS	17 9 20 10	IJ I IF	292 312 95 JUICE 295 81 GEL 296

198

The following pages provide a guide to various diet ideas that are based on the benefits of natural foods. These diet ideas are not remedies or treatments, please consult a medical practitioner for a diagnosis and advice. The main aim of these diet ideas is to show how natural foods, in the daily diet contribute specific nutrients or ingredients that may provide improved health benefits, when taken regularly. In most cases, natural foods are recognized as being safe and essential for human health. As the research on natural foods continues, more benefits seem to be discovered.

If we forget the 'art of using natural foods', and, let our taste buds be dictated by advertising, packaging, additives, flavours and cooked oils, plus take away, drive-in and fast foods, the society and future generations of processed fast food addicts are likely to end up with recurrent health problems. Is that worth all the temporary taste stimulation from a repetitive intake of 2 minute meals and fast acting sugar drinks. Natural foods provide all human nutritional needs and they are presented in unique packages. Natural foods are the undisputable king of nutrition and generous health benefits.

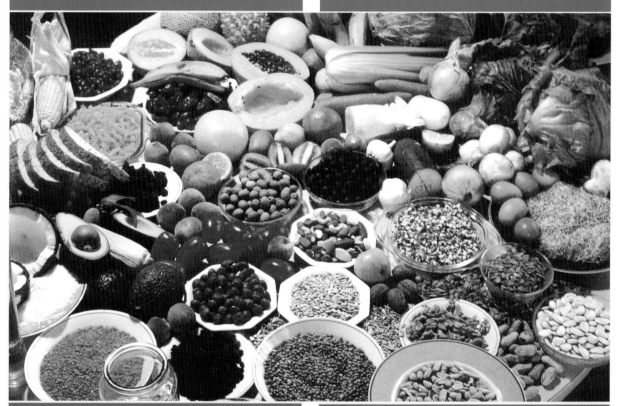

In this era, factories are manufacturing food products that are nearly always based on natural foods. This food processing is basically on the move for profit and advertising costs are just a tax deduction. Colourful, shiny packets with approx. one finely sliced potato, cooked oils, free radicals, salt and flavours, providing no health benefits and they 'cost the earth'. Factory foods take the place of the 'real thing'; properly prepared natural meals, they can be quick, simple, cheap, nutritious and delicious!

This book provides over 200 different meal ideas that are all full of flavour, nutritional benefits and positive future health benefits.

Discover a new meal idea, prepare yourself with a shopping list (page 221) of natural foods, based on the Recipe Ideas on pages 216 - 218. Most recipe ideas take less time to make than a trip to the drive - through, waiting in the queue with the smells of car exhaust and paying through the nose for packaging with a life span of 5 minutes.

NOTE: All amounts in this book are measured in milligrams (mg) per 100 grams, unless stated otherwise.

199

ANTI - CANCER DIET IDEAS

This information is provided only as a guide. Please consult your medical practitioner for a proper diagnosis and treatment. Cancer comes in many forms, some of the ideas mentioned may suit one type of cancer but be less helpful for other types. Natural foods in their natural state provide safe nutrition and there are numerous possible healing benefits, if they are obtained regularly.

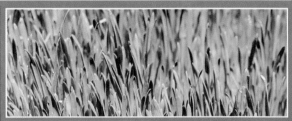

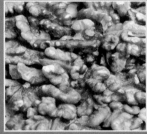
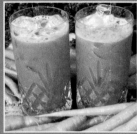

BREAKFAST:

A papaya for breakfast provides anti-colon cancer qualities, due to the fibre, folate, vitamin C and beta carotene. The kiwi fruit supplies a good amount of vitamin C, antioxidant power, reducing free radicals. Lemon and lime juice supply flavonoids: flavonol glycosides that help to reduce cell division in many cancer cells, plus they supply vitamin C. Grapefruit contain phytochemicals: limonoids that inhibit tumour formation by producing an enzyme that helps eliminate toxins from the liver. Pineapple juice, provides manganese, vital for antioxidant defence against free radicals. A rockmelon will provide vitamin C and A, for antioxidant power and anti - free radical activity. Berries, especially blue berries are full of antioxidant power as they contain phenols, promoting anticancer power as they prevent oxygen damage in body organs. Blueberries and strawberries also supply ellagic acid, an antioxidant that can block cancer development. Blueberries are the ultimate source of phytonutrients that neutralize free radical cell damage and promote the action of vitamin C. A fruit breakfast is a positive way to start a day.

MORNING TEA

Start with a freshly extracted carrot and parsley juice for an excellent dose of carotene to inhibit tumour growth and for help with lung and pancreatic cancer. Sulphur in carrots assists to eliminate toxins. Parsley supplies anti cancer benefits such as myristicin, a volatile oil and the flavonoid: luteolin in parsley is an antioxidant, plus with the excellent vitamin C, parsley heals. Try 90% carrot juice with 10% parsley, every two days.

LUNCH

For colon cancer, try a legume meal, refer recipes page 216 - 218. For other cancers, steamed brown rice with broccoli, sliced Brussels sprouts, carrots, onions, corn and red capsicum. Rice is alkaline, it helps healing, add garlic in the last seconds and ground pepitas, especially for prostate cancer. Or for a simple snack, asparagus with soy mayonnaise and baked tofu. Or a fresh salad with walnut oil.

AFTERNOON SNACK

Wheat grass juice, the ultimate blood rebuilder and anti-cancer tonic due to the super beta carotene power, super lycopene antioxidant power and chlorophyll content, refer to page 112 for details. Without a regular wheat grass juice, blood based cancers are hard to beat.

EVENING MEAL

Baked pumpkin with broccoli and fish / lemon for help with lung cancer. Tabouli salad with grilled tofu for help with colon cancer. Pasta with lots of ground pepitas, chopped parsley and parmesan to help blood based cancer. Serve with a sip of red wine. Brussells sprouts with honey carrots and salmon, with red chili peppers for help with skin cancer. For sweets, acidophillus yoghurt with honey for colon health. Black cherries contain ellagic acid, flavonoids and perrillyl alcohol, anti-carcinogenic and they stunt the growth of cancer cells.

ANTI - STRESS DIET IDEAS

BREAKFAST:

Watermelon juice or apple juice, both provide alkaline balance to the blood, plus melons are full of bromine, vital for emotional stability and also as an anti-depressant. Tahini on toast, as tahini is full of *magnesium* (320 mg) the nerve mineral, plus *calcium* (330 mg) for the nerves and a peaceful sleep. Vegemite or yeast extract on toast, a very good source of vitamins *B1*: nerves, *B2*: anti stress, anti fatigue *B3*: nourishes the nerves, anti depression, fatigue, *B5*: anti stress, depression, *B6*: anti stress, irritability, nervousness, folate: nerves, brain, anti-fatigue, most of these B vitamins are water soluble and required daily. A B complex tablet daily is beneficial.

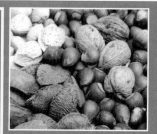
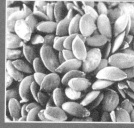
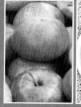
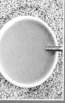
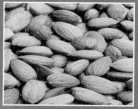

MORNING TEA

Try a handfull of almonds: *phosphorus* 490 mg: strength and repair of nerves, improves concentration and memory, *magnesium* 260 mg: protects against hardened arteries and high blood pressure and *calcium* 250 mg: regular heart action, and digestion. Have an apple or 2 peaches with the almonds.

AFTERNOON SNACK

Handfull of cashews with the cup of tea, cashews are rich in *zinc* 5.7 mg protects against fatigue and is required for the action of B vitamins and for mental alertness. Cashews are a good source of *manganese* 0.8 mg required for memory, *magnesium* 250 mg, *phosphorus* 530 mg for energy production, concentration, nerves and brain health. Cashews and a crisp apple for a nourishing nerve snack.

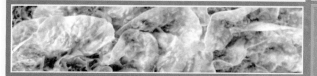

LUNCH

Salad sandwich: lettuce is an excellent source of *silicon*: 1,500 mg protects against nervous exhaustion, mental fatigue and baldness. Lettuce also supplies *folate* 15 mg nerve functioning, *sulphur* 580 mg brain functioning and *chlorine* regulates blood pressure. Add some sliced red capsicum for an excellent supply of *vitamin C* anti stress and headache vitamin. Add a few walnuts rich in *Omega 3*: nerve functioning and *biotin* for sleep, anti-depression and nervousness with a few slices of cheddar cheese: *protein*: nerve cell building, adrenaline production, brain hormone transfer, on rye bread for *potassium* (460 mg) strengthens the heart muscles and vital for mental function, nervous system and brain.

EVENING MEAL:

Pepita pasta: Add 4 tbl.sp. of ground pepitas to the pasta sauce, or sprinkle on top of the pasta with cheese. Pepitas are an excellent source of *iron* 11.3 mg protects against fatigue, promotes endurance and resistance to stress. Pepitas are also an excellent source of *zinc* 7.5 mg required for the action of B vitamins, alcohol conversion and protection from fatigue and mental stress, *magnesium* 535 mg, controls the central nervous system, protects against mental exhaustion and irritability, plus with the excellent balance of *phosphorus* 1174 mg essential for the nervous system and brain function, as it promotes memory and concentration, copper 1.4 mg promotes vitamin C absorption, protects the nerve fibres and promotes iron utilization. Add ground pepitas to a soup, vegetable burgers for the ultimate regenerating balance to the nervous system. Pepitas are the greatest anti stress food.

ATHLETES DIET IDEAS

BREAKFAST:

Grape juice freshly extracted provides the ultimate source of *dextrose*, easily absorbed into the bloodstream, providing nearly instant energy for that early morning workout or aerobics session.

Sunflower butter is easy to make, mix one cup of sunflower kernels in a blender or grinder, place in a large bowl, hand mix with a fork 1tbl.sp. honey and 2 tbls.sp. soft butter, mix together into a smooth consistency, serve on rye bread toast, sunflower butter will provide an excellent source of *vitamin E* (34 mg) promoting the endurance, stamina and power of muscles, *protein* (23 g) for muscle growth: as muscle fibres are collections of protein molecules. repair of damaged tissues and for hormones to regulate body functions. *Vitamin B1*(2.3 mg) essential during strenuous exercise, oxygen absorption and for energy conversion, *iron* (6.8 mg) for muscle endurance, tissue repair and blood oxygen levels, *phosphorus* (705 mg) for energy distribution and blood circulation *zinc* (5.1 mg) tissue growth and insulin-glucose activity, *selenium* (60 mcg) for vitamin E activity, *vitamin B3* (4.5 mg) for protein effectiveness, energy production in muscle cells and B3 is depleted during bouts of strenuous exercise.

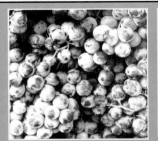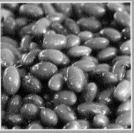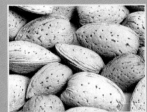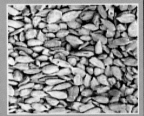

MORNING TEA

Banana smoothie the banana is an ideal provider of *energy* (22 g) and a good source of *potassium* (358 mg) the muscle mineral as it is vital for repair of muscles, strength of muscles and it is the foundation mineral of muscular tissue, *chlorine* (270 mg) for heart muscle action, *sulphur* (120 mg) for heart muscles, carbohydrate metabolism and insulin manufacture. Milk will provide a fair amount of *calcium* (115 mg) for muscle action, tissue development, heart muscle function and bone strength and repair.

AFTERNOON SNACK

2 serves of hazel nuts with 2 apples, for an excellent supply of *protein* (30-42 g) vitamin E (30mg), carbohydrate (34g) magnesium (320 mg) calcium (220 mg) unsaturated fats (100 g) for lasting energy.

LUNCH

Kidney bean tacos, kidney beans provide excellent *carbohydrate* value (60 g) with a low g.i. and an energy supply to last all afternoon, the excellent *potassium* (1,406 mg) for muscles, *iron* (8 mg) for oxygen supply, *folate* (394 mcg) for physical endurance and protein formation, *calcium* (143 mg.) bone strength, *phosphorus* (407 mg) bone strength and energy production, *magnesium* (140 mg) muscle function, protection from muscular cramps, *copper* (1 mg) heart muscles, *molybdenum* for iron-oxygen utilization. The lettuce, carrot, onion and tomato sauce will provide numerous nutrients and the cheese will add increased protein value to the kidney bean *complete protein* (24-40 g) plus excellent *calcium* (700-900 mg) for bone strength and muscle action.

EVENING MEAL

Fish and chips fish will supply excellent *protein* (20-25 g) for muscle growth, *cobalt* for body cell activity, growth and energy, *selenium* for growth, skin elasticity, *vanadium* for blood circulation, potatoes, chips will provide quick carbohydrate energy with the fat content providing slower release of energy. About 2-3 hours after the fish meal, have a large serve of yoghurt to promote a peaceful nights sleep and to relax your muscles, as yoghurt helps to break down lactic acid which builds up during strenuous exercise.

CHILDREN'S DIET IDEAS

BREAKFAST:

Pineapple, apple & mango juice in summer.
Grape juice in autumn.
Mandarin & strawberry juice in winter,
Apple & peach juice in spring.

Allow children to have a choice from a variety of in-season fruits to make a freshly extracted juice. Start with small serves of approx. 120ml. or half a cup, serve in a glass and in hot weather, add a few cubes of ice. The fresh juice in the morning will provide children with a fair dose of *vitamin C*, depending on the juice, plus a variety of *other vitamins and minerals* that are lacking from cooked and processed foods. Freshly made fruit juices provide *natural sweetness* that children crave, as fructose-fruit sugars are converted into glucose. Over 90% of all glucose is used for the nervous system and for brain activity. Give your children a head start, everyday.

Cereal, toast, pancakes, muffins, scrambled eggs, croissants, rolled oats, fruit salad or yoghurt,

Allow children to choose from at least a few of the above, even set-up a small blackboard, whiteboard on the kitchen wall, pretend it's a classy restaurant. Nearly everyday, children have slightly different nutritional needs and by giving a choice, once a child has experienced a variety of foods, their body and taste buds will go for the foods that may provide the specific nutrients that are required for their current development. Processed cereals of good quality are ok once or twice a week, try the blackboard choice idea and utilize natural foods and canned apricots or peaches on cereal, or a sprinkle of finely cracked macadamia or pecan nuts. Pancakes with stewed apples and cream, or toast with honey, vegemite or peanut butter. Breakfast is vital for growing children.

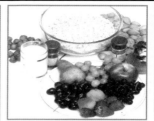
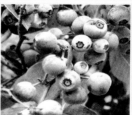
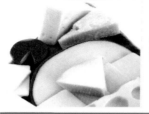
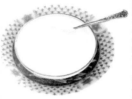

MORNING PLAY TIME AT SCHOOL

Children are keen to run and play after a morning of sitting down, they have little time to eat, so give them quick snacks and make up for the nutrition factor at home. Make the serves small, their hand size, a *cheese sandwich* in quarters is ample and excellent, *biscuits and cheese*, a small *tub of yoghurt*, a *muesli bar*, *sesame bar*, an *apple juice*, a fresh *crisp small apple*, *dried apricots*, *apples* provide compact nutrition, time for the bell!

LUNCHTIME

Give your children the choice, it's their lunch, use the blackboard idea at home for lunch ideas, depending on the season and temperature, always give them pure water and a *choice* of sandwich, salad or cheese or chicken or ham or egg. Or biscuits with cheese, or some muffins, snack bar or tub of yoghurt. In winter a milk drink can last till lunch, in summer a frozen fruit juice will be refreshing. Lunch time is also play time!

AFTER SCHOOL & EVENING MEAL

A milkshake and toasted baked bean jaffle or a chocolate drink and pancake, or a toasted cheese sandwich will give children ample nourishment till the evening meal whilst doing their home work. For evening meal ideas, as a family, choose from the variety of recipe ideas on pages 212 - 216. For sweets, yoghurt is ideal as it provides essential calcium during their sleep.

Our Home Menu
- [ ] pancakes with apple and cream
- [ ] scrambled eggs on toast
- [ ] rye toast with vegemite
- [ ] toast with cheese
- [ ] rolled oats with peaches, apricots
- [ ] cereal with macadamia nuts
- [ ] yoghurt with waffles and strawberries
- [ ] croissants with blueberry jam, cream.

IRON DIET IDEAS

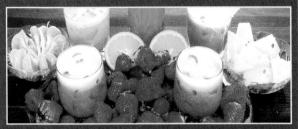

BREAKFAST:
Apple (0.2 mg) and strawberry (0.6mg) juice: TOTAL IRON approx. (0.8 mg)
Rolled oats (3.7mg) with 50 gram of raisins (2.2 mg.) plus a tblsp. of wheat germ (2 mg), serve with a cup of milk (0.05 mg) or soy milk (0.5mg): TOTAL BREAKFAST IRON approx. (8.4 mg).

MORNING TEA
Date dip: dried dates (2.6 mg) dipped into Tahini 50 g (3 mg) or, walnuts (2.5 mg) on rye bread (2.7 mg) with honey, or sunflower seed butter 50 g (2 mg) on wholemeal bread (2.2 mg).

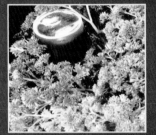
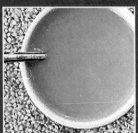

LUNCH
Tabouli salad, parsley 50 gram (4.5 mg), tomato 50 gram (0.2mg) with raw spinach 50 gram (3.2 mg) with tahini dressing 30 gram (1.7 gram) on rye bread (2.7 mg) TOTAL LUNCH IRON: 12.3 mg. Seafood mix with mussels (14 mg) or clams (8 mg) Hummus dip: chick peas (2.5 mg) with tahini 30 mg (1.8 mg) on rye cracker biscuits (2 mg). TOTAL LUNCH IRON: 6.3 mg.
Iron protects against colds and infections.

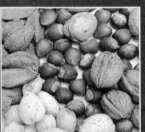
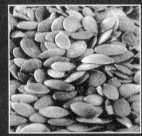

AFTERNOON TEA
Carob milkshake, mix 50 gram carob powder (2.3 mg) with 2 cups soy milk (1.1 mg) TOTAL IRON 3.4 mg.
Carrot and parsley juice, 200 gram carrot (2.2 mg) with 50 mg. parsley (4.7 mg). TOTAL IRON 6.9mg.

EVENING MEAL:
Stir fry: Mix first into stir fry: tofu cubes (7.9 mg) with peas 50 g (1.6 mg), broccoli (1mg) parsley 50 mg. (4.7 mg) 50 mg onions (0.27 mg) capsicum (0.7mg) and 50 gram cashews (1.9 mg) TOTAL IRON 18 mg.
Pepita burgers: Mix in a bowl, ground pepitas (11.2 mg) 30 mg finely chopped parsley (3.2 mg), spinach (3.2 mg) and onions 20 mg (1.2mg) with 100 g cooked rice (0.4mg), mix together and form into patties, fry with canola oil, serve with garden fresh salad (3mg). TOTAL IRON: 19.2 mg.

RDA: DAILY IRON INTAKE

GENDER/ STAGE	AGE	IRON mg. per day
children	1 - 10	10 mg.
male	11 - 18	12 mg.
male	19 - 50	10mg
female	11 - 50	15 mg.
female	51 +	10 mg.
pregnancy		30 mg.
lactation		15 mg.

IRON DIET DAILY SUPPLY VALUES

MEAL	TOTAL	AVERAGE
breakfast	8.4	8.4
morning snack	5	5
lunch	6.3 -14	10
afternoon snack	3.4 - 6.9	5
evening meal	18-19.2	18.5
TOTAL DAILY IRON AVERAGE		46.9 mg.

REJUVENATING DIET IDEAS

BREAKFAST:

Papaya slices with a squeeze of lemon juice, promotes cleansing and healing, the papaya provides *lutein* and *zeaxanthin* for eyesight restoration, *carpain* for heart healing, *beta cryptoxanthin* for colon health and *vitamin C* (62 mg) - the youth vitamin, for supple skin, reduced skin cell oxidation, good eyesight and for collagen-skin formation. Lemon juice will provide *vitamin C*, *sulphur* (125mg) for cleansing and elimination of bacteria.

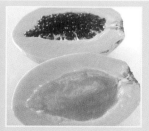
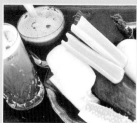

MORNING TEA

Walnuts and Swiss cheese on rye with green tea. Walnuts are an excellent source of *Omega 3*, for healthy skin and eyes, *vitamin B6* (0.7mg) the vitality vitamin, for antibody production and the pituitary gland function, *copper* (2 mg) skin pigment and vitamin C activity, *folate* (98 mcg) reproduction of cells, *biotin* for cellular rejuvenation and conversion of fats into energy, green tea provides *flavonoids* that promote antioxidant benefits and healthy skin. Swiss cheese provides excellent *protein* for cellular production and excellent *calcium* to offset osteoporosis and for elasticity of the skin.

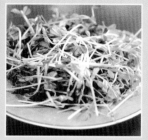
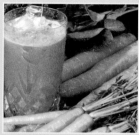

LUNCH

Tahini with sprout salad tahini is a very good source of *vitamin E* (40 mg), protects cells from oxidation, promotes healing of damaged skin and promotes normal cell life and skin nourishment, *vitamin T* for brain nourishment and improved memory, *zinc* (4.6 mg) for healing, healthy skin and hair, *calcium* (420 mg) for good sleep, skin cell and tissue development.

The sprouts will provide numerous active enzymes to promote the digestive, glandular and immune system functions, plus vitamin C and numerous trace nutrients to rejuvenate the body.

For a super rejuvenating sprout salad add 2 tb.sp. of ground pepitas to obtain an excellent supply of *iron*, for cell development, tissue repair and body cleansing, *protein* for cellular repair and a wide variety of minerals for a complete balance of body needs.

AFTERNOON SNACK

Carrot and cucumber juice, the ultimate skin cleansing and rejuvenating juice, the excellent carotene supply from carrots (11,000 mg) promotes soft skin and healing of damaged skin, the excellent sulphur content (445 mg) and chlorine content (318 mg) promote liver and skin cleansing like no other food. Carrot and cucumber are a good source of silicon, vital for healthy hair growth and a good complexion.

EVENING MEAL

Salmon with a fresh garden salad, salmon is a very good source of Omega 3, for improved skin condition and healing, protection from dry skin. The lettuce will provide the ultimate source of silicon for hair growth and condition, plus chlorophyll for body cleansing and numerous active enzymes for rejuvenation. Red capsicum will provide an abundance of vitamin C for skin rejuvenation, improved eyesight and bioflavonoids for prevention of cell oxidation and premature ageing. Asparagus will provide an abundance of *fluoride* for skin and eye health and bladder cleansing, folate 120 mcg for the cellular system and skin health, *rutin* to strengthen blood vessels and protect against varicose veins. Later in the evening, have a serve of acidophillus yoghurt for a peaceful sleep and to balance and cleanse the digestive system of bad bacteria and toxins.

TEENAGER'S DIET IDEAS

BREAKFAST:

Start the day with any freshly extracted fruit juice to kick off the brain power, as the fruit sugar will quickly get to work, feeding the brain and just in case you have a hangover, naughty, fructose will eliminate excess alcohol quicker than any other substance. Vitamin C eliminates toxins and boosts the immune system with antioxidant power. Try pineapple, orange and strawberry juice for a delicious fruit, non alcoholic cocktail! For further brain power, if you are a student, try some slithered almonds on the basic breakfast cereal, full of magnesium and stacks of brain minerals, or try some tahini, the memory food with rye toast for super brain power, or add a few lecithin granules to your scrambled eggs to feed the 'grey matter' as 28% of a healthy brain is comprised of lecithin and processed and nearly all foods contain no lecithin. If you are a hard physical working teenager, check the 'athletes diet' for breakfast ideas. Give your body the *'breakfast habit'*, it's the foundation to brain stability.

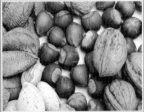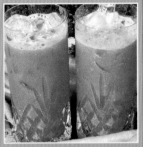
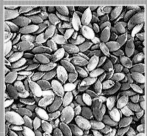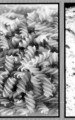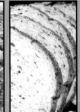

MORNING TEA

Try a walnut cream bun, or an almond cake with a cup of mixed cereal beverage with coffee, half-half, for a mild but steady caffeine hit. If you have an acne skin problem, have a glass of water, one apple or peach and a handfull of raw almonds, a rich source of vitamin E, an antioxidant and required regularly. Take a mild B complex tablet to help the skin and brain, as there are 12 B vitamins and 5 are required daily plus they are 'hard to get' from takeaway and cooked foods.

LUNCH

Depending on the climate, a serve of fish with chips will provide heaps of *protein* and *carbohydrate* energy, or try a kebab with lots of salad. If you have a skin problem, carrot juice is really tops as it provides abundant *sulphur* for eliminating toxins from the skin plus heaps of *carotene* for the skin. Have a carrot juice 3 times a week and watch spots disappear. A salad sandwich is easy, cheap and beneficial.

AFTERNOON SNACK

If you are stuck in the city or near a big shopping centre, the variety of snacks is amazing, but, choose wisely for true value. If you have not had a fresh juice, make it the priority, then, add on the calories knowing your body will be obtaining great benefits from the juice: cleansing the skin, antioxidant power and brain energy. A handfull of almonds, brazil and cashew nuts with an apple will keep you going for ages and provide excellent protein and nutrients. A good quality pie provides 600 calories, about the same as the nuts and will keep you going for 3 hours, you need 2,700 - 3,000 calories a day.

EVENING MEAL

Rice and pasta are simple to prepare and depending on the additions, they can be a very good base for a complete meal. For a real protein and iron boost, add a tbl.sp. of ground pepitas to the pasta and cheese, or sauce mix, or stir fry and gain the best Omega 3 and iron boost in the world, to promote healthy skin and resistance to bugs, flues, infections, viruses and fatigue. Tacos with salad is easy and nutritious, fish and baked vegetables or check any of the recipe ideas on pages 212 - 216. It's the *natural foods you add* that make all the difference in flavour and nutrition.

ANTI-AILMENT DIET IDEAS & RECIPE GUIDE

The chart below provides a list of diet ideas for help in the prevention of particular ailments. This chart is not to be used as a treatment of a specific ailment. Please consult a medical practitioner or naturopath for diagnosis and treatment of an illness.

The code system below refers to the Recipe Guide Ideas Charts on pages 214 - 219. For example; anti-ageing diet: 9L, refer to page 214: Fruits, 9: melons or papaya, L: lunch: fresh papaya entree.

These simple recipe ideas are based on numerous nutritional benefits that may be obtained from specific natural foods. Feed your 'nutritional appetite' daily with natural foods.

DIET IDEAS	BREAK FAST	MORNING SNACK	LUNCH	AFTER-NOON SNACK	EVENING MEAL	OTHER BENEFICIAL FACTORS	POSSIBLE DETRMENTAL FACTORS
Anti-ageing diet	9 L	57 B	21 L	12 L	47 E	papaya flax oil swimming	excess sunlight smoking, stress
Anti-arthritis diet	8 B	1 M	23 L	33 E	60 E	celery, grapefruit almonds	refined wheat stress, worry excess work
Anti-asthma diet	1 B	1 PL	1 M	1 AS	1 ES	apples pineapple pumpkin	pollen, dust stress strenuous work
Anti-baldness diet	33 B	25 L	33 L	33 L	25 E	lettuce juice cucumber juice b complex vit.	heridatary factors. excess meat. smoking. stress
Anti-bowel cancer diet	30 B	9 M	35 L (2)	59 B (3)	30 L	pears dates legumes	refined foods meat chicken
Anti-high blood pressure diet	7 B	13 M	23 L (1 & 2)	48 L (1)	41 E	grapes, lecithin pineapple celery, flax oil	saturated fats margarine, stress
Anti-cold diet	8 B 11 B	9 PL	21 (1) 21 E	13 M	28 E	sunlight ,lemons rest, capsicum garlic, peppers.	milk, dairy foods stress, processed foods.
Anti-osteoporosis diet.	48 B (1)	33 L (1)	59 L (1)	60 E (3)	48 E (1)	sunlight almonds cheese, yoghurt	refined wheat lack of exercise
Anti -Diabetes diet	49 B	58 B (1)	40 L	33 L (1)	33 E (2)	rolled oats celery pepitas	refined foods sugar soft drinks
Menopause diet	9 B	35 B (1)	57 L (1)	21 L (1)	15 E (1 & 2)	melons, rye cantaloup pineapple	lack of melons obesity poor diet
Pregnancy Lactation diet	57 B	6 AS	48 E	6 ES	57 L	walnuts dates sunlight	stress, obesity poor diet, drugs smoking, alcohol
Weight loss diet	9 B	30 B	41 E	14 B	15 E	fresh fruits, rice exercise, juices water,	animal fats dairy produce big breakfast

FOOD COMBINATION CHART

MAIN FOOD GROUPS		1 SWEET FRUITS	2 SUB-ACID FRUITS	3 ACID FRUITS	4 MELONS	5 VEGE TABLES	6 STARCH VEG.	7 GRAINS	8 LEGUMES	9 NUTS & SEEDS	12 MEAT, FISH, POULTRY	11 DAIRY PRODUCE
SWEET FRUITS	1	F	V	F	B	P	B	F	B	B	B	F
SUB ACID FRUITS	2	V	E	V	P	F	P	G	P	F	F	G
ACID FRUITS	3	F	V	E	P	F	P	G	F	G	F	G
MELONS	4	B	P	P	V	B	B	B	B	B	B	B
VEGETABLES	5	P	F	F	B	E	V	E	E	G	E	V
STARCH VEGETABLES	6	B	P	P	B	V	G	P	P	B	F	G
GRAINS & PRODUCTS	7	F	G	G	B	E	P	F	G	F	F	G
LEGUMES	8	B	P	F	B	E	P	G	G	P	P	G
NUTS & SEEDS	9	B	F	G	B	G	P	P	P	B	P	F
MEAT, FISH, POULTRY	10	B	F	F	B	E	F	F	P	P	F	F
DAIRY PRODUCE	11	F	G	G	B	V	G	G	G	F	F	V

Legend:

EXCELLENT COMBINATION	E
VERY GOOD COMBINATION	V
GOOD COMBINATION	G
FAIR COMBINATION	F
POOR COMBINATION	
BAD COMBINATION	B

This food combination chart provides a guide to the various main food groups and their ability to promote proper digestion and subsequent supply of nutrients. The difference between a diet with good to excellent combinations, compared to a diet with fair to poor combination is remarkable.

A great increase in health benefits is possible just by understanding and utilizing proper food combinations with every meal.

Obviously the simple meals with only one or two foods are usually easy to digest, but it really depends on the individual meal combinations.

On pages 123-124 a detailed guide to the reasons behind food combination is provided. Simply speaking, continued intake of meals with poor food combination is one of the main reasons behind obesity, or more specifically the distended stomach image. This is due to the fact that poor combinations promote the formation of intestinal gas which over many years causes the lower intestine area to expand.

In addition, the loss of food value from meals may lead to excess eating in order to satisfy the 'nutritional appetite.'

Also, once the body becomes used to the intake of large meals, it continually requires an intake to support the 'additional fat cells' even though they are not required.

To reverse the problem, proper natural food combinations and a strong will power to offset the 'hunger demands' is required on a regular basis.

SWEET FRUITS:

Sweet fruits, especially all dried fruits are a concentrated source of energy- fruit sugars (fructose) and they require unique digestion. Simple combinations are best, such as a few dried fruits as a snack are ideal, however when combining other fruits, it is best to have apple or peach. Bananas are a concentrated food and should not be combined with any dried fruit but can be combined with apple, apricot, peach or pear. Do not combine dried fruits with nuts, peanuts or any other food group as poor digestion and gas may develop. Simple banana milk shakes are a fair combination and can be nutritious. It is best not to include too many varieties of dried fruits in a fruit salad. Dried fruits need to be chewed very well and preferably taken with a glass of water or herbal tea, to ensure that digestion goes smoothly.

SUB ACID FRUITS:

Sub acid fruits combine very well with one another and therefore a complete fruit salad can be made with them and be most nutritious. Obviously a few of the sub-acid fruits would not be included due to their unfavourable taste combinations.

Avocado on toast, or with a salad with olives is good. Apples or peaches with almonds is an excellent, delicious simple snack. Paw paw with banana is an excellent snack. Grapes are best eaten alone or just a few in fruit salad or muesli. A fruit salad with ice-cream is delicious and alright.

ACID FRUITS:

Simple combinations of acid fruits is excellent, such as orange, pineapple and mandarin. Or, kiwi, strawberry, tangerine and pineapple. The tomato is an acid fruit and it is widely used in various combinations, however they are not always nutritionally favourable. Tomato with pasta, eaten regularly can lead to ulcers in the digestive tract. Tomato in salads is common and alright, due to the benefits of fresh salads. Ideally, tomato should not be combined with starches and may be replaced with red capsicum. Acid fruits do combine well with small portions of sub acid fruits and such combinations as orange and almonds is a good combination.

MELONS:

Melons require no digestion in the stomach and are basically the simplest food to assimilate, due to their very high water content and very simple structure. Melons are best thought of as a drink and should not be eaten after a large meal, as fermentation and gas may develop. They are an ideal breakfast food, make a melon fruit salad with no other foods and that will provide maximum benefits and taste sensation. A small quantity of melon with a fruit salad is alright occasionally.

LEAFY & OTHER VEGETABLES:

The variety of vegetables is abundant and this provides the widest range of very suitable food combinations. Fresh garden salads are optimum nutritionally and combine very well with all grains, or nuts and seeds, or animal proteins, or legumes. Ideally, fresh vegetables and cooked vegetables are not the best combinations, especially when including due to the group of starch vegetables. The taste and colours of vegetables enhances the appetite of any protein meal and combines very well. Some vegetables mixed with dairy foods also combines very well. Ideally, you can combine any leafy vegetable with any single protein food or grain and legume meal for an excellent combination.

BRASSICA & STARCH VEGETABLES:

Brassica vegetables combine very well with leafy vegetables and they are alright to add to simple meals such as pasta, rice or with legumes. Starch vegetables should not be combined with nuts, seeds, grains, legumes and animal proteins. It is common for the starch vegetables to be combined with meat, fish, eggs, chicken but it is likely to complicate protein digestion, due to the different requirements of starch vegetables compared to proteins. Starch vegetables when cooked are prepared into less complex starches and require the action of the enzyme ptyalin within the stomach to continue the breakdown of starch, however the addition of a protein food will retard the action of the alkaline enzyme ptyalin. It is best to eat most of the starch vegetables first. Starch vegetables combine fairly well with other cooked vegetables and dairy foods such as milk, cheese, or yoghurt.

FOOD COMBINING INFORMATION

GRAINS & PRODUCTS:
Generally, the use of whole grains is very limited. Rolled oats, brown rice and sweet corn are the most common whole grain foods. Such whole grains combine very well with vegetables, especially rice and corn. Rolled oats combine very well with most sub acid fruits and milk. The variety of bread is increasing to include mixtures of wheat, rye, oats and corn, all of which combine very well with fresh vegetables or dairy produce. Pasta is very suitable when combined with some vegetables. Pizza varieties are numerous and for best digestion the vegetarian with cheese is alright. Pies and pastries are best when combined with spinach, asparagus, cabbage, onion, carrot, leek or zucchini.

LEGUMES:
The best single combination with legumes is leafy vegetables. The simple baked beans on toast is a good, cheap, simple combination. Legumes should not be combined with any protein foods as their concentrated starch needs very different digestion to meat, fish, eggs, poultry, nuts or seeds. Legumes combine well with dairy foods. The peanut is an ideal snack food when eaten alone or as peanut butter on bread or peanut sauce with rice. Corn chips and beans is a very good combination. Carob powder is ideal with milk drinks. Soy milk combines well with oats or cereals. Ideally, most legumes can be pre-soaked 'sprouted' for 2 days, for improved digestion and supply of nutrients.

NUTS & SEEDS:
The best combination for nuts is with other nuts especially almonds, brazil and cashew nuts as a complete protein snack. Simple snacks of almonds with apple or peach is very good. Nuts with seeds are not the best combination, due to their different protein and lipid structure. Nuts or seeds with leafy vegetables is very good. Do not combine nuts with starch vegetables, legumes, animal proteins or sweet fruits. Simple combinations of nuts with cookies are alright. A fruit salad with acid fruits and nuts or seeds is very good. Sunflower seeds combine well with oats/milk for breakfast. Ground pepitas with rice or pasta is very good especially with leafy vegetables. Tahini is ideal with salads, bread, hummus or sub acid fruits.

ANIMAL PROTEINS:
Compared to all other food groups the animal protein foods require the most complex digestion, especially in the stomach. The best combination for animal protein foods is with salads or cooked leafy vegetables, not starch vegetables. A seafood combination is alright if no other food group is eaten at the same time, apart from salads. A mixed grill is a very complicated meal to digest especially when starch vegetables are combined. Meat with leafy vegetables is a very good combination. Fish combines very well with cooked leafy or brassica vegetables, or a garden salad. Eggs should not be combined with other animal proteins. Eggs in cakes, cookies and vegetable omelette's is alright. Avoid combining animal protein foods with one another or with cheese. Fish and chips is a fair combination. Chicken and salads, leafy or brassica vegetables is a good combination. Keep the meals simple and you will be assured of better digestion.

DAIRY & OTHER PRODUCTS:
Cheese is the most concentrated dairy food. It combines well with salads, bread, pasta or with both starch and brassica vegetables. Cheese and milk will inhibit the secretion of essential digestive enzymes required for protein digestion. It may feel like a satisfying meal but the result is often gas, indigestion and aches a few hours later. Butter with bread or vegetables is good. Yoghurt is best eaten alone or with a simple addition of apple, apricot or peach. Due to the high fat content of dairy foods, they provide a very satisfying taste combination with other foods, especially when sugar is added, such as with ice cream. Small portions are fine but best not eaten directly after a large protein meal. Chocolate is concentrated milk fats and should be treated as an occasional snack, not as a meal.

FOOD COMBINATION SUMMARY:
Proper food combination is primarily based on the varying digestive processes the body performs to convert and utilize individual food groups.

Poor food combination causes improper digestion and loss of food value.

Relax and enjoy the art of dining.

QUESTION 59	What is a diet?	regular eating routine

Everybody has a diet and every diet includes at least a few foods. The most simple way to evaluate a diet is based on the proportion of the three main foods groups that are consumed on a regular basis. Most diets are also based on a proportion of three main meals per day: breakfast, lunch and evening meal, plus morning snack and afternoon snack. On the following pages the Laugh with Health Diet will be explained in detail with recipe ideas for a wide variety of primary produce natural foods.

QUESTION 60	What are the main dietary requirements?	CARBS. PROTEIN LIPIDS

The main dietary requirements are for the three main food groups: Carbohydrates, Protein & Lipids . The chart below provides a guide to the daily requirements for calories and grams from the three main food groups. The chart is based on the Laugh with Health diet and is very similar to the standard USDA Recommended Daily Allowances of 45-65% carbohydrates, 10-35% protein and 20-35% lipids, as explained on pages 212. Generally speaking, very few people measure their daily meal intake in calories or grams. The important factors are to obtain an approximate balance per day of 50% carbohydrate foods, 30 - 40% protein foods and 15-20% Lipids. On the following pages, a more detailed guide to the individual food groups will show how the daily or weekly intake of foods is best obtained for a balanced diet, including the supply of minerals, vitamins, fibre, enzymes and antioxidants.

DAILY CALORIE & GRAMS INTAKE OF THE MAIN FOOD GROUPS CHART

AGE GROUP years.	TOTAL calories per day. approx.	CARBOHYDRATES 4 calories per gram. 50% DAILY DIET		PROTEIN 4 calories per gram 30-40% DAILY DIET		LIPIDS 9 calories per gram 15-20% DAILY DIET	
CHILDREN							
1-3	1300	650 calories	162 grams	390 calories	97 grams	260 calories	28 grams
4-6	1800	900 calories	225 grams	540 calories	137 grams	360 calories	40grams
7-10	2000	1000 calories	250 grams	600 calories	150 grams	400 calories	44grams
MALE							
11-14	2500	1250 calories	312 grams	750 calories	187 grams	500 calories	55 grams
15-18	3000	1500 calories	375 grams	900 calories	225 grams	600 calories	66 grams
18-50	2900	1450 calories	362 grams	870 calories	217 grams	580 calories	64 grams
51 +	2300	1150 calories	287 grams	690 calories	172 grams	460 calories	51 grams
FEMALE							
11-50	2200	1100 calories	275 grams	660 calories	165 grams	440 calories	48 grams
51 +	1900	950 calories	237 grams	570 calories	142 grams	380 calories	42 grams
PREG.	2500	1250 calories	312 grams	750 calories	187 grams	500 calories	55 grams
LACT.	2700	1350 calories	337 grams	810 calories	202 grams	540 calories	60 grams

NUTRITION & DIET SUMMARY

<table>
<tr><td>QUESTION
61</td><td>*What is the*
Laugh with Health
diet?</td><td>50% - Carbs.
30-35% - Protein
15-20% - Lipids</td></tr>
</table>

For over 20 years, the Laugh with Health diet, designed by the Australian author of this book has recommended a 50% carbohydrate, 30 - 35% protein and 15 - 20% lipids diet. This simple dietary balance of the main food groups is designed to provide a complete supply of all nutrients, based on the benefits of natural foods. The USDA National Academy of Science Report, 2002, recommends a similar dietary balance of the three main food groups: 45-65% carbohydrates, 10 - 35% protein and 20 - 35% lipids. Obviously, when the USDA figures are averaged, they become: 55% carbohydrates, protein 22.5%, lipids 27.5%.

The Laugh with Health diet suggests less lipids, in particular, compared to the USDA diet, mainly due to the fact that the food group nuts are promoted as a regular part of the Laugh with Health diet, as a protein food, even though they also contain a good percentage of beneficial unsaturated fats. In addition, the Laugh with Health diet suggests less protein than the USDA diet, mainly due to the fact that legumes are suggested as a staple food in the Laugh with Health diet. Kidney beans, chick peas, mung beans are classed in the carbohydrate group, but they also provide a fair percentage of complete protein. Further charts in this summary section will detail the specific ratio of all food groups and it will be evident that the Laugh with Health diet provides a complete balance of all natural foods as well as the three main food groups. Other variations for the main food groups occur due to such factors as climate, for example, in a cold climate more fats are required, also, for very athletic people, extra protein is required and for people who use a lot of brain power, extra carbohydrates are required, as approx. 90% of all carbohydrate-glucose is used for brain function. Another factor is that generally speaking, nobody calculates their exact meal to the percentage, these dietary balance charts are provided as a guide for your daily and weekly balance and to consider when planning a balanced diet.

Numerous other factors, such as the type of foods: natural or processed are far more important than the exact ratio of the three main food groups. Furthermore, the balance between raw foods and cooked foods is vital. Ideally 70% of all foods are eaten raw. Foods such as nuts, seeds, fruits, vegetables, natural cheese, sprouts, dairy and oats. The balance of 30% cooked foods includes natural foods such as vegetables, whole grains in bread, legumes, eggs, fish and animal produce. Throughout this summary, the Laugh with Health diet will detail the best possible human nutrition information.

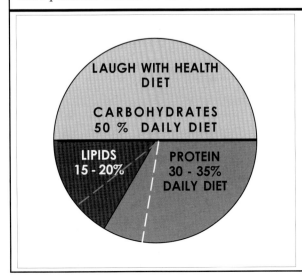

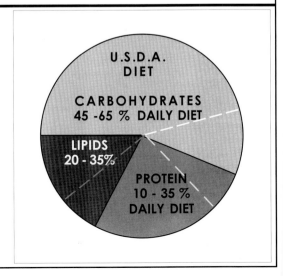

NUTRITION & DIET SUMMARY

What foods does the Laugh with Health diet suggest?

a variety of natural food groups

The Laugh with Health diet suggests a full range of natural foods, including the 13 food groups listed in the chart below. The Laugh with Health diet also suggests a diet with at least 50% fresh foods, ideally 70%. Due to the fact that all natural foods contain at least one of the main food groups and often two or all three food groups, most foods are grouped into portions of the three main food groups, except for fruits and vegetables which are nearly all pure carbohydrates. Such foods as whole grains provide mainly carbohydrates but they also supply protein and a low fat content. The chart below provides a guide to the 13 natural food groups and their supply of the three basic food groups, plus, minerals and vitamins, fibre, water, enzymes and antioxidants. The Laugh with Health diet recommends a diet that includes the intake of the full range of natural food groups, over a period of one week. By referring to the chart on page 211, a detailed evaluation of individual food intake, calorie balance and the balanced diet is provided. The Laugh with Health diet is ready to satisfy any healthy appetite.

THE BALANCED DIET - WEEKLY INTAKE OF MAIN FOOD GROUPS & NUTRIENT SUPPLY

MAIN FOOD GROUPS	CARB.	PROTEIN	LIPIDS	MINERALS	VITAMINS	FIBRE	WATER	ENZYMES	ANTI-OXIDANTS
GRAINS	20%	5%	3%	5%	5%	10%	0%	0%	0%
LEGUMES	20%	15%	2%	5%	5%	40%	0%	0%	0%
FRUITS & FRUIT JUICES	20%	0%	0%	10%	15%	10%	55%	45%	50%
VEGETABLES & VEG. JUICES	20%	0%	0%	15%	15%	15%	30%	35%	40%
NUTS	5%	25%	25%	15%	15%	15%	0%	0%	0%
SEEDS	5%	10%	10%	10%	10%	10%	0%	0%	0%
SPROUTS	5%	0%	0%	5%	5%	0%	5%	10%	10%
FISH	0%	20%	10%	5%	5%	0%	0%	0%	0%
SEAFOOD	0%	5%	5%	5%	5%	0%	0%	0%	0%
MEAT	0%	5%	10%	5%	5%	0%	0%	0%	0%
POULTRY	0%	5%	10%	5%	5%	0%	0%	0%	0%
EGGS	0%	5%	5%	5%	5%	0%	0%	0%	0%
DAIRY FOODS	5%	5%	20%	10%	5%	0%	10%	10%	0%
TOTAL	100%	100%	100%	100%	100%	100%	100%	100%	100%

NUTRITION & DIET SUMMARY

How do I obtain more fruits in my diet?

try a new breakfast idea.

FRUITS DAILY RECIPE GUIDE IDEAS & BENEFITS CHART

FRUITS	BREAKFAST (B)	MORNING TEA (M)	PRE (PL) LUNCH	AFTERNOON SNACK (AS)	EVENING SWEETS (ES)	MAIN BENEFITS
1 APPLES	JUICE with pineapple	Crisp Apple with raw almonds	JUICE with strawberry	CRISP with cashews	STEWED with yoghurt	promotes a healthy digestive system, provides over 12 nutrients, plus an alkaline blood balance.
2 APRICOTS	JUICE fresh or canned nectar	DRIED or fresh in season	JUICE from shop	DRIED with fresh apple	CANNED with icecream	rich in vitamin a, vital for the respiratory system, ideal snack for smokers
3 AVOCADO	RIPE on rye toast	RIPE on cracker biscuits	DIP with biscuits or celery .	on bread roll with cheese	guacamole with corn chips	good source of omega 3, helps reduce cholesterol, supplies over 12 nutrients.
4 BANANA	RIPE on cereal	banana smoothie	banana with fruit salad	banana cake	banana on icecream	provides abundant energy, lots of potassium and numerous nutrients.
5 BERRIES CHERRIES CURRANTS PRUNES SULTANAS RAISINS	FRESH or dried with cereal	Currant or blueberry muffin.	JUICE with apple	cookies with slivered almonds	strawberries with cream	full of antioxidants, especially blueberries, protects the brain from stress. Rich in vitamin c.
6 DATES FIGS	finely cut served with cereal	scones or dried or fresh	dipped in tahini	date slice	dates with custard	compact energy food, abundant potassium, fibre, and iron. Ideal food to relieve tiredness.
7 GRAPES	JUICE	fresh fruit	pre lunch juice	fresh fruit snack	red wine	ideal for blood cleansing, supplies antioxidants, manganese and energy.
8 GRAPEFRUIT LEMONS	fresh JUICE	lemon merangue slice	squeezed on fish	lemon tea	squeezed on seafood	cleansing the blood and joint system, good supply of vitamin c and sulphur.
9 MELONS PAPAYA	melon JUICE	dried papaya slices	fresh papaya entree	watermelon juice	papaya with fruit salad	very alkaline foods, ideal for healing, relax the skin, nerves, ideal for glands.
10 OLIVES	oil on toast	with cheese	greek salad	on pizza	salad dressing	mono unsaturated oil.
11 ORANGES	fresh JUICE	orange tea cake	orange pineapple juice	marmalade on crackers	orange tea	good source of vitamin c, magnesium, potassium, vitamin a,
12 PEACHES PEARS	served on cereal	fresh fruit snack	peaches and almonds	peach pear pineapple juice	with icecream or yoghurt	ideal for the skin, hair, digestion, supplies fibre, antioxidants, vitamin a.
13 PINEAPPLE	fresh juice with orange	juice with apple	on pizza or fresh juice	pineapple fritter	served with fish	ideal for the respiratory system, full of sulphur, chlorine, manganese.
14 TOMATO	on toast	juice	in salad	on sandwich	pasta sauce	antioxidant-lycopene. numerous nutrients.

NUTRITION & DIET SUMMARY

<table>
<tr><td>QUESTION
64</td><td>How do I obtain
more vegetables
in my diet?</td><td>try them
for lunch</td></tr>
</table>

VEGETABLES DAILY RECIPE GUIDE IDEAS & BENEFITS CHART

VEGETABLES	LUNCH (L)	EVENING MEAL (E)	MAIN BENEFITS
5 ASPARAGUS	Asparagus on toast with avocado or grilled cheese. Asparagus with egg mayonnaise and salad.	Asparagus, cottage cheese and grilled fish with baked pumpkin. Asparagus soup with rye bread	*cleansing the bladder and kidneys, eyesight, glands,blood vessels, nerves and brain.*
6 BEETROOT	Beetroot juice with carrot. Grated beetroot with salad sandwich.	Baked beetroot, sweet potato with roast chicken and peas. Grated beetroot in lentil burgers.	*blood building, anti cancer, antioxidants, numerous nutrients.*
7 BROCCOLI	Broccoli in stir fry with cashews, bean shoots, onion, rice and garlic.	Broccoli with melted cheese and baked potatoes, baked fish and tartare sauce.	*anti-cancer, anti peptic ulcers, anti-viral, chromium, vitamin a, calcium.*
8 BRUSSEL SPROUTS	Brussel sprouts steamed, served with butter, chips and a salad.	Brussel sprouts sliced in quarters, steamed with mashed potato and chicken fillets marinated and char-grilled.	*sulphur for cleansing, indoles as cancer inhibitors, folic acid, fibre.*
9 CABBAGE	Coleslaw salad with kidney bean burgers.	Cabbage rolls, filled with rice, sesame seeds, onion, garlic, parsley, deep fried.	*chlorine, sulphur, vitamin u, cleansing , enzymes.*
0 CAPSICUM	Add to salad sandwiches, garden salads, pasta.	Baked capsicum filled with rice, tomatoes, cabbage and cheese.	*vitamin c, bioflavonoids for strong blood vessels.*
1 CARROTS	Carrot juice Grated carrot with mayonnaise on rye bread.	Steamed carrots with pepita burgers, rice, chilli sauce and papadams.	*excellent carotene, anti cancer, anti colds, liver cleansing, eyes, lungs.*
2 CAULIFLOWER	Cauliflower pieces finely chopped in garden salad with pasta and cheese.	Cauliflower slightly steamed, baked in oven with onions, garlic grilled cheese served with garlic prawns.	*sulphur, chlorine, cleansing the blood, anti ulcers, silicon for hair growth.*
3 CELERY	Celery Juice Waldorf salad with walnuts, celery, apple, mayonnaise.	Garden salad with finely chopped celery, cottage cheese, red capsicum, served with fried tofu or zucchini.	*decreased blood pressure, anti tumor, eyes, joint system, glands, diabetics.*
4 CUCUMBER	Cucumber Juice Cucumber, cottage cheese dip with crackers.	Cucumber on rye bread with smoked salmon fillets served with grilled tomato and cheese.	*silicon, hair growth, skin condition, diuretic, blood cleansing, digestion.*
5 LETTUCE	Kebab with lettuce, onion, tomato, tahini sauce and falafels.	Tacos with sliced lettuce, grated carrot, cheese, tomato, onion, capsicum, garlic, kidney beans and sweet chilli sauce.	*excellent silicon, hair growth, chlorophyl, iron, folate, vitamin k, sulphur.*
6 LEEK ONIONS	Leek soup with whole grain barley bread. Leeks / onions with burgers.	Add leeks or onions to any baked dish, barbecue meal, vegetable soup, stir fry or finely cut in a fresh garden salad .	*antiseptic oils, sulphur, antioxidants, cleansing anti bacteria, colds.*
7 POTATOES	Potato mashed with tuna in patties, add onion, peas and serve with chili sauce pan fried with fresh garden salad	Potato soup with finely cut carrots, onions parsley and cabbage, serve with cream or yoghurt. Potato bake with grilled zucchini, tomatoes, cheddar cheese and onions.	*potassium, energy provider but has a very high glycemic index when obtained baked, add oils or cheese to lower g.i.*
3 PUMPKIN	Pumpkin soup with toasted rye bread.	Roast pumpkin with veal cutlets, fried mushrooms, garlic and onions.	*beta cryptoxanphin respiratory system, smokers.*
9 SILVERBEET SPINACH	Spinach/ silverbeet and ricotta cheese baked rolls. Spinach leaves in a fresh garden salad.	Steamed spinach/ s.b. in a quiche, or omlette. Spinach or s.b. leaves with fettuccine pasta and lasagne.	*chlorophyl, lutein and zeaxanthin, eyes, folate, potassium, vitamin k, iron. anti cancer, muscles.*

NUTRITION & DIET SUMMARY

<table>
<tr><td>QUESTION
65</td><td>*How do I obtain
more whole grains
in my diet?*</td><td>obtain a
new
variety</td></tr>
</table>

GRAINS DAILY RECIPE GUIDE IDEAS & BENEFITS CHART

GRAINS	BREAKFAST (B)	LUNCH (L)	EVENING MEAL (E)	MAIN BENEFITS
30 BARLEY	Barley toast with honey. Barley beverage.	Barley soup with vegetables and cottage cheese.	Barley and mushroom baked casserole, onions, chives, parsley.	*energy providing, body warmth, low gluten content.*
31 CORN	Add lecithin granules and slithered almonds to makethe corn flakes a healthy breakfast	Try corn chips with an avocado dip or have corn on the cob as a simple lunch.	Corn taco shell with salad, tomato, kidney beans, onion, garlic. Corn tortillos, add minced beef, or kidny beans with salads.	*Fresh corn is rich in vitamin a, folate, ideal sweet food for children. Corn bread and chips are low in nutrient value but added foods can make it nutritious.*
32 MILLET	Use rolled millet with honey, sunflower seed meal, or almond meal as a regular breakfast or in winter, millet flakes cooked like oats.	Millet salad, with boiled millet, cooked onions fresh chopped parsley, basil, capsicum, brazil nuts, sprinkley with balsamic vinegar	Millet pudding, as a sweet, with nutmeg, butter, flour, eggs,. Millet pilaf with wine, vegetables, egg plant, and tomato paste.	*no gluten content, alkaline food, rich in silicon, iron, folate and various nutrients,ideal food to add to the diet.*
33 OATS	Rolled oats or oat flakes for breakfast with a sprinkle of slivered almonds, a few tinned apricots and a dash of cream and honey. muesli bar snack.	Oat bread with tahini, or peanut butter. Oat salad sandwich with lettuce, cheese, celery, mayonnaise, pepper and salt.	Oat bread rolls with a french garden salad. Original fresh muesli with grated apples, hazel nuts, fruits, milk, or fruit juice and rolled oats.	*promote a steady metabolism, ideal breakfast food, low gluten, rich in silicon and many nutrients, body building food.*
34 RICE	Rice flakes with rice milk, honey and sultanas. Rice pudding with steamed rice, vanilla pods, milk, cream, salt, honey or sugar.	Rice cakes with tahini. Steamed rice with grilled fish and veg. Fried rice chinese style with mushrooms, egg, onions, parsley.	Stir fry rice with prawns, or chicken and vegetables. Rice and kidney beans with grilled tomatoes and cheese.	*alkaline grain, easy to digest, cheap, fair source of nutrients, no gluten content ideal food for recipes sweet and spicy.*
35 RYE	Rye bread toasted with honey and tahini. Rye flakes with milk, apricots or peaches and honey or sultanas. Sourdough rye bread with avocado.	Rye crackers with avocado dip and cheese. Rye bread salad sandwich with egg or avocado or salmon.	Pumpernickel bread as entree with camembert, brie or soft cheese and olives. Rye bread with omlette or quiche and salad.	*body building food, good source of minerals, potassium, excellent fibre, ideal food during menopause.*
36 WHEAT	Whole wheat bread with vegemite, tahini or peanut butter. Whole wheat breakfast cereal with a sprinkle of wheat germ, or almond meal or sunflower meal. Wheat pancakes with honey, maple syrup, tahini and stewed apples. Home made bread rolls with cheese. Cereal with lecithin, hazel nuts and cream. Croissants with tahini or avocado or honey. Sourdough wheat bread with jam or hazelnut spread.	Whole wheat bread salad sandwich with tahini sauce. Pasta with tuna, tomatoes and garlic. Vegetable pastie with wheat pastry. Wheat bread with walnuts and honey. Pizza with olives, mushrooms, capsicum, onions and cheese. Wheat cracker biscuits with cottage cheese. Hamburger bun with onion and lettuce, beef, tomato Turkish bread with tuna and olive oil.	Wheat pastry for quiche, family size vegetable or chicken pie with onions, mushrooms, peas, zucchini and spices. Pizza with ham, cheese and pineapple. Fresh bread rolls with garlic, garden salad and avocado spread. Pasta with vegetables and cheese. Lasagne with kidney beans and cheese. Spaghetti bolognaisse. Macaroni, tuna and cheese with salad.	*Whole wheat is a fair source of many nutrients, iron, b vitamins, vitamin e good energy food. Processed, refined wheat products are depleted in nutrients, full of gluten and acid forming. The foods that combine with the wheat can really make it nutritious, such as salads, walnuts, avocado etc. Try other grains for breakfast, otherwise it's wheat all day long.*

216

NUTRITION & DIET SUMMARY

<table>
<tr><td>QUESTION
66</td><td>*How do I obtain
more legumes
in my diet?*</td><td>dine at a
traditional
restaurant</td></tr>
</table>

LEGUMES DAILY RECIPE GUIDE IDEAS & BENEFITS CHART

		LUNCH **(L)**	EVENING MEAL **(E)**	*MAIN BENEFITS*
37	CAROB BEAN	Carob milkshake. Carob smoothie with icecream	Carob sprinkled on icecream. Hot carob soy milk drink.	*alkaline, pectin, removes toxins, rich in calcium, potassium.*
38	CHICK PEAS	Hummous dip with rye bread triangles.	cooked chick peas, fried with beef and veg.	*complete protein, rich in iron, copper.*
39	GREEN BEANS	steamed with butter and spices added and served with grilled fish or seafood recipes.	Green beans in quiche, or vegetable soup, as a side serve with chicken or with rice dishes.	*folate, potassium, magnesium, vitamin k, fibre, phosphorus, good diabetic food.*
40	KIDNEY BEANS	Tacos with salad, kidney beans, chilli sauce, salad, tomato, garlic and onions.	Kidney beans with steamed rice, tomatoes and cheese. Kidney bean burgers.	*complete protein, excellent fibre, to stabilize blood sugar levels, potassium.*
41	LENTILS	Lentil patties with fresh salad. Lentils with fried rice and chicken. Lentil sprout soup.	Lentil soup with carrots, celery, bay leaves, vinegar, vegetable stock, onion, olive oil.	*complete protein, very rich in iron, low fat content, helps lower cholesterol.*
42	LIMA BEANS	Lima bean soup with onions, carrot, parsley, oil, pepper, basil, thyme, garlic.	Lima bean loaf with sesame seeds, carrot, onions, veg. salt. flour, soy sauce and garlic.	*excellent iron, complete protein rich in molybdenum, folate, magnesium.*
43	MUNG BEANS	Mung bean sprouts in garden salad with mayonnaisse. Mung bean sprout soup with yoghurt.	Mung bean dal with mustard, pepper, tumeric, curry powder on flat bread with oil. Mung bean patties.	*complete protein, excellent fibre, magnesium, folate, potassium and copper.*
44	PEANUT	Peanut butter on whole grain rye bread with chopped celery. Peanuts in the shell, roasted.	Peanut sauce over rice dishes with stir fried vegetables. Roasted peanuts as an appetiser, with beer.	*excellent supply of protein, vitamin b5, b3, copper, folate, vit. e. manganese. magnesium.*
45	PEAS	Green peas or snow peas fresh from the pod, served with garden salad.	Pea soup with garlic. Fried rice with peas. Snow peas with fish. Peas with roast vegs.	*excellent supply of fibre, potassium, magnesium, folate, vit. k, copper.*
46	SOYA BEANS	Garden salad with fried tofu cubes. Soy milk shake. Soy mayonnaise with vegetable burgers.	Soy sauce with stir fried vegetables and rice. Soy pastry apple pie. Soy burgers. Soy vegetable soup.	*excellent complete protein, fibre, lecithin, unique source of genistein , iron, molybdenum, phosphorus, folate.*

SPROUTS DAILY RECIPE GUIDE IDEAS & BENEFITS CHART

47	SPROUTS	Wheat or buckwheat sprouts with cinnamon, nutmeg in pancake mix with honey. Wheat sprouts in home made bread served with a variety of soft cheese.	Sunflower sprouts in garden salad with tahini dressing. Sprouts in soup. Alfalfa sprouts with tahini on rye bread. All sprouts in garden salad with cheese cubes and mayonnaise.	*Excellent source of enzymes, good source of trace minerals, b vitamins, antioxidants, protitamin e, k,u,folate, rutin, zinc, phytoestrogens.*

NUTRITION & DIET SUMMARY

<table>
<tr><td>QUESTION
67</td><td>How do I obtain
more nuts
in my diet?</td><td>try a new
recipe
every week</td></tr>
</table>

NUTS DAILY RECIPE GUIDE IDEAS & BENEFITS CHART

NUTS	BREAKFAST (B)	LUNCH (L)	EVENING MEAL (E)	*MAIN BENEFITS*
48 ALMONDS	Ground almonds sprinkled on breakfast cereal with milk. Ground almonds mixed into pancake mix with stewed apples and cream.	Almonds with crisp apple or peaches. Halva as lunch sweet. Almonds slivered in fresh garden salad. Craked almonds in stir fry with vegetables.	Slivered almonds with grilled fish and fresh salad. Roasted almond pieces with chicken breasts. Almond butter with roast vegetables. Almonds on rice custard sweet.	*alkaline food, excellent complete protein, magnesium, calcium, phosphorus, iron, zinc, omega 6, vitamin e, fibre, copper, potassium, b vit, mono unsaturated.*
49 BRAZIL NUTS	ground brazil nut in muesli with cream. cracked brazil nuts with cereal. brazil nut butter on toast with honey.	Brazil nuts with almonds and cashews and crisp apple. Cracked brazil nuts on fresh garden salad or on pasta and cheese.	Ground brazil nuts sprinkled on seafood entree. Cracked roasted brazil nut pieces with boiled rice and honey chicken. Brazil nuts cracked on ice cream.	*excellent source of selenium, antioxidant, essential for diabetics, very good supply of phosphorus, potassium, magnesium, fibre, methionine - protein.*
50 CASHEWS	cashew nuts raw cracked and sprinkled on toast with honey, or on the breakfast cereal, or mixed into peach, apple, apricot fruit salad.	Cashew butter on whole grain rye bread with garden salad. Cashews raw in fried rice with steamed vegetables and peas. Cashews and apple.	Roasted cashews in crisp garden salad. Cracked raw cashews sprinkled on broccoli and melted cheese. Roast cashews in curried vegetables. Cashews on ice cream.	*excellent source of copper for the brain, joint system, good source of complete protein, magnesium, phosphorus, omega 6, oleic acid, monounsaturates.*
51 CHESTNUT	Roasted chestnuts with morning cereal beverage. Chestnut pieces roasted on muesli.	Roasted chestnut pieces with garden salad and soy mayonnaise. Chestnut pieces with satay sauce and rice.	Roasted chestnut pieces on salmon fillets with egg mayonnaise. Roasted chestnuts by the camp fire with a glass of red wine or apple cider.	*low calories, good carbohydrate food, potassium, magnesium, folic acid, fibre, vit. c low fat content.*
52 HAZEL NUTS	Hazel nut spread on whole grain toast. Cracked hazel nuts with original fresh muesli recipe. Ground hazel nuts in pancakes.	Cracked roasted hazel nuts with garden salad. Hazel nuts with crisp apple and peach. Ground hazel nuts with yoghurt.	Roasted hazel nut pieces with steamed vegetables and cheese sauce. Cracked hazel nuts with beef steaks and mustard. Hazel nuts and ice cream.	*complete protein, very good source of vitamin e, iron, copper, calcium, manganese, b vitamins, zinc, magnesium, fibre.*
53 MACADAMIA NUTS	Cracked macadamia nut pieces with breakfast cereal or mixed into pancake. Macadamia butter on rye toast or croissants.	Macadamia pieces raw with french salad. Macadamia oil on salad. Roasted macadamia with sweet and sour vegs.	Cracked macadamia with baked fish fillets. Roasted macadamia with rice and beef. Ground macadamia sprinkled on tofu ice cream and cherries or strawberries.	*excellent source of monounsaturated oleic acid and palmitoleic acid, good source of copper, protein, fibre, vitamin e.*
54 PECAN NUTS	Cracked pecan nuts sprinkled on pancakes with maple syrup. Ground pecan nuts with breakfast cereal or oat muesli.	Pecan nuts with peaches. Roasted pecan nut pieces with baked green beans and tomato with a paprika sauce.	Cracked pecan nuts with baked zucchini, shallots, garlic and spinach with cheese sauce. Pecan nut pie with ice cream or fresh fruits and cream.	*excellent source of copper, good source of phosphorus, magnesium, fibre, complete protein, may help reduce cholesterol.*
55 PINE NUTS	Pine nuts with grilled tomatoes. Pine nuts with ricotta cheese on whole grain toast. Pine nuts with grated apple/ yoghurt.	Pine nuts with garden salad or Greek salad. Pine nuts with grilled fish and tomatoes. Pesto or Pine nuts with avocado salad.	Roasted pine nuts with fresh smoked salmon and fried mushrooms. Pine nuts with Asian noodles and stir fry vegetables. Pine nuts with chocolate cake.	*Excellent supply of phosphorus, magnesium, complete protein, iron, fibre, manganese, good brain food and for the blood system.*
56 PISTACIO	Pistachio nut pieces with grilled cheese on rye bread. Pistachio nut pieces sprinkled on scrambled eggs, with toast.	Pistachio nut pieces with honey chicken. Pistachio nuts ground with fresh Greek salad or with cottage cheese on rye bread.	Cracked pistachio nut pieces sprinkled on baked fish with fresh salad. Ground pistachio mixed into sweet pastry. Pistachio cracked on ice cream.	*very good source of phytosterols, anti-cancer and cholesterol, very good source of potassium, magnesium, copper, zinc, calcium and vitamin e.*
57 WALNUTS	Walnuts on toast with honey. Walnuts with fruit salad or original fresh muesli. Walnuts with tahini on rye toast.	Walnuts in Waldorf salad. Walnuts with grilled cheese on toast. Walnut pieces in carrot cake or muffins. Walnuts and cream cheese on wheat biscuits.	Walnuts ground and mixed into fish batter with steamed vegetables. Walnuts baked into bread mix served with continenal soft cheese and wine.	*excellent source of the hard to obtain omega 3, also supplies good amounts of omega 6, folate, iron, phosphorus, manganese, copper.*

NUTRITION & DIET SUMMARY

<table>
<tr><td>QUESTION
68</td><td>*How do I obtain
more seeds
in my diet?*</td><td>grind them
and add
to meals.</td></tr>
</table>

SEEDS DAILY RECIPE GUIDE IDEAS & BENEFITS CHART

SEEDS	BREAKFAST (B)	LUNCH (L)	EVENING MEAL (E)	MAIN BENEFITS
PUMPKIN SEEDS (PEPITAS)	Pepitas ground and served on top of grilled tomatoes with cheddar cheese. Pepitas ground into savoury crepes mix with mushrooms and cream cheese sauce, cracked pepitas in muesli mix with fresh grated red apples.	Ground pepitas sprinkled on fresh garden salad served with pasta. Ground pepitas mixed into pasta sauce served over pasta with parmesan cheese. Ground pepitas served on top of pumpkin cream soup.	Roasted pepitas served over grilled zucchini, tomatoes served with melted cheese or yoghurt. Ground pepitas mixed into fish bread crumbs or served over cauliflower cheese sauce. Cracked pepitas sprinkled over omelette with vegetables.	*excellent complete protein, excellent iron content, excellent omega 3 content, zinc, phosphorus, cucurbitabins for prostate gland health plus anti-inflammatory power against arthritis and rheumatism.*
SESAME SEEDS (TAHINI)	Sesame seeds paste - tahini on toasted whole grain bread with honey. Tahini on pancakes with honey. Tahini on fruit salad.	Fresh garden salad with tahini salad dressing. Tahini cake with tea. Spinach rolls with sesame seeds, sesame seed buns with salad.	Hummous with tahini served with corn chips or rye bread and Greek salad. Tahini in halva as a sweet. Sesame seeds toasted sprinkled on steamed vegetables wiith grilled fish.	*excellent complete protein rich in methionine, excellent calcium, copper, iron, zinc, vit. e, lecithin, phytosterols and special fibre-lignans to lower blood cholesterol.*
SUNFLOWER SEEDS	Ground sunflower seeds in pancake mix, serve with maple syrup and pears. Sunflower seeds in muesli or sprinkle on standard breakfast cereal. Sunflower seeds ground in half butter mix spread on toast with honey.	Roasted sunflower seeds on french garden salad. Sunflower oil in salad dressing. Ground sunflower seeds in vegetable burger mix with carrot, beetroot, onions, parsley, spices.	Sunflower seed paties with onion, spinach and celery served with soy mayonnaise. Sunflower meal mixed into cream sauce served over grilled fish or fresh smoked salmon. Sunflower seeds sprinkled over ice cream or mixed into a cake, with coffee.	*excellent complete protein, vitamin e, magnesium, phosphorus, silicon, selenium, zinc, full of antioxidant power and fibre plus b group vitamins plus monounsaturates plus omega 6 and omega 3.*

<table>
<tr><td>QUESTION
69</td><td>*How do I obtain
more supplements
in my diet?*</td><td>refer to
chart and
health store</td></tr>
</table>

SUPPLEMENTS DAILY RECIPE GUIDE IDEAS & BENEFITS CHART

SUPPLEMENTS	BREAKFAST(B)	LUNCH (L)	EVENING MEAL (E)	MAIN BENEFITS
APPLE CIDER VINEGAR	Served as an ingredient in fresh juices, or use as a gargle for sore throats.	Cider vinegar in salad dressing with olive oil or soy oil, or mix cider vinerar with tahini and honey.	Mix a tbl. sp. of cider vinegar into a standard salad dressing or mix with lemon for a seafood cocktail with tartare sauce.	*digestive aid, acid-alkaline blood balance, potassium, healthy skin condition, phosphorus, iron, sodium,*
BREWERS YEAST	Sprinkle a dash into pancake mix or omelette or bread mix.	Sprinkle a dash over salads or into quiche or in patties.	Mix a dash into gravy or bread crumb mix or in soups or curry.	*excellent source of nearly all b group vitamins.*
DANDELION	Use as beverage instead of coffee.	Make dandelion tea or coffee	Make dandelion plunger coffee.	*vitamin a, iron, potassium, liver tonic, bladder health.*
KELP	add kelp sea salt to scrambled eggs or bread.	Sprinkle kelp over salads or try kelp cracker biscuits.	Use kelp finely sliced in stir fried vegetables or with noodles.	*60 trace elements, excellent source of iodine, 13 vitamins.*
LECITHIN	Add to any egg breakfast or pancake mix.	Sprinkle over garden salads or add to soups or stews.	Add to gravy or sprinkle into cheese sauce or pasta sauce.	*excellent to reduce high cholesterol, brain food.*
WHEAT GERM	Add to a pancake mix, bread mix, or sprinkle over cereals.	Mix into bread crumbs with fish meals or use in cakes.	Sprinkle into stir fried vegetables, or over a fresh garden salad.	*excellent protein, vitamin e, minerals and vitamins.*

NUTRITION & DIET SUMMARY

<table>
<tr><td>QUESTION
70</td><td>How do I obtain a
healthy and happy
balanced life?</td><td>obtain more
positive
life factors</td></tr>
</table>

The healthy balanced life requires many factors and the chart below provides a guide to some of the best health, lifestyle and food factors possible. You can photocopy this chart. Add up the positive and negative factors per week or day and see how your life is balanced. Throughout life, various factors on the negative side deplete our health and happiness. Whenever you are affected by negative factors, add a few extra positive factors to your life balance and discover that with regular effort, your life will feel and be positive. Just imagine a life with only the positive factors, it would certainly be above and beyond the average lifestyle. The life balance chart is the summary to this book. Whenever you need help with your health and happiness, refer to this chart to check on what factors you can add to your daily life. Everyone has different needs due to age, health, gender and various other factors but generally speaking, this chart is designed to show that life is full of choices, the real challenge is to obtain the lifestyle that maintains a stable, healthy and happy life. "see ya"!

LIFE BALANCE CHART

AVOID NEGATIVE LIFE FACTORS				OBTAIN POSITIVE LIFE FACTORS			
NEGATIVE HEALTH FACTORS	x	**NEGATIVE FOOD FACTORS**	x	**POSITIVE HEATH FACTORS**	✓	**POSITIVE FOOD FACTORS**	✓
stress, nervousness		cooked oils		laughing		wheat grass juice	
smoking		deep fried foods		walking moderatedly		fresh vegetable juices	
excess alcohol		sugar		swimming, water exercises		fresh fruit juices	
obesity		soft drinks		sleeping regularly		pepitas	
no exercise		white flour products		relaxation time outside		cold pressed flax oil	
anger		salt and salty foods		exercise on a daily basis		sunflower seed kernels	
pollution		cholesterol rich foods		gardening every few days		walnuts, almonds	
chemicals		trans fatty acids		mountain air, bush walks		blueberries	
drug taking		caffeine and cola drinks		riding a bicycle, or horse		tahini	
excess television		sausages and bacon		reading a good book		papaya	
toxins in bad foods		take away foods		going to church regularly		apples	
rushing around		processed foods, drinks		helping people, family time		avocado	
virus, infection, injury		potato chips		listening to relaxing music		fish, salmon, tuna	
food poisoning		refined foods		regular moderate sunlight		rolled oats	
overeating, indigestion		processed meat		love and friendship time		lettuce, spinach	
lack of sleep		gluten, yeast products		proper chewing of food		kidney beans	
excess computer time		food additives, colours		regular bathing, showers.		garlic	
micro wave meals		lollies, excess sweets		fasting and body cleansing		carrots, broccoli	
bad news		poor food combination		comfortable happy home		pure water	
no fresh food		excess chocolate		regular holidays, free days.		acidophillus yoghurt	
TOTAL NEGATIVE HEALTH FACTORS		**TOTAL NEGATIVE FOOD FACTORS**		**TOTAL POSITIVE HEALTH FACTORS**		**TOTAL POSITIVE FOOD FACTORS**	
TOTAL WEEKLY NEGATIVE FACTORS				**TOTAL WEEKLY POSITIVE FACTORS**			

NATURAL FOODS SHOPPING LIST

GRAINS		LEGUMES		FRUITS		FRUITS		VEGETABLES		FISH	
BARLEY - grain		CAROB - powder		APPLES - red fresh		MANGO - canned		ARTICHOKE - fresh		FISH - fresh ocean	
BARLEY - bread		CAROB - sweets		APPLES - golden		MELONS		ARTICHOKE - bottled		FISH - fresh river	
CORN - chips		CAROB - beans		APPLES - green		NECTARINE		ASPARAGUS - fresh		FISH - frozen	
CORN - sweet		CAROB - flour		APPLES - dried		OLIVES - black		ASPARAGUS - canned		FISH - canned	
CORN - flour		CHICK PEAS - whole		APRICOT - fresh		OLIVES - green		BEETROOT - fresh		TUNA - canned	
MILLET		CHICK PEAS - canned		APRICOT - dried		ORANGES		BEETROOT - canned		FISH - products	
OATS - rolled		CHICK PEAS - hummus		AVOCADO		PEACHES -fresh		BROCCOLI - fresh		**SEAFOOD**	
OAT - bread		GREEN BEANS - fresh		BANANA - fresh		PEACHES - canned		BROCCOLI - frozen		CRAB - fresh	
OAT - muesli		GREEN BEANS - frozen		BANANA - chips		PEACHES - dried		BRUSSEL SPROUTS		CRAB - frozen	
RICE - brown		GREEN BEANS - can		BANANA - dried		PEARS - fresh		CABBAGE		CRAYFISH	
RICE - white		KIDNEY BEANS - whole		BLUEBERRIES - fresh		PEARS - canned		CABBAGE - saurekraut		OYSTERS	
RICE - flour		KIDNEY BEANS - can		BLUEBERRIES - can		PEARS - dried		CARROTS - fresh		PRAWNS / SHRIMPS - fresh	
RICE - cakes		LENTILS - brown, whole		BERRIES - fresh		PINEAPPLE - fresh		CARROTS - canned		PRAWNS / SHRIMPS - frozen	
RICE - flakes		LENTILS - red, whole		BERRIES - canned		PINEAPPLE - canned		CARROTS - frozen		SCALLOPS	
RYE - grain		LENTILS - canned		CANTALOUP		PINEAPPLE - dried		CAPSICUM - red		MUSSELS	
RYE - bread		MUNG BEANS - whole		CHERRIES - fresh		PLUMS - fresh		CAPSICUM - green		CALAMARI - fresh	
RYE - flour		MUNG BEANS - sprouts		CHERRIES - can		PLUMS - canned		CELERY		SEAFOOD - other products	
WHEAT - grain		PEAS - fresh		CHERRIES - glazed		PRUNES		CUCUMBER		**OILS & SPREADS**	
WHEAT - w.grain bread		PEAS - canned		CURRANTS - fresh		STRAWBERRIES		EGG PLANT		AVOCADO OIL	
WHEAT - white bread		PEAS - frozen		CURRANTS - can		TOMATO - fresh		LEEK		ALMOND OIL	
WHEAT - flour w.grain		PEANUT - in shell raw		CURRANTS - dried		TOMATO - dried		MUSHROOMS		APRICOT OIL	
WHEAT - flour self raising		PEANUT - in shell, roast		DATES - fresh		WATERMELON		MUSHROOMS - can		CANOLA OIL	
WHEAT - flour plain		PEANUT - raw		DATES - dried		**FRUIT DRINKS**		LETTUCE		COCONUT OIL	
WHEAT - pastry		PEANUT - roasted		FIGS - fresh		APPLE JUICE		ONIONS		CORN OIL	
WHEAT - bread rolls		PEANUT - butter		FIGS - dried		APRICOT NECTAR		PARSNIPS		LINSEED /FLAX OIL	
WHEAT - spaghetti		SOY BEANS - whole		GRAPEFRUIT		BLACKCURRANT		PEPPERS		MACADAMIA OIL	
WHEAT - lasagne sheets		SOY BEANS - canned		GRAPES		GRAPE JUICE		POTATO -fresh		OLIVE OIL	
WHEAT - plain pasta		SOY - milk		GUAVA		ORANGE JUICE		POTATO - chips frozen		PEANUT OIL	
WHEAR - w.g. pasta		SOY - flour		KIWI FRUIT		PEACH NECTAR		POTATO - canned		SAFFLOWER OIL	
WHEAT - veg. pasta		SOY - grits		LEMONS		PINEAPPLE JUICE		PUMPKIN		SOY OIL	
WHEAT - noodles		SOY - sauce		LIMES		TOMATO JUICE		RADISH		SESAME OIL	
WHEAT - baking prod.		SOY - tofu		MANGO - fresh		FRUIT COCKTAIL		SPINACH -fresh		TAHINI	
WHEAT - other products		SOY - other products		MANGO - dried		FRUIT CORDIAL		SPINACH - canned		SUNFLOWER OIL	
NUTS		**NUTS**		**SPROUTS / SEEDS**		**DAIRY FOODS**		SPINACH - frozen		WALNUT OIL	
ALMONDS - raw		HAZEL NUTS - raw		ALFALFA		CREAM - pure		SWEET POTATO		WHEAT GERM OIL	
ALMONDS - blanched		HAZEL NUTS - roasted		BUCKWHEAT		CREAM - thickened		TURNIPS		**FOODS & SUPPLEMENTS**	
ALMONDS - roasted		HAZEL NUT - spread		LENTIL SPROUTS		MILK - full cream		ZUCCHINI		APPLE CIDER VINEGAR	
ALMONDS -slivered		HAZEL NUT - products		MUNG BEAN		MILK - low fat		**MEAT & POULTRY**		BRAN	
ALMONDS - products		MACADAMIA - raw		SUNFLOWER		MILK - calcium		BEEF - steak, rump,		BREWERS YEAST	
BRAZIL NUTS		MACADAMIA - roasted		**CHEESE**		MILK - goats		BEEF - sausages.		DANDELION- coffee	
CASHEW NUTS - raw		PECAN NUTS		CHEESE - mild		MILK - products		BEEF - other products		KELP - salt and products	
CASHEW NUTS - roasted		PINE NUTS		CHEESE - tasty		**YOGHURT**		CHICKEN - frozen		LECITHIN - granules	
CASHEW - butter		PISTACHIO NUTS		CHEESE - cream		ACIDOPHILLUS - plain		CHICKEN - roasted		WHEAT GERM	
CHESTNUT		WALNUTS		CHEESE - ricotta		ACIDOPHILLUS - fruit		CHICKEN - other prod.		HERBAL DRINKS	
COCONUT - raw		**SEEDS**		CHEESE - soft		YOGHURT - plain		EGGS		HERBS	
COCONUT - desiccated		PEPITAS		CHEESE - CONTINENTAL		YOGHURT - low fat		LAMB		OTHER SUPPLEMENTS	
COCONUT - milk		SESAME		CHEESE - slices		YOGHURT - Greek		TURKEY / POULTRY		SPICES, YEAST, SALT	
COCONUT - other prod.		SUNFLOWER		CHEESE - grated		YOGHURT - other		OTHER PRODUCTS		TABLETS	

OTHER SHOPPING ITEMS

BIBLIOGRAPHY

Anatomy and Physiology for Nurses W. Gordon Sears
Introduction to Nutrition Henrietta Heck. McMillan Publishing.
Healthful Eating Without Confusion - Paul G. Bragg, N.D.P.H.D. Health Science Books
Protein for Vegetarians - Garry Null. Jove Books.
Scientific Vegetarianism, Book of Natures Healing Grasses - H.E. Kirshner. H.C. White Publications
Become Young - N.W. Walker, M.D.D.S.C. Norwalk Press.
Food Combining Made Easy - H.M. Shelton.
Food Remedies - M. Blackmore, N.D.D.C.
Laurels Kitchen - L. Robertson, C. Hinders, B. Godfrey - Nilgri Press.
Family Health Care - Readers Digest.
Concise Oxford Dictionary - Clarendon Press.
Relax and Survive - Anne Wigmore, D.D.N.D. Naturama - Anne Wigmore.
Energy, Evolution, Universe, The Mind, The Body, Health & Disease, Water, Time, The Cell, Growth - Time Life Books - Publication.
Vitamin C and the Common Cold. Linus Pauling - Bantam Books.
Diet & Nutrition, R. Ballentine M.D. The Himalayan Int. Institute.
Lets Get Well, Lets Have Healthy Children, Lets Eat Right to Keep Fit Adelle Davis. C.H. Robinson - MacMillan Publishing.
Basic Nutrition in Health and Disease. Goodhart and M.E. Shils - Lea and Febiger Publishing.
Beware of the Food You Eat - Ruth Winter. Signet Books.
Fit for Anything - Kekir Sidhwa - Health for all Publishing.
Proteins - Their Chemistry and Politics. A.M. Altschul - Basic Books Publishing
Nutrition Almanac - Nutrition Research Inc. Lavon J. Dunne. McGraw-Hill Book Company.
The Wholefood Catalogue - Vicki Peterson.
The Natural Health Book - Dorothy Hall. Thomas Nelson Australia Pty Ltd.
The Healing Power of Natural Foods - May Bethel Wilshire Book Company.
Diet and Nutrition - Rudolph Ballentine, M.D.
The Natural Foods and Nutrition Handbook. Rafael Marcia Harper & Row Publishing.
Nutrition and Physical Fitness - L.J. Saunders Publishing
The World's Healthiest Foods. George Mateljan Foundation.
Nutritional Factors in foods, David A Phillips, Ph.D.

MEASURES

OVEN TEMPERATURES

Celsius	F'heit	Gas Mark
110	225	1/4
130	250	1/2
140	275	1
150	300	2
170	325	3
180	350	4
190	375	5
200	400	6
220	425	7
230	450	8
240	475	9

LIQUID MEASURES

Metric	Imperial
150 ml	1/2 pint
300 ml	1/2 pint
450 ml	3/4 pint
600 ml	1 pint
900 ml	1 & 1/2 pints
1 litre	1 & 3/4 pints
1.2 litres	2 pints
1.5 litres	2 & 1/2 pints
1.75 litres	3 pints
2.00 litres	3 & 1/2 pints

Australian pint = 16 fluid oz
Imperial pints = 20 fluid oz
Australian cup = 8 fluid oz
Imperial cup = 10 fluid oz

1 quart = 4 cups
1 pint = 2 cups
1 cup = 1/2 pint
1 cup = 8 fluid ounces
1 cup = 16 tablespoons

2 tablespoons = 1 fluid oz
1 serve = approx. 4 ounces
1 ounce fluid = approx. 28 g
1 cup of honey = 325 grams
1 cup of milk = 240 grams
1 cup of oil = 200 grams
1 cup of water = 220 grams
1 cup of sugar = 200 grams
1 cup of flour = 100 grams
1 cup of soup = 240 grams